ATS-47 ADMISSION TEST SERIES

This is your PASSBOOK for...

National Pharmacy Boards (NPB)

Test Preparation Study Guide Questions & Answers

NLC®

NATIONAL LEARNING CORPORATION®

National Learning Corporation

212 Michael Drive, Syosset, NY 11791
(516) 921-8888 • www.passbooks.com
E-mail: info@passbooks.com

PASSBOOK® SERIES

THE *PASSBOOK® SERIES* has been created to prepare applicants and candidates for the ultimate academic battlefield – the examination room.

At some time in our lives, each and every one of us may be required to take an examination – for validation, matriculation, admission, qualification, registration, certification, or licensure.

Based on the assumption that every applicant or candidate has met the basic formal educational standards, has taken the required number of courses, and read the necessary texts, the *PASSBOOK® SERIES* furnishes the one special preparation which may assure passing with confidence, instead of failing with insecurity. Examination questions – together with answers – are furnished as the basic vehicle for study so that the mysteries of the examination and its compounding difficulties may be eliminated or diminished by a sure method.

This book is meant to help you pass your examination provided that you qualify and are serious in your objective.

The entire field is reviewed through the huge store of content information which is succinctly presented through a provocative and challenging approach – the question-and-answer method.

A climate of success is established by furnishing the correct answers at the end of each test.

You soon learn to recognize types of questions, forms of questions, and patterns of questioning. You may even begin to anticipate expected outcomes.

You perceive that many questions are repeated or adapted so that you can gain acute insights, which may enable you to score many sure points.

You learn how to confront new questions, or types of questions, and to attack them confidently and work out the correct answers.

You note objectives and emphases, and recognize pitfalls and dangers, so that you may make positive educational adjustments.

Moreover, you are kept fully informed in relation to new concepts, methods, practices, and directions in the field.

You discover that you are actually taking the examination all the time: you are preparing for the examination by "taking" an examination, not by reading extraneous and/or supererogatory textbooks.

In short, this PASSBOOK®, used directedly, should be an important factor in helping you to pass your test.

NATIONAL PHARMACY BOARDS (NPB)

Developed by the National Association of Boards of Pharmacy (NABP), the National Pharmacy Boards is multiple-choice examination designed to determine whether candidates have the knowledge, judgment and skill necessary to practice pharmacy at entry-level competence. The computerized exam tests three fundamental areas: managing drug therapy, safely and accurately preparing and dispensing medications, and providing drug information and promoting public health.

A majority of the questions on the examinations are scenario-based, meaning they are based on patient profiles. These questions require both a fundamental knowledge of pharmacy as well as the ability to interpret and analyze patient information. Most other questions are of standard multiple-choice format.

The candidate is allowed 4 hours and 15 minutes to complete the questions on the test computer. There is a mandatory 10-minute break in the middle of the exam. Thirty-five of the exam questions are pretest items that will not factor into the final test score

There are three fundamental areas that the exam covers. Area 1, the assurance of safe and effective pharmacotherapy and optimizing therapeutic outcomes, makes up approximately 54% of the exam. The assurance of safe and accurate preparation and dispensing of medications makes up 35%, and the providing of health care information and promotion of public health covers the other 11% of the exam. A strong understanding of these areas and their components will aid in test preparation.

HOW TO TAKE A TEST

You have studied long, hard and conscientiously.

With your official admission card in hand, and your heart pounding, you have been admitted to the examination room.

You note that there are several hundred other applicants in the examination room waiting to take the same test.

They all appear to be equally well prepared.

You know that nothing but your best effort will suffice. The "moment of truth" is at hand: you now have to demonstrate objectively, in writing, your knowledge of content and your understanding of subject matter.

You are fighting the most important battle of your life—to pass and/or score high on an examination which will determine your career and provide the economic basis for your livelihood.

What extra, special things should you know and should you do in taking the examination?

I. YOU MUST PASS AN EXAMINATION

A. WHAT EVERY CANDIDATE SHOULD KNOW

Examination applicants often ask us for help in preparing for the written test. What can I study in advance? What kinds of questions will be asked? How will the test be given? How will the papers be graded?

B. HOW ARE EXAMS DEVELOPED?

Examinations are carefully written by trained technicians who are specialists in the field known as "psychological measurement," in consultation with recognized authorities in the field of work that the test will cover. These experts recommend the subject matter areas or skills to be tested; only those knowledges or skills important to your success on the job are included. The most reliable books and source materials available are used as references. Together, the experts and technicians judge the difficulty level of the questions.

Test technicians know how to phrase questions so that the problem is clearly stated. Their ethics do not permit "trick" or "catch" questions. Questions may have been tried out on sample groups, or subjected to statistical analysis, to determine their usefulness.

Written tests are often used in combination with performance tests, ratings of training and experience, and oral interviews. All of these measures combine to form the best-known means of finding the right person for the right job.

II. HOW TO PASS THE WRITTEN TEST

A. BASIC STEPS

1) Study the announcement

How, then, can you know what subjects to study? Our best answer is: "Learn as much as possible about the class of positions for which you've applied." The exam will test the knowledge, skills and abilities needed to do the work.

Your most valuable source of information about the position you want is the official exam announcement. This announcement lists the training and experience qualifications. Check these standards and apply only if you come reasonably close to meeting them. Many jurisdictions preview the written test in the exam announcement by including a section called "Knowledge and Abilities Required," "Scope of the Examination," or some similar heading. Here you will find out specifically what fields will be tested.

2) Choose appropriate study materials

If the position for which you are applying is technical or advanced, you will read more advanced, specialized material. If you are already familiar with the basic principles of your field, elementary textbooks would waste your time. Concentrate on advanced textbooks and technical periodicals. Think through the concepts and review difficult problems in your field.

These are all general sources. You can get more ideas on your own initiative, following these leads. For example, training manuals and publications of the government agency which employs workers in your field can be useful, particularly for technical and professional positions. A letter or visit to the government department involved may result in more specific study suggestions, and certainly will provide you with a more definite idea of the exact nature of the position you are seeking.

3) Study this book!

III. KINDS OF TESTS

Tests are used for purposes other than measuring knowledge and ability to perform specified duties. For some positions, it is equally important to test ability to make adjustments to new situations or to profit from training. In others, basic mental abilities not dependent on information are essential. Questions which test these things may not appear as pertinent to the duties of the position as those which test for knowledge and information. Yet they are often highly important parts of a fair examination. For very general questions, it is almost impossible to help you direct your study efforts. What we can do is to point out some of the more common of these general abilities needed in public service positions and describe some typical questions.

1) General information

Broad, general information has been found useful for predicting job success in some kinds of work. This is tested in a variety of ways, from vocabulary lists to questions about current events. Basic background in some field of work, such as sociology or economics, may be sampled in a group of questions. Often these are principles which have become familiar to most persons through exposure rather than through formal training. It is difficult to advise you how to study for these questions; being alert to the world around you is our best suggestion.

2) Verbal ability

An example of an ability needed in many positions is verbal or language ability. Verbal ability is, in brief, the ability to use and understand words. Vocabulary and grammar tests are typical measures of this ability. Reading comprehension or paragraph interpretation questions are common in many kinds of civil service tests. You are given a paragraph of written material and asked to find its central meaning.

IV. KINDS OF QUESTIONS

1. Multiple-choice Questions

Most popular of the short-answer questions is the "multiple choice" or "best answer" question. It can be used, for example, to test for factual knowledge, ability to solve problems or judgment in meeting situations found at work.

A multiple-choice question is normally one of three types:

- It can begin with an incomplete statement followed by several possible endings. You are to find the one ending which best completes the statement, although some of the others may not be entirely wrong.
- It can also be a complete statement in the form of a question which is answered by choosing one of the statements listed.
- It can be in the form of a problem – again you select the best answer.

Here is an example of a multiple-choice question with a discussion which should give you some clues as to the method for choosing the right answer:

When an employee has a complaint about his assignment, the action which will best help him overcome his difficulty is to

A. discuss his difficulty with his coworkers
B. take the problem to the head of the organization
C. take the problem to the person who gave him the assignment
D. say nothing to anyone about his complaint

In answering this question, you should study each of the choices to find which is best. Consider choice "A" – Certainly an employee may discuss his complaint with fellow employees, but no change or improvement can result, and the complaint remains unresolved. Choice "B" is a poor choice since the head of the organization probably does not know what assignment you have been given, and taking your problem to him is known as "going over the head" of the supervisor. The supervisor, or person who made the assignment, is the person who can clarify it or correct any injustice. Choice "C" is, therefore, correct. To say nothing, as in choice "D," is unwise. Supervisors have and interest in knowing the problems employees are facing, and the employee is seeking a solution to his problem.

2. True/False

3. Matching Questions

Matching an answer from a column of choices within another column.

V. RECORDING YOUR ANSWERS

Computer terminals are used more and more today for many different kinds of exams.

For an examination with very few applicants, you may be told to record your answers in the test booklet itself. Separate answer sheets are much more common. If this separate answer sheet is to be scored by machine – and this is often the case – it is highly important that you mark your answers correctly in order to get credit.

VI. BEFORE THE TEST

YOUR PHYSICAL CONDITION IS IMPORTANT

If you are not well, you can't do your best work on tests. If you are half asleep, you can't do your best either. Here are some tips:

1) Get about the same amount of sleep you usually get. Don't stay up all night before the test, either partying or worrying—DON'T DO IT!
2) If you wear glasses, be sure to wear them when you go to take the test. This goes for hearing aids, too.
3) If you have any physical problems that may keep you from doing your best, be sure to tell the person giving the test. If you are sick or in poor health, you relay cannot do your best on any test. You can always come back and take the test some other time.

Common sense will help you find procedures to follow to get ready for an examination. Too many of us, however, overlook these sensible measures. Indeed, nervousness and fatigue have been found to be the most serious reasons why applicants fail to do their best on civil service tests. Here is a list of reminders:

- Begin your preparation early – Don't wait until the last minute to go scurrying around for books and materials or to find out what the position is all about.
- Prepare continuously – An hour a night for a week is better than an all-night cram session. This has been definitely established. What is more, a night a week for a month will return better dividends than crowding your study into a shorter period of time.
- Locate the place of the exam – You have been sent a notice telling you when and where to report for the examination. If the location is in a different town or otherwise unfamiliar to you, it would be well to inquire the best route and learn something about the building.
- Relax the night before the test – Allow your mind to rest. Do not study at all that night. Plan some mild recreation or diversion; then go to bed early and get a good night's sleep.
- Get up early enough to make a leisurely trip to the place for the test – This way unforeseen events, traffic snarls, unfamiliar buildings, etc. will not upset you.
- Dress comfortably – A written test is not a fashion show. You will be known by number and not by name, so wear something comfortable.
- Leave excess paraphernalia at home – Shopping bags and odd bundles will get in your way. You need bring only the items mentioned in the official notice you received; usually everything you need is provided. Do not bring reference books to the exam. They will only confuse those last minutes and be taken away from you when in the test room.

- Arrive somewhat ahead of time – If because of transportation schedules you must get there very early, bring a newspaper or magazine to take your mind off yourself while waiting.
- Locate the examination room – When you have found the proper room, you will be directed to the seat or part of the room where you will sit. Sometimes you are given a sheet of instructions to read while you are waiting. Do not fill out any forms until you are told to do so; just read them and be prepared.
- Relax and prepare to listen to the instructions
- If you have any physical problem that may keep you from doing your best, be sure to tell the test administrator. If you are sick or in poor health, you really cannot do your best on the exam. You can come back and take the test some other time.

VII. AT THE TEST

The day of the test is here and you have the test booklet in your hand. The temptation to get going is very strong. Caution! There is more to success than knowing the right answers. You must know how to identify your papers and understand variations in the type of short-answer question used in this particular examination. Follow these suggestions for maximum results from your efforts:

1) Cooperate with the monitor

The test administrator has a duty to create a situation in which you can be as much at ease as possible. He will give instructions, tell you when to begin, check to see that you are marking your answer sheet correctly, and so on. He is not there to guard you, although he will see that your competitors do not take unfair advantage. He wants to help you do your best.

2) Listen to all instructions

Don't jump the gun! Wait until you understand all directions. In most civil service tests you get more time than you need to answer the questions. So don't be in a hurry. Read each word of instructions until you clearly understand the meaning. Study the examples, listen to all announcements and follow directions. Ask questions if you do not understand what to do.

3) Identify your papers

Civil service exams are usually identified by number only. You will be assigned a number; you must not put your name on your test papers. Be sure to copy your number correctly. Since more than one exam may be given, copy your exact examination title.

4) Plan your time

Unless you are told that a test is a "speed" or "rate of work" test, speed itself is usually not important. Time enough to answer all the questions will be provided, but this does not mean that you have all day. An overall time limit has been set. Divide the total time (in minutes) by the number of questions to determine the approximate time you have for each question.

5) Do not linger over difficult questions

If you come across a difficult question, mark it with a paper clip (useful to have along) and come back to it when you have been through the booklet. One caution if you do this – be sure to skip a number on your answer sheet as well. Check often to be sure that you have not lost your place and that you are marking in the row numbered the same as the question you are answering.

6) Read the questions

Be sure you know what the question asks! Many capable people are unsuccessful because they failed to read the questions correctly.

7) Answer all questions

Unless you have been instructed that a penalty will be deducted for incorrect answers, it is better to guess than to omit a question.

8) Speed tests

It is often better NOT to guess on speed tests. It has been found that on timed tests people are tempted to spend the last few seconds before time is called in marking answers at random – without even reading them – in the hope of picking up a few extra points. To discourage this practice, the instructions may warn you that your score will be "corrected" for guessing. That is, a penalty will be applied. The incorrect answers will be deducted from the correct ones, or some other penalty formula will be used.

9) Review your answers

If you finish before time is called, go back to the questions you guessed or omitted to give them further thought. Review other answers if you have time.

10) Return your test materials

If you are ready to leave before others have finished or time is called, take ALL your materials to the monitor and leave quietly. Never take any test material with you. The monitor can discover whose papers are not complete, and taking a test booklet may be grounds for disqualification.

VIII. EXAMINATION TECHNIQUES

1) Read the general instructions carefully. These are usually printed on the first page of the exam booklet. As a rule, these instructions refer to the timing of the examination; the fact that you should not start work until the signal and must stop work at a signal, etc. If there are any special instructions, such as a choice of questions to be answered, make sure that you note this instruction carefully.

2) When you are ready to start work on the examination, that is as soon as the signal has been given, read the instructions to each question booklet, underline any key words or phrases, such as least, best, outline, describe and the like. In this way you will tend to answer as requested rather than discover on reviewing your paper that you listed without describing, that you selected the worst choice rather than the best choice, etc.

3) If the examination is of the objective or multiple-choice type – that is, each question will also give a series of possible answers: A, B, C or D, and you are called upon to select the best answer and write the letter next to that answer on your answer paper – it is advisable to start answering each question in turn. There may be anywhere from 50 to 100 such questions in the three or four hours allotted and you can see how much time would be taken if you read through all the questions before beginning to answer any. Furthermore, if you

come across a question or group of questions which you know would be difficult to answer, it would undoubtedly affect your handling of all the other questions.

4) If the examination is of the essay type and contains but a few questions, it is a moot point as to whether you should read all the questions before starting to answer any one. Of course, if you are given a choice – say five out of seven and the like – then it is essential to read all the questions so you can eliminate the two that are most difficult. If, however, you are asked to answer all the questions, there may be danger in trying to answer the easiest one first because you may find that you will spend too much time on it. The best technique is to answer the first question, then proceed to the second, etc.

5) Time your answers. Before the exam begins, write down the time it started, then add the time allowed for the examination and write down the time it must be completed, then divide the time available somewhat as follows:
   - If 3-1/2 hours are allowed, that would be 210 minutes. If you have 80 objective-type questions, that would be an average of 2-1/2 minutes per question. Allow yourself no more than 2 minutes per question, or a total of 160 minutes, which will permit about 50 minutes to review.
   - If for the time allotment of 210 minutes there are 7 essay questions to answer, that would average about 30 minutes a question. Give yourself only 25 minutes per question so that you have about 35 minutes to review.

6) The most important instruction is to read each question and make sure you know what is wanted. The second most important instruction is to time yourself properly so that you answer every question. The third most important instruction is to answer every question. Guess if you have to but include something for each question. Remember that you will receive no credit for a blank and will probably receive some credit if you write something in answer to an essay question. If you guess a letter – say "B" for a multiple-choice question – you may have guessed right. If you leave a blank as an answer to a multiple-choice question, the examiners may respect your feelings but it will not add a point to your score. Some exams may penalize you for wrong answers, so in such cases only, you may not want to guess unless you have some basis for your answer.

7) Suggestions
   a. Objective-type questions
      1. Examine the question booklet for proper sequence of pages and questions
      2. Read all instructions carefully
      3. Skip any question which seems too difficult; return to it after all other questions have been answered
      4. Apportion your time properly; do not spend too much time on any single question or group of questions
      5. Note and underline key words – all, most, fewest, least, best, worst, same, opposite, etc.
      6. Pay particular attention to negatives
      7. Note unusual option, e.g., unduly long, short, complex, different or similar in content to the body of the question
      8. Observe the use of "hedging" words – probably, may, most likely, etc.

9. Make sure that your answer is put next to the same number as the question
10. Do not second-guess unless you have good reason to believe the second answer is definitely more correct
11. Cross out original answer if you decide another answer is more accurate; do not erase until you are ready to hand your paper in
12. Answer all questions; guess unless instructed otherwise
13. Leave time for review

b. Essay questions
1. Read each question carefully
2. Determine exactly what is wanted. Underline key words or phrases.
3. Decide on outline or paragraph answer
4. Include many different points and elements unless asked to develop any one or two points or elements
5. Show impartiality by giving pros and cons unless directed to select one side only
6. Make and write down any assumptions you find necessary to answer the questions
7. Watch your English, grammar, punctuation and choice of words
8. Time your answers; don't crowd material

8) Answering the essay question

Most essay questions can be answered by framing the specific response around several key words or ideas. Here are a few such key words or ideas:

M's: manpower, materials, methods, money, management
P's: purpose, program, policy, plan, procedure, practice, problems, pitfalls, personnel, public relations

a. Six basic steps in handling problems:
1. Preliminary plan and background development
2. Collect information, data and facts
3. Analyze and interpret information, data and facts
4. Analyze and develop solutions as well as make recommendations
5. Prepare report and sell recommendations
6. Install recommendations and follow up effectiveness

b. Pitfalls to avoid
1. Taking things for granted – A statement of the situation does not necessarily imply that each of the elements is necessarily true; for example, a complaint may be invalid and biased so that all that can be taken for granted is that a complaint has been registered
2. Considering only one side of a situation – Wherever possible, indicate several alternatives and then point out the reasons you selected the best one
3. Failing to indicate follow up – Whenever your answer indicates action on your part, make certain that you will take proper follow-up action to see how successful your recommendations, procedures or actions turn out to be
4. Taking too long in answering any single question – Remember to time your answers properly

EXAMINATION SECTION

EXAMINATION SECTION
TEST 1

DIRECTIONS: Each question or incomplete statement is followed by several suggested answers or completions. Select the one that BEST answers the question or completes the statement. *PRINT THE LETTER OF THE CORRECT ANSWER IN THE SPACE AT THE RIGHT.*

1. One of the ingredients of Compound Sodium Cyclamate Solution is 1.____

   A. calcium cyclamate
   B. glycerol
   C. saccharin sodium
   D. sorbitol

2. The one of the following galenicals which is NOT official at present is 2.____

   A. Anthralin Ointment
   B. Arnica Tincture
   C. Belladonna Liniment
   D. Taraxacum Fluidextract

3. Belladonna Ointment is prepared from 3.____

   A. Belladonna Leaf Fluidextract
   B. Belladonna Root Fluidextract
   C. Pilular Belladonna Extract
   D. Powdered Belladonna Extract

4. Of the following official galenicals, the one which is a supersaturated solution in water is 4.____

   A. Aluminum Subacetate Solution
   B. Boric Acid Solution
   C. Mannitol Injection
   D. Potassium Iodide Solution

5. Ethyl Aminobenzoate is MOST soluable in 5.____

   A. ethanol
   B. glycerol
   C. olive oil
   D. water

6. The process of lypophilization involves 6.____

   A. alpha hemolysis
   B. electrophoresis
   C. freeze drying
   D. plasmoptysis

7. The pH of a solution of Tetracycline Hydrochloride for Injection is between 7.____

   A. 2 and 3
   B. 4 and 5
   C. 6 and 7
   D. 8 and 9

8. Of the following, the compound which is MOST soluble in water at 25° C. is 8.____

   A. codeine sulfate
   B. dihydromorphinone hydrochloride
   C. ethylmorphine hydrochloride
   D. quinine sulfate

9. Thiamine hydrochloride is INCOMPATIBLE with 9.____

   A. ferrous gluconate
   B. glycerol
   C. sodium citrate
   D. sorbitol solution

10. The PRINCIPAL solvent used in the preparation of Medicinal Soft Soap Liniment is 10.____

A. chloroform
B. ethanol
C. glycerol
D. isopropanol

11. The solubility of codeine phosphate compared with that of codeine sulfate, at room temperature, is ______ times greater. 11.____

A. four
B. six
C. eight
D. twelve

12. Glycerin is a constituent of 12.____

A. Chalk Mixture
B. Compound Sarsaparilla Syrup
C. Liquid Petrolatum Emulsion
D. Phenobarbital Elixir

13. Of the following acids, the one LEAST soluble in water at 25° C. has the formula 13.____

A. $HC_2H_3O_2$
B. $HC_7H_5O_2$
C. $H_2C_4H_4O_6$
D. H_3BO_3

14. Romilar Syrup is INCOMPATIBLE with 14.____

A. Elixir Three Bromides
B. Sedulon Syrup
C. Syrup Hydriodic Acid
D. Thephorin Syrup

15. Wild Cherry Syrup U.S.P. is made from the bark of 15.____

A. Cassia acutifolia
B. Prunus cerasus
C. Prunus serotina
D. Rhamnus purshiana

16. Myciguent is an ointment containing as the PRINCIPAL ingredient 16.____

A. Griseofulvin
B. Neomycin
C. Novabiocin
D. Nystatin

17. Monoethanolamine is a pharmaceutical NECESSITY in 17.____

A. Nitrofurazone Ointment
B. Nitromersal Solution
C. Thiomersal Ointment
D. Thiomersal Solution

18. The ointment base used in the preparation of Phenol Ointment N.F. is 18.____

A. Hydrophilic Ointment
B. White Ointment
C. White Petrolatum
D. Yellow Petrolatum

19. Thephorin Syrup is INCOMPATIBLE with 19.____

A. ammonium chloride
B. ephedrine sulfate
C. ethylmorphine hydrochloride
D. potassium guaiacolsulfonate

20. A eutectic mixture will be obtained when camphor is triturated with an EQUAL weight of 20.____

A. mannitol
B. saccharin
C. saligenin
D. thymol

21. The ointment base used in the preparation of the official Ichthammol Ointment consists of Wool Fat and _______. 21.____

A. Hydrophylic Ointment
B. Liquid Petrolatum
C. White Ointment
D. Yellow Petrolatum

22. The percentage range of isopropanol present in the official Isopropyl Alcohol Rubbing Compound is _______ percent. 22.____

A. 55 - 60
B. 68 - 72
C. 82 - 88
D. 92 - 99

23. In the preparation of Yellow Mercuric Oxide Ointment, the Yellow Mercuric Oxide is rubbed with Liquid Petrolatum until the mixture is smooth. This process is called 23.____

A. alligation
B. comminution
C. levigation
D. maceration

24. The OFFICIAL synonym for Noscapine Hydrochloride is 24.____

A. Naepaine Hydrochloride
B. Naphazoline Hydrochloride
C. Narcotine Hydrochloride
D. Nylidrin Hydrochloride

25. A substance NO LONGER permitted legally as a denaturant of ethyl alcohol is 25.____

A. acetone
B. boric acid
C. camphor
D. isopropyl alcohol

KEY (CORRECT ANSWERS)

1. C
2. C
3. C
4. C
5. A
6. C
7. A
8. B
9. C
10. B
11. D
12. D
13. B
14. C
15. C
16. B
17. D
18. B
19. D
20. D
21. D
22. B
23. C
24. C
25. B

TEST 2

DIRECTIONS: Each question or incomplete statement is followed by several suggested answers or completions. Select the one that BEST answers the question or completes the statement. *PRINT THE LETTER OF THE CORRECT ANSWER IN THE SPACE AT THE RIGHT.*

1. A substance used as a preservative for galenicals is 1.____
   A. benzalkonium chloride
   B. methyl parahydroxybenzoate
   C. parachlorophenol
   D. phenylmercuric nitrate

2. The ACTIVE component of Liquor Carbonis Detergens is 2.____
   A. Coal Tar
   B. Juniper Tar
   C. Pine Tar
   D. Rectified Tar Oil

3. Methadon hydrochloride is INCOMPATIBLE with 3.____
   A. Aromatic Elixir
   B. Orange Syrup
   C. Peppermint Water
   D. Wild Cherry Syrup

4. Persic Oil is an ingredient used in the preparation of 4.____
   A. Calamine Lotion
   B. Chrysarobin Ointment
   C. Lime Liniment
   D. Rose Water Ointment

5. Cherry Syrup is INCOMPATIBLE with 5.____
   A. ascorbic acid
   B. codeine phosphate
   C. potassium citrate
   D. thiamine hydrochloride

6. Sulfur Ointment is NOT prepared by the fusion method because the 6.____
   A. ointment base becomes rancid
   B. sulfur is precipitated
   C. sulfur reacts with the ointment base
   D. sulfur is volatilized

7. Of the following, the one which is a component used in the preparation of Chalk Mixture is 7.____
   A. Bentonite Magma
   B. Bismuth Magma
   C. Methylcellulose
   D. Sodium Alginate

8. The formula CH_3CHNH_2COOH represents the compound 8.____
   A. alanine
   B. fumaric acid
   C. glutamic acid
   D. tryptophane

9. A compound permitted for use as an antibacterial agent in opthalmic solutions has the formula 9.____
   A. $C_6H_5C_2H_4OH$
   B. $C_6H_8\,(OH)_6$
   C. C_6H_5CHO
   D. $C_6H_4\,(OH)\,COOH$

10. A proteolytic enzyme obtained from the pancreas gland of the ox is 10.____

A. lipase B. pepsin C. rennin D. trypsin

11. Ethylcellulose is characterized as an 11.____

A. alcohol B. ester C. ether D. inner oxide

12. An alkaloid which is a DERIVATIVE of ecgonine is 12.____

A. atropine B. brucine
C. cocaine D. lobeline

13. An antibacterial substance produced by the growth of Bacillus brevis is 13.____

A. Nystatin B. Polymyxin
C. Tetracycline D. Tyrothricin

14. A solution of formaldehyde in concentrated sulfuric acid is used as a reagent to test for the presence of 14.____

A. atropine B. marijuana C. morphine D. phenobarbital

15. Of the following compounds, the one which has the HIGHEST vapor pressure at room temperature is 15.____

A. amphetamine B. atropine
C. ephedrine D. epinephrine

16. Of the following alkaloids, the one which is a liquid at 25° C. is 16.____

A. emetine B. lobeline
C. papaverine D. scopolamine

17. Of the following, the one employed as a gaseous fumigant has the formula 17.____

A. CH_3Br B. $(C_2H_5)_2O$ C. CH_3COOH D. C_6H_5CHO

18. When a prescription calls for $C_6H_4OOCH_3COOH$, the substance required is 18.____

A. acetaminophenol B. acetylsalicylic acid
C. benzoic acid D. phenyl salicylate

19. Chloropropamide is a DERIVATIVE of 19.____

A. ethylenediamine B. oxazolidine
C. pyrrolidine D. sulfonylurea

20. Nordefrin hydrochloride is ISOMETRIC with ______ hydrochloride. 20.____

A. ephedrine B. epinephrine
C. norephedrine D. phenylephrine

21. Peritrate is a DERIVATIVE of 21.____

A. pentaerythritol B. phenobarbital
C. sorbitol D. tartaric acid

22. A NATURAL source of an official steroid glycoside is 22.____

    A. Brassica nigra
    B. Digitalis purpurea
    C. Fagopyrum esculentum
    D. Prunus serotina

23. Peanut Oil is obtained from the seed kernels of 23.____

    A. Arachis hypogaea
    B. Aralis racemosa
    C. Gossypium hirsutum
    D. Zea mays

24. A balsam obtained from the trunk of Liquidambar orientalis is an ingredient of Compound ______. 24.____

    A. Colocynth and Jalap Pills
    B. Resorcinol Ointment
    C. Tincture of Benzoin
    D. White Pine Syrup

25. An OFFICIAL natural source of Santonin is 25.____

    A. Aralia racemosa
    B. Artemisia cina
    C. Candida utilis
    D. Smilaz regelii

KEY (CORRECT ANSWERS)

1. B
2. A
3. D
4. D
5. C
6. B
7. A
8. A
9. A
10. D
11. C
12. C
13. D
14. C
15. A
16. B
17. A
18. B
19. D
20. B
21. A
22. B
23. A
24. C
25. B

TEST 3

DIRECTIONS: Each question or incomplete statement is followed by several suggested answers or completions. Select the one that BEST answers the question or completes the Statement. *PRINT THE LETTER OF THE CORRECT ANSWER IN THE SPACE AT THE RIGHT.*

1. The botanical source of Mexican Scammony Resin is 1.____

   A. Exogonium purga
   B. Ipomaea orizabensis
   C. Pistacia lentiscus
   D. Phamnus purshiana

2. The seed of Anamirta cocculus is the source of the active *principle* 2.____

   A. pavatrine
   B. phenylalanine
   C. picrotoxin
   D. pilocarpine

3. The following prescription is to be compounded: 3.____
   Rx

Atropine Sulfate	0.300 gram
Sodium Chloride	q.s.
Distilled water to make	30.0 ml.

   Prepare an isotonic solution.
   The sodium chloride equivalent for atropine sulfate is 0.12. The weight of sodium chloride required is ______ milligrams.

   A. 36
   B. 117
   C. 234
   D. 306

4. Blood plasma contains 5.0 milliequivalents of combined potassium per liter. Assuming that all the potassium is present as KCl, the corresponding weight of potassium chloride is, MOST NEARLY, ______ grams. 4.____
   (The formula weight for potassium chloride is 74.6 the atomic weight for potassium is 39.1.)

   A. 3.73
   B. 0.373
   C. 0.0373
   D. 0.00373

5. The volume of a sodium hydroxide solution having a specific gravity of 1.530 and containing 49.0% of NaOH (by weight) required to prepare 2500 milliliters of a 0.2000 Normal solution of NaOH is, MOST NEARLY, ______ ml. 5.____
   (Molecular weight of NaOH = 40.0)

   A. 10.6
   B. 13.3
   C. 26.6
   D. 37.5

6. A pesticide formula contains 25 grams of ethohexadiol (specific gravity 0.940) in 100 ml. of solution. The volume of ethohexadiol required to prepare one gallon of this preparation is, MOST NEARLY, ______ ml. 6.____

   A. 889
   B. 946
   C. 1006
   D. 1064

7. The hydrogen ion concentration of a solution with a pOH equal to 10 is ______ molar. 7.____

   A. 1×10^{-4}
   B. 8×10^{-6}
   C. 4×10^{-10}
   D. 2×10^{-12}

8. The weight of H_2SO_4 (formula weight = 98.06) required to prepare 2500 ml. of a solution with a pH of 3 is, MOST NEARLY, _______ milligrams. 8.____

A. 61.3 B. 122.6 C. 245.2 D. 490.4

9. The weight in milligrams of a ten per cent (by weight) triturate of atropine sulfate required to prepare 100 capsules, each to contain 1/200 grain of atropine sulfate, is 9.____

A. 648 B. 405 C. 324 D. 162

10. The molar concentration of a 1:5000 solution of potassium permanganate is _______. (The molecular weight of potassium permanganate is 158.) 10.____

A. 0.0630 B. 0.00126 C. 0.00025 D. 0.00002

11. An effective surface anaesthetic useful in ophthalmology is 11.____

A. Benoxinate Hydrochloride
B. Hydroxydione Sodium Succinate
C. Pramoxine Hydrochloride
D. Thiamyal Sodium

12. Plasmolysis is caused by a solution which is 12.____

A. hypertonic B. hypotonic
C. isohydric D. mutagenic

13. A compound possessing the properties of an ozytocic is 13.____

A. Ephedrine sulfate B. Homatropine hydrobromide
C. Lanatoside C. D. Sparteine sulfate

14. Mannitol is used as a 14.____

A. diagnostic agent for kidney function
B. pharmaceutical necessity in ointments
C. preservative for sucrose solutions
D. solvent for volatile oils

15. Gout is ESSENTIALLY a disease caused by 15.____

A. deposit of uric acid derivatives
B. increase in renin excretion
C. reduction of exchangeable phosphorus
D. streptococcus endotoxin

16. Ascorbic acid is CLOSELY related to 16.____

A. benzoic acid B. cyclic amines
C. monosaccharide sugars D. phosphopyruvic acid

17. The microorganism Streptomyces fradiae is the source of the antibiotic 17.____

A. Chloroamphenicol B. Neomycin
C. Streptomycin D. Tetracycline

18. The PRIMARY therapeutic use of Salicylanilide is as a(n) 18.____

A. analgesic
B. anthelmintic
C. antifungal
D. keratolytic

19. A compound classified as a cholinergic blocking agent is 19.____

A. diphenhydramine hydrochloride
B. methylergonovine tartrate
C. papaverine hydrochloride
D. propantheline bromide

20. The NATURAL habitat of enteric organisms is the 20.____

A. axillae
B. digestive tract
C. epidermis
D. oral cavity

21. Moniliasis is a disease caused by infection with 21.____

A. Candida albicans
B. Cryptococcus neoformans
C. Pseudomonas aeruginosa
D. Treponema pallidum

22. Sodium Radiochromate Injection is used 22.____

A. as a biological tracer to tag erythrocytes
B. as a means of detecting brain tumors
C. as a neoplastic suppressant
D. in measuring absorption of vitamin B_{12}

23. Sodium Radioiodide solution is used as a diagnostic aid in 23.____

A. determining thyroid function
B. determining kidney function
C. estimating total body water
D. evaluating liver function

24. A drug used in the treatment of motion sickness is 24.____

A. apomorphine hydrochloride
B. bentyl hydrochloride
C. hexamethonium chloride
D. meclizine hydrochloride

25. The use of reserpine in daily doses above 250 mg. is CONTRAINDICATED in cases of 25.____

A. hyperglycemia
B. hypertension
C. migraine
D. peptic ulcer

KEY (CORRECT ANSWERS)

1. B
2. C
3. C
4. B
5. C

6. C
7. A
8. B
9. C
10. B

11. A
12. A
13. D
14. A
15. A

16. C
17. B
18. C
19. D
20. B

21. A
22. A
23. A
24. D
25. D

TEST 4

DIRECTIONS: Each question or incomplete statement is followed by several suggested answers or completions. Select the one that BEST answers the question or completes the statement. *PRINT THE LETTER OF THE CORRECT ANSWER IN THE SPACE AT THE RIGHT.*

1. Of the following, the one used as an antitussive is 1.____

   A. carbetapentane citrate
   B. hydroxychloroquine sulfate
   C. hydroxyzine hydrochloride
   D. metabutethamine hydrochloride

2. The USUAL adult dose for Levorphanol Tartrate is ______ milligrams. 2.____

   A. 0.5 B. 3 C. 10 D. 30

3. Of the following insecticides, the one LEAST toxic to humans is 3.____

   A. allethrin B. dieldrin
   C. lindane D. parathion

4. The USUAL adult dose of ethylmorphine hydrochloride is ______ gram. 4.____

   A. 0.001 B. 0.005 C. 0.020 D. 0.050

5. Of the following, the one which is used in the treatment of hyperglycemia is 5.____

   A. Ethoxzolamide B. Isocarboxazid
   C. Mepazine D. Tolbutamide

6. Smallpox Vaccine consists of 6.____

   A. dead bacteria B. live bacteria
   C. dead virus D. live virus

7. Warfarin Sodium is used as a(n) 7.____

   A. anticoagulant B. hemostatic
   C. insect repellant D. scabicide

8. The microorganism Clostridium perfringens is responsible for the disease known as 8.____

   A. botulism B. gas gangrene
   C. lockjaw D. whooping cough

9. A vaccine prepared from a saline suspension of a pure culture of the bacteria responsible for an individual's own infection is called 9.____

   A. autogenous B. heterologous
   C. opsonic D. pyrogenic

10. Isofluorphate is used in the treatment of 10.____

    A. dental caries B. glaucoma
    C. hypertension D. otitis media

11. The name *Spansule* identifies a product manufactured by 11.____

A. Eli Lilly & Company
B. Parke Davis & Company
C. Smith, Kline & French Laboratories
D. Wallace Laboratories

12. A drug subject to the law governing the dispensing of narcotic preparations is _______ hydrochloride. 12.____

A. eucatropine
B. bentyl
C. marezine
D. meperidine

13. Perphenazine is the GENERIC name for 13.____

A. Compazine
B. Librium
C. Stelazine
D. Trilafon

14. The one of the following which is NOT a trade name for Tetracycline U.S.P. is 14.____

A. Achromycin
B. Panmycin
C. Pen-Vee
D. Steclin

15. Sulfamethoxypyridazine is the GENERIC name for the product marketed under the name 15.____

A. Compazine
B. Exna
C. Kynex
D. Sandrel

16. A PROPRIETARY tablet containing hydroxyzine pamoate is manufactured by 16.____

A. Pfizer Laboratories
B. Roche Laboratories
C. Smith, Kline & French Laboratories
D. Wallace Laboratories

17. The name *Kapseal* identifies a product manufactured by 17.____

A. Burroughs, Wellcome & Co.
B. Eli Lilly & Company
C. Merck, Sharp & Dohme
D. Parke Davis & Company

18. The following prescription is to be compounded: 18.____

R_x

Ethyl aminobenzoate	3.60 gm
Resorcinol	7.00 gm
Bismuth Subgallate	14.00 gm
White Petrolatum	70.00 gm

The MOST expensive component of this prescription, as written, is

A. Bismuth Subgallate
B. Ethyl aminobenzoate
C. Resorcinol
D. White Petrolatum

19. Of the following, the one which is the LOWER limit of the temperature range required for the storage of bacterial vaccines is 19.____

A. -10° C B. 2° C C. 12° C D. 18° C

20. The expiration date for Smallpox Vaccine is NOT MORE THAN ______ months after the date of issue. 20.____

A. eighteen
B. six
C. three
D. twelve

21. Triethanolamine must be preserved in tight, light-resistant containers in order to minimize 21.____

A. absorption of carbon dioxide
B. conversion to ammonium acetate
C. reduction to carbamide
D. volatilization of ammonia

22. In considering storage temperature, a cold place is officially defined in the U.S.P. as one having a temperature NOT EXCEEDING 22.____

A. 15° C B. 20° C C. 32° C D. 49° C

23. Lime Water is directed to be stored at a temperature not exceeding 25° C in order to prevent 23.____

A. deposition of calcium carbonate
B. formation of calcium bicarbonate
C. formation of calcium silicate
D. precipitation of calcium hydroxide

24. The PREFERRED glass container for the storage of Injections is Type ______. 24.____

A. I B. II C. III D. IV

25. Ephedrine MUST be stored in a cold place because it 25.____

A. decomposes rapidly at 40° C
B. has a low melting point
C. is deliquescent at room temperature
D. volatilizes at 30° C

KEY (CORRECT ANSWERS)

1. A
2. B
3. A
4. B
5. D

6. D
7. A
8. B
9. A
10. B

11. C
12. D
13. D
14. C
15. C

16. A
17. D
18. A
19. B
20. C

21. A
22. A
23. D
24. A
25. B

EXAMINATION SECTION
TEST 1

DIRECTIONS: Each question or incomplete statement is followed by several suggested answers or completions. Select the one that BEST answers the question or completes the statement. *PRINT THE LETTER OF THE CORRECT ANSWER IN THE SPACE AT THE RIGHT.*

1. Arachis Oil is available under the name of ______ oil. 1.____

   A. Peach Kernel
   B. Peanut
   C. Persic
   D. Sweet Almond

2. A pharmacist filling a prescription that requires Methylrosaniline Chloride should use 2.____

   A. Gentian Violet
   B. Merbromin
   C. Methylene Blue
   D. Scarlet Red

3. In filling a prescription calling for Witch Hazel Extract, the pharmacist should use 3.____

   A. Chondrus Extract
   B. Dakin's Solution
   C. Fluidextract Buchu
   D. Hamamelis Water

4. A proprietary product corresponding to Benzethonium Chloride is 4.____

   A. Etamon Hydrochloride
   B. Methedrine Hydrochloride
   C. Phemerol Chloride
   D. Zephiran Chloride

5. Sulfisoxazole is the OFFICIAL title for the proprietary product identified by the name 5.____

   A. Diamox
   B. Gantrisin
   C. Thalamyd
   D. Tricombisul

6. Thiomersal is the OFFICIAL title of a product sold under the name of 6.____

   A. Meralluride
   B. Mercurochrome
   C. Merthiolate
   D. Metaphen

7. The OFFICIAL equivalent for Ilotycin is 7.____

   A. Erythromycin
   B. Fumagillin
   C. Neomycin
   D. Tetracycline

8. The U.S.P. equivalent for the x-ray contrast agent Diodrast is 8.____

   A. Iodobrassid
   B. Iodophthalein
   C. Iodopyracet
   D. Iopanoic Acid

9. A certain prescription calls for 9.____

   R_x

Camphor	8.0 grams
Sulfathiozole	5.0 grams
Thymol Iodide	3.5 grams
Boric Acid	83.5 grams

   The ingredient in this prescription which is MOST expensive is

   A. Boric Acid
   B. Camphor
   C. Sulfathiazole
   D. Thymol Iodide

10. Antimony and Potassium Tartrate is an ingredient of 10.____

A. Brown Mixture
B. Chalk Mixture
C. Rhubarb and Soda Mixture
D. Stoke's Expectorant

11. Einkle's Pills is the OFFICIAL synonym for 11.____

A. Aloin, Belladonna, Cascara, and Podophyllum Pills
B. Aloin, Strychnine, Belladonna, and Cascara Pills
C. Aloin, Strychnine, Belladonna, and Ipecac Pills
D. Compound Pills of Aloe and Podophyllum

12. Mild Mercurous Chloride is an ingredient of 12.____

A. Compound Cathartic Pills
B. Mercury and Chalk
C. Mercury Bichloride Opthalmic Ointment
D. Mild Mercurial Ointment

13. The OFFICIAL title for Tincture of Green Soap is 13.____

A. Camphor and Soap Liniment
B. Hexachlorophene Liquid Soap
C. Medicinal Soft Soap Liniment
D. Saponated Benzyl Benzoate

14. Hydrochloric Acid is used in the preparation of 14.____

A. Belladonna Leaf Fluidextract
B. Compound Pepsin Elixir
C. Nux Vomica Tincture
D. Thimerosal Solution

15. Cholesterol is used in the preparation of 15.____

A. Benzyl Benzoate Lotion
B. Coal Tar Ointment
C. Hydrophilic Petrolatum
D. Polyethylene Glycol Ointment

16. Wild Cherry Syrup is INCOMPATIBLE with 16.____

A. Ammonium Chloride
B. Codeine Phosphate
C. Potassium Acetate
D. Sodium Citrate

17. Sodium Perborate is INCOMPATIBLE with 17.____

A. Boric Acid
B. Potassium Bicarbonate
C. Potassium Permanganate
D. Sodium Chloride

18. Thiamine Hydrochloride is INCOMPATIBLE with 18.____

A. Citric Acid
B. Ethanol
C. Sodium Chloride
D. Tannin

19. The official title of the substance defined as a native, hydrous magnesium silicate, sometimes containing a small proportion of aluminum silicate, is 19.____

A. Bentonite B. Kaolin C. Pumice D. Talc

20. The proportions of fixed oil, water, and dry Acacia used to prepare emulsions by the Continental method are 20.____

A. 1 part dry Acacia, 2 parts fixed oil, 4 parts water
B. 1 part dry Acacia, 2 parts water, 4 parts fixed oil
C. 1 part fixed oil, 2 parts water, 4 parts dry Acacia
D. 1 part water, 2 parts dry Acacia, 4 parts fixed oil

21. Boric Acid is used to stabilize 21.____

A. Aluminum Acetate Solution
B. Apomorphine Hydrochloride Injection
C. Calamine Lotion
D. Starch Glycerite

22. Isopropyl Alcohol is NOT used as a solvent in the preparation of Iodine Tincture because 22.____

A. Iodine is insoluble in Isopropyl Alcohol
B. Iodine solutions in Isopropyl Alcohol are not bactericidal
C. Iodine will react with Isopropyl Alcohol forming irritant compounds
D. Isopropyl Alcohol will oxidize Potassium Iodide

23. The OFFICIAL diluent used in the preparation of Powdered Belladonna Extract is 23.____

A. Anhydrous Dextrose
B. Exhausted Belladonna Leaves
C. Powdered Glycyrrhiza
D. Starch dried at 100°C

24. Boulton's Solution is an OFFICIAL synonym for 24.____

A. Antiseptic Solution B. Carbol-Fuchsin Solution
C. Castellani's Point D. Phenolated Iodine Solution

25. A non-aqueous solvent suitable for injections is ______ Oil. 25.____

A. Betula B. Cade C. Mineral D. Sesame

KEY (CORRECT ANSWERS)

1. B
2. A
3. D
4. C
5. B
6. C
7. A
8. C
9. D
10. A
11. A
12. A
13. C
14. C
15. C
16. B
17. C
18. D
19. D
20. B
21. A
22. C
23. D
24. D
25. D

TEST 2

DIRECTIONS: Each question or incomplete statement is followed by several suggested answers or completions. Select the one that BEST answers the question or completes the statement. *PRINT THE LETTER OF THE CORRECT ANSWER IN THE SPACE AT THE RIGHT.*

1. Potassium Citrate is used to increase the solubility in water of 1.____

   A. Acetophenetidin B. Acetylsalicylic Acid
   C. Benzyl Benzoate D. Iodochlorhydroxyquin

2. Calciferol is insoluble in 2.____

   A. edible vegetable oil B. Polysorbate 80
   C. Propylene Glycol D. Purified Water

3. The Ointment base used in Zinc Oxide Ointment U.S.P. is a mixture of 3.____

   A. Liquid Petrolatum and White Ointment
   B. Stearyl Alcohol and Benzoinated Lard
   C. White Petrolatum and White Wax
   D. White Wax and White Ointment

4. A water-soluble ointment is prepared from a mixture of 4.____

   A. Cholesterol and White Petrolatum
   B. Polyethylene Glycol 400 and Polyethylene Glycol 4000
   C. Spermaceti, Sodium Borate, and Persic Oil
   D. Stearyl Alcohol and White Wax

5. In the preparation of Sulfur Ointment, the Precipitated Sulfur is levigated with 5.____

   A. Glycerin B. Liquid Petrolatum
   C. Peanut Oil D. Propylene Glycol

6. A flavoring agent useful in masking the saline taste of bromides is 6.____

   A. Cherry Syrup B. Cinnamon Water
   C. Iso-Alcoholic Elixir D. Phenylethyl Alcohol

7. If a fatty acid is desired as a component of an injection the acid used is ______ acid. 7.____

   A. butyric B. oleic C. palmitic D. stearic

8. An example of a solubilizing agent capable of increasing the solubility of Cresol in water is 8.____

   A. ammonium chloride B. calcium stearate
   C. magnesium carbonate D. sodium oleate

9. A 10% solution of a potassium soap is used as a solvent for 9.____

   A. Chlorophenothane B. Dienestrol
   C. Hexachlorophene D. Propylparaben

10. Potassium Iodide is insoluble in 10.____

A. benzol
B. ethanol
C. glycerol
D. water

11. A class of liquid galenicals NO LONGER represented in *either* the U.S.P. or the N.F. is 11.____

A. Infusions
B. Mucilages
C. Oleoresins
D. Vinegars

12. Bentonite is classified as a 12.____

A. native clay
B. purified carbohydrate
C. synthetic product
D. water-soluble gum

13. Amaranth Solution is used as a 13.____

A. coloring agent for pharmaceutical preparations
B. diagnostic reagent in determining liver function
C. flavoring agent for bitter medicinals
D. topical antiseptic in surgery

14. Calcium Cyclamate is used as a 14.____

A. non-caloric sweetener
B. preservative in syrups
C. source of dietary calcium
D. vitamin synergist

15. To insure MAXIMUM buffer capacity in the preparation of a buffer solution, it is best to 15.____

A. add a high concentration of sodium chloride to the buffer mixture after the mixture has been prepared
B. be certain that the weak acid selected is an inorganic rather than an organic compound
C. have the compounds employed in the solution in concentration less than 0.02 ml
D. select a weak acid with an ionization constant approximately equal to the pH at which the buffer is to be used

16. An isotonic solution is one having the *same* 16.____

A. absorption index as a body fluid
B. normal concentration as a body fluid
C. mitotic pressure as a body fluid
D. pH as a body fluid

17. The U.S.P. states that the adult rectal suppository shall weigh, most nearly, ______ grams. 17.____

A. five
B. four
C. two
D. one

18. If the pH of a solution is stated to be 6.0, the hydrogen ion concentration of the solution is ______ molar. 18.____

A. 6×10^{-1}
B. 3×10^{-2}
C. 1.5×10^{-4}
D. 1×10^{-6}

19. The MINIMUM concentration of Phenol in Liquefied Phenol is 19.____

A. 98% B. 88% C. 78% D. 68%

20. The adult dose of a given drug is 1/25 grain per kilogram of body weight. The weight, in milligrams, of the drug to be administered to a person weighing 165 pounds is, *most nearly,* ______ milligrams. 20.____

A. 195 B. 95 C. 75 D. 26

21. If one gram of Ammonium Chloride is soluble in 2.6 milliliters of water, then the quantity of Ammonium Chloride that 100 milliliters of water will dissolve is, *most nearly,* ______ grams. 21.____

A. 38.46 B. 26.00 C. 19.23 D. 13.00

22. The formula for the preparation of Phenol Ointment is: 22.____

Phenol	20.0 grams
Glycerin	20.0 grams
White Ointment	960.0 grams

The quantity of Phenol required to prepare one pound (avoirdupois) of Phenol Ointment is, *most nearly,* ______ grams.

A. 9.08 B. 9.60 C. 18.16 D. 19.20

23. The MAXIMUM number of tablets, each containing 1/50 grain of Atropine Sulfate, that can be obtained from 1/8 ounce avoirdupois of Atropine Sulfate is, *most nearly,* 23.____

A. 2734 B. 3000 C. 4800 D. 5468

24. A prescription calls for 2 fluid ounces of a 3% (weight/ volume) solution of Gentian Violet in water. 24.____
The weight of Gentian Violet required for this prescription is, *most nearly,* ______ grams.

A. 26.0 B. 27.3 C. 28.8 D. 29.2

25. The weight of Potassium Permanganate which is required to prepare 500 milliliters of a 1:4000 solution of Potassium Permanganate is ______ milligrams. 25.____

A. 125 B. 250 C. 500 D. 750

KEY (CORRECT ANSWERS)

1. B
2. D
3. A
4. B
5. B
6. A
7. B
8. D
9. C
10. A
11. A
12. A
13. A
14. A
15. D
16. B
17. C
18. D
19. B
20. A
21. A
22. A
23. A
24. B
25. A

TEST 3

DIRECTIONS: Each question or incomplete statement is followed by several suggested answers or completions. Select the one that BEST answers the question or completes the statement. *PRINT THE LETTER OF THE CORRECT ANSWER IN THE SPACE AT THE RIGHT.*

1. A formula for a preparation used as a diagnostic agent calls for 250 milliliters of 0.5 Normal Sodium Carbonate Solution. 1.____
The weight of Sodium Carbonate Monohydrate required in this preparation is, *most nearly*, _______ grams.

   A. 62.005 B. 31.003 C. 15.501 D. 7.750

   (Formula Weight for Sodium Carbonate Monohydrate is 124.01)

2. The formula weight of Potassium Chloride is 74.56. If 9.320 grams of Potassium Chloride is dissolved in enough water to make 250 milliliters of solution, EACH milliliter of the solution will contain, *most nearly*, ______ milliequivalent of Potassium Chloride. 2.____

   A. 0.2500 B. 0.3750 C. 0.5000 D. 1.000

3. Tincture of Ferric Chloride contains 14 grams of $FeCl_3$ in each 100 milliliters. 3.____
The weight of Fe in 5 milliliters of Tincture of Ferric Chloride is, *most nearly*, _______ milligrams.

   A. 120 B. 241 C. 482 D. 700

   (Formula Weight of $FeCl_3$ = 162.22)
   (Atomic Weight of Fe = 55.85)

4. Chromium Trioxide is characterized as a(n)(the) 4.____

   A. chelating agent
   B. strong oxidizing agent
   C. active reducing agent
   D. anhydride of a strong base

5. The compound 2-hydroxypropionic acid is *also* known as ______ acid. 5.____

   A. Folic B. Gluconic C. Lactic D. Tartaric

6. Potassium Iodide is READILY oxidized in aqueous solution by 6.____

   A. Arsenous Acid
   B. Ferric Chloride
   C. Mercuric Chloride
   D. Sodium Bisulfite

7. The MAJOR constituent of Beeswax is ______ Palmitate. 7.____

   A. Cetyl B. Glyceryl C. Myricyl D. Stearyl

8. The millicurie is a unit for measuring 8.____

   A. activity of radioactive isotopes
   B. concentration of isotonic solutions
   C. effects of cosmic rays on humans
   D. mitotic activity of human cells

9. The PRINCIPAL pancreatic hormone is 9.___

A. insulin B. rennin C. secretin D. vasopressin

10. The *only* OFFICIAL vitamin that contains a metal atom in its structure is 10.___

A. Cyanocobalamin
B. Pyridoxine Hydrochloride
C. Riboflavin
D. Thiamine Hydrochloride

11. Amylolytic enzymes are active constituents of 11.___

A. Beef, Iron and Wine
B. Malt Extract
C. Pepsin and Rennin Elixir
D. Soluble Liver Fraction

12. The chemical structure of Amphetamine is 12.___

A. 1-phenyl-2-aminopropanol
B. 1-phenyl-2-aminopropane
C. 1-phenyl-2-methylaminopropanol
D. 2-phenyl-1-methylaminopropane

13. The one of the following antihistamines which is a derivative of ethylenediamine is 13.___

A. Clistine Maleate
B. Perazil
C. Pyribenzamine
D. Trimeton

14. Derivatives of malonylurea are classified as 14.___

A. barbiturates
B. carbamates
C. hydantoins
D. purines

15. The sodium chloride equivalent of Boric Acid is 0.55. The weight of sodium chloride required to be added in the preparation of 30 milliliters of an isotonic 1% (weight/volume) solution of Boric Acid is ______ milligrams. 15.___

A. 30 B. 105 C. 165 D. 270

16. The euphoriant marijuana is obtained from 16.___

A. Cannabis sativa
B. Cocculus indicus
C. Papaver somniferum
D. Viburnum opulus

17. The OFFICIAL synonym for Myristica Oil is ______ Oil. 17.___

A. Bergamot
B. Clove
C. Nutmeg
D. Pimenta

18. Aspidium Oleoresin is obtained from 18.___

A. Cephaelis acuminata
B. Dryopteris Felix-mas
C. Foeniculum vulgare
D. Prunus serotina

19. Caster Oil is derived from the seed of 19.____

A. Exogonium purga
B. Plantago ovata
C. Podophyllum peltatum
D. Ricinus communis

20. Of the following, the one that is an example of a steroid glycoside is 20.____

A. Aloin
B. Corticosterone
C. Coumarin
D. Digitoxin

21. The rind of citrus fruits is a source of 21.____

A. Bentonite
B. Citric Acid
C. Methylcellulose
D. Pectin

22. Rescinnamine is an alkaloid which occurs in certain species of 22.____

A. Cinnamomum
B. Myristica
C. Papaver
D. Rauwolfia

23. The target organ of the hormone Corticotropin is the 23.____

A. adrenal cortex
B. mammary gland
C. ovary
D. thyroid

24. Folic Acid is used PRIMARILY in the treatment of 24.____

A. agranulocytosis
B. certain megaloblastic anemias
C. menopausal syndrome
D. nutritional achromotrichia

25. A specific antidote in acute narcotic intoxication is 25.____

A. Mercurophylline
B. Nalorphine Hydrochloride
C. Potassium Iodide
D. Theobromine Calcium Salicylate

KEY (CORRECT ANSWERS)

1. D
2. C
3. B
4. B
5. C

6. B
7. C
8. A
9. A
10. A

11. B
12. B
13. C
14. A
15. B

16. A
17. C
18. B
19. D
20. D

21. D
22. D
23. A
24. B
25. B

TEST 4

DIRECTIONS: Each question or incomplete statement is followed by several suggested answers or completions. Select the one that BEST answers the question or completes the statement. *PRINT THE LETTER OF THE CORRECTANSWER IN THE SPACE AT THE RIGHT.*

1. A compound used as an antidote in cyanide poisoning is 1.____

   A. Ferrous Sulfate
   B. Magnesium Hydroxide
   C. Potassium Iodide
   D. Sodium Thiosulfate

2. A compound employed in solution as a dental prophylactic is 2.____

   A. Boric Acid
   B. Potassium Bitartrate
   C. Sodium Fluoride
   D. Sorbitol

3. Rabies Vaccine is an example of a ______ vaccine. 3.____

   A. bacterial
   B. protozoal
   C. rickettsial
   D. viral

4. Haemophilus pertussis is the microorganism used to prepare ______ vaccine. 4.____

   A. cholera
   B. plague
   C. typhoid
   D. whooping cough

5. The Schick test is used to ascertain susceptibility to 5.____

   A. diphtheria
   B. scarlet fever
   C. syphilis
   D. tuberculosis

6. The PRINCIPAL use of Primaquine is in the treatment of 6.____

   A. amebiasis
   B. malaria
   C. schistosomiasis
   D. trypanosomiasis

7. An OFFICIAL compound used in therapy as an antihistamine is 7.____

   A. Mephenesin
   B. Pentylenetetrazol
   C. Pyrilamine Maleate
   D. Tolazoline Hydrochloride

8. The action of Menadione is counteracted by 8.____

   A. Ascorbic Acid
   B. Dicumarol
   C. Pepsin
   D. Pyridoxine

9. Liver damage may be brought about by poisoning with 9.____

   A. Carbon Tetrachloride
   B. Choline
   C. Oleic Acid
   D. Sodium Chloride

10. A substance which is used PRINCIPALLY as a fungistat is 10.____

    A. Dimethylphthalate
    B. Para-aminobenzoic acid
    C. Sodium Morrhuate
    D. Zinc undecylenate

11. A diagnostic agent used for determining kidney function is 11.____

    A. Fluorescein Sodium
    B. Iodipamide Sodium
    C. Phenolsulphonphthalein
    D. Sulphbromophthalein

12. A compound found to be of value as an anthelmintic is 12.___

A. para-aminosalicylic acid
B. piperazine citrate
C. procaine amide
D. promethiazine

13. An *official* drug which has been demonstrated to produce a MARKED increase in the renal elimination of potassium ion is 13.___

A. Acenocumarol
B. Acetazolamide
C. Acetylsulfisooxazole
D. Aniliridine hydrochloride

14. Using Young's Rule, the usual dose of Ferrous Sulfate for a child eight years old is, *most nearly*, _______ milligrams. 14.___

A. 240
B. 650
C. 800
D. 960

15. The dose of Meperidine Eydrochloride USUALLY recommended for adults is _______ milligrams. 15.___

A. 2
B. 100
C. 250
D. 500

16. The dose of Strychnine Sulfate USUALLY recommended for adults is _______ milligrams. 16.___

A. 2
B. 20
C. 40
D. 100

17. Lead Acetate must be packaged and stored in tight containers because on exposure to air Lead Acetate 17.___

A. becomes sensitive to light
B. is extremely deliquescent
C. is oxidized to Lead Peracetate
D. reacts with carbon dioxide forming Lead Carbonate

18. The stability of Aromatic Ammonia Spirit is NOT affected by 18.___

A. concentration of volatile oils
B. exposure to light
C. temperatures above 30°C.
D. tightness of closure

19. A pharmaceutical preparation which may be dispensed *without* a written prescription, according to the provisions of the Federal Food, Drug and Cosmetic Act, is 19.___

A. Desoxycorticosterone Acetate Pellets
B. Phenobarbital Elixir
C. Propylthiouracil Tablets
D. Terpin Hydrate Elixir

20. The substance dl-alpha-Tocopherol is employed as a stabilizing agent in 20.___

A. Peruvian Balsam
B. Petrolatum
C. Phenol
D. Polyethylene Glycol 400

21. Methanol is added to Formaldehyde Solution in order to prevent 21.____

A. evaporation
B. hydrolysis
C. oxidation
D. polymerization

22. The direction in the U.S.P. for the packaging and storage of Eydrocortisone Acetate read as follows: Preserve Hydrocortisone Acetate in 22.____

A. a cold place
B. tight, light- resistant containers
C. half-filled containers
D. well-filled, tight containers

23. The Pyrogen Test is applied to 23.____

A. capsules
B. injections
C. suppositories
D. tablets

24. An example of an exempt narcotic included in Class M preparations is 24.____

A. Dihydrocodeinone
B. Meperidine
C. N-allylnormorphine
D. Morphine

25. If a pharmacist wishes to obtain the wholesale price of a pharmaceutical product, it would be MOST advisable for him to consult the 25.____

A. American Druggist Blue Book
B. Chemical Week Buyers' Guide
C. Drug Trade News
D. Soap and Chemical Specialties Blue Book

KEY (CORRECT ANSWERS)

1. D
2. C
3. D
4. D
5. A
6. B
7. C
8. B
9. A
10. D
11. C
12. B
13. B
14. A
15. B
16. A
17. D
18. A
19. D
20. B
21. D
22. B
23. B
24. C
25. A

EXAMINATION SECTION
TEST 1

DIRECTIONS: Each question or incomplete statement below is followed by several suggested answers or completions. Select the one that BEST answers the question or completes the statement. *PRINT THE LETTER OF THE CORRECT ANSWER IN THE SPACE AT THE RIGHT.*

1. Boiling a drug with water is a process known as 1.____

   A. decoction B. infusion C. maceration D. percolation

2. The solvent used in the process of crude drug extraction is called the 2.____

   A. extractive B. marc C. menstruum D. percolate

3. If Burow's Solution contains a precipitate, the solution should be 3.____

   A. diluted with water
   B. discarded
   C. filtered off
   D. rewarmed to dissolve it

4. The alcohol in Potassium Arsenite Solution is a 4.____

   A. preservative
   B. reactant
   C. solvent
   D. vehicle

5. Of the following, the one which can be dispensed only on prescription is ______ liniment. 5.____

   A. belladonna
   B. camphor
   C. chloroform
   D. turpentine

6. Camphor Liniment has the official caution: 6.____

   A. Camphor liniment is extremely poisonous.
   B. Should be used no later than one year after preparation.
   C. This liniment should not come in contact with metal.
   D. This preparation is not intended for parenteral use.

7. Hard Soap in N.F. Dentifrice is used primarily as a(n) 7.____

   A. abrasive
   B. detergent
   C. emulsifier
   D. antiseptic

8. The range of the ethyl alcohol content of Terpin Hydrate Elixir is from ______ percent to ______ percent. 8.____

   A. 7; 9 B. 24; 27 C. 39;44 D. 66; 71

9. Of the following, the one which is an ingredient of Brown Mixture is 9.____

   A. antimony potassium tartrate
   B. senega fluidextract
   C. terpin hydrate
   D. thyme syrup

10. Ipecac Fluid extract contains the alkaloids 10.____

A. brucine and strychnine
B. emetine and cephaeline
C. gelsemine and colchicine
D. hyoscine and hyoscyamine

11. Potassium Iodide is present in Lugol's Solution in order to 11.____

A. increase the solubility of iodine
B. increase the volatility of the iodine
C. neutralize hydriodic acid
D. promote germicidal activity

12. In the preparation of Medicinal Soft Soap, the vegetable oil that is NOT permitted is _______ oil. 12.____

A. coconut B. corn C. peanut D. sesame

13. $KHCO_3$ is used in Magnesium Citrate Solution to 13.____

A. act as an antacid laxative
B. ensure complete solution of the oils
C. neutralize excess citric acid
D. produce CO_2 for palatability

14. The precipitate formed on exposing Calcium Hydroxide Solution to air is 14.____

A. calcium carbonate
B. calcium hydroxide
C. calcium oxide
D. calcium silicate

15. A mucilage MOST compatible with ethyl alcohol is made from 15.____

A. acacia B. althea C. mimosa D. tragacanth

16. Epinephrine Solution U.S.P. is obtained by dissolving epinephrine in distilled water with the aid of _______ acid. 16.____

A. acetic
B. hydrochloric
C. phosphoric
D. tartaric

17. In labelling vitamin-containing preparations, the vitamin content expressed in micrograms per dosage form unit is applied to Vitamin _______. 17.____

A. A B. B_1 C. B_{12} D. C

18. The official English title for Compound Digestive Elixir is _______ elixir. 18.____

A. compound pepsin
B. pepsin
C. pepsin and rennin
D. saccharated pepsin

19. Hebra's Itch Ointment is an official synonym for _______ ointment N.F. 19.____

A. compound resorcinol
B. compound sulfur
C. mild mercurous chloride
D. phenolated calamine

20. That part of the prescription that gives the required directions to the patient as to its use is called the 20.____

A. inscription
B. subscription
C. superscription
D. transcription

21. A prescription calls for Merbromin in Cacao Butter suppositories. 21.____
The MOST suitable solvent for the Merbromin is

A. chloroform
B. coconut oil
C. distilled water
D. ethanol

22. An example of a thixotropic gel is 22.____

A. aluminum hydroxide gel
B. bentonite magma
C. bismuth magma
D. pectin paste

23. An example of a nonionic emulsifying agent is 23.____

A. dioctylsodium sulfonate
B. hydroxystearin sulfate
C. polyethylene glycol 400 monostearate
D. sodium lauryl sulfonate

24. Sippy Powder No. 2 contains sodium bicarbonate and 24.____

A. acetylsalicylic acid
B. magnesium oxide
C. potassium sodium tartrate
D. precipitated calcium carbonate

25. A solution recommended as a substitute for Cudbear Tincture is ______ solution. 25.____

A. amaranth
B. merbromin
C. methylrosaniline chloride
D. thiomerosal

KEY (CORRECT ANSWERS)

1. A
2. C
3. B
4. A
5. A
6. D
7. B
8. C
9. A
10. B
11. A
12. A
13. D
14. A
15. B
16. B
17. C
18. A
19. B
20. D
21. C
22. B
23. C
24. B
25. A

TEST 2

DIRECTIONS: Each question or incomplete statement is followed by several suggested answers or completions. Select the one that BEST answers the question or completes the statement. *PRINT THE LETTER OF THE CORRECT ANSWER IN THE SPACE AT THE RIGHT.*

1. The ointment base employed in the preparation of Compound Undecylenic Acid Ointment is 1.____

   A. hydrophylic petrolatum
   B. polyethylene glycol ointment
   C. rose water ointment
   D. white ointment

2. Triethanolamine must be preserved in tight containers because it is 2.____

   A. dehydrated
   B. efflorescent
   C. hygroscopic
   D. volatile

3. A solution prepared by boiling sublimed sulfur with lime in water is called 3.____

   A. Basham's Mixture
   B. Dobell's Solution
   C. Goulard's Extract
   D. Vleminckx's Solution

4. The solvent employed in the preparation of Tribromoethanol Solution U.S.P. is 4.____

   A. amylene hydrate
   B. chloroform
   C. ethanol
   D. sesame oil

5. The ointment base employed in the preparation of Coal Tar ointment is 5.____

   A. anhydrous lanolin
   B. hydrophilic ointment
   C. rose water ointment
   D. zinc oxide paste

6. A substance added to Magma Magnesia in order to minimize action of the glass container is 6.____

   A. citric acid
   B. potassium bitartrate
   C. sodium citrate
   D. tartaric acid

7. Oils used in preparing injections should 7.____

   A. be colorless
   B. be unsaturated
   C. have a high ester value
   D. have a limited fatty acid content

8. Chloroform is used in the preparation of ______ ointment. 8.____

   A. capsicum
   B. chrysarobin
   C. coal tar
   D. scarlet red

9. Neocalamine Lotion N.F. is prepared with B 9.____

   A. bentonite magma
   B. carboxymethyl cellulose
   C. polyethylene glycol 400
   D. stearyl alcohol

10. Camphor is classified as a(n) 10.____

    A. aldehyde
    B. glycoside
    C. inner anhydride
    D. ketone

11. Of the following, the compound classified as a disaccharide is 11.____

A. dextrose B. d-fructose C. maltose D. rhamnose

12. Of the following substances, the one which is LEAST soluble in water is 12.____

A. $CuSO_4$ B. K_2SO_4 C. $MgSO_4$ D. $SrSO_4$

13. In qualitative analysis, potassium thiocyanate is used to test for 13.____

A. Al^{+++} B. Cu^{++} C. Fe^{+++} D. Ni^{++}

14. Dimethylglyoxime is used as a specific reagent for the detection of 14.____

A. Ca^{++} B. Ni^{++} C. NO_3^- D. SO_4^{--}

15. One liter of a 2M HCl solution will readily dissolve 10 grams of 15.____

A. Ag_2S B. CuS C. S D. ZnS

16. A colorless solution is treated with dilute HCl giving a white precipitate. When the precipitate is treated with $6MNH_3$, the white precipitate turns black. 16.____
The original solution must have contained

A. Ag^+ B. Hg^{++} C. Hg_2^{++} D. Pb^{++}

17. A mixture of $BaCla_2$, LiCl, NaCl, and NE_4Cl is heated in an evaporating dish over a strong Bunsen flame. 17.____
The cloud of white vapor which is observed is due to the

A. $BaCl_2$ B. LiCl C. NaCl D. NH_4Cl

18. A violet color obtained in a flame test indicates the presence of 18.____

A. copper B. lead C. potassium D. sodium

19. A solution of $KMnO_4$, may be standardized by titration against 19.____

A. oxalic acid B. potassium acid phthalate
C. sodium bicarbonate D. sulfuric acid

20. A solution of sodium hydroxide may be standardized by titration against 20.____

A. barium diphenylamine sulfonate
B. potassium acid phthalate
C. sodium carbonate
D. sodium thiosulfate

21. Cellulose is a 21.____

A. mineral deposit in plant cells
B. mixture of proteins
C. polysaccharide
D. synthetic rubber

22. The heat of combustion of an organic compound is generally measured by means of a 22.____

    A. bomb calorimeter
    B. Carius tube
    C. pyrometer
    D. Victor Meyer apparatus

23. The amount of nitrogen in an organic compound may be measured by means of 23.____

    A. an emission spectroscope
    B. a polarimeter
    C. the Hell-Volhard-Zelinsky reaction
    D. the Kjeldahl method

24. Small amounts of soluble solid impurities in solution of organic compounds are frequently removed by boiling with 24.____

    A. activated charcoal
    B. boiling stones
    C. glass beads
    D. small scraps of rubber tubing

25. Enzymes are 25.____

    A. an essential part of the diet
    B. biological catalysts
    C. hormones
    D. vitamins

KEY (CORRECT ANSWERS)

1. B
2. C
3. D
4. A
5. D
6. A
7. D
8. B
9. A
10. D
11. C
12. D
13. C
14. B
15. D
16. C
17. D
18. C
19. A
20. B
21. C
22. A
23. D
24. A
25. B

TEST 3

DIRECTIONS: Each question or incomplete statement is followed by several suggested answers or completions. Select the one that BEST answers the question or completes the statement. *PRINT THE LETTER OF THE CORRECT ANSWER IN THE SPACE AT THE RIGHT.*

1. In quantitative analysis, a precipitate of silver chloride is generally separated from the supernatant solution by 1.____

   A. a Gooch crucible
   B. a powder funnel
   C. a separatory funnel
   D. mixing with strong NH_3 solution and then decanting

2. The amount of rise of a liquid in a capillary is used to measure 2.____

   A. conductivity
   B. diffusion coefficient
   C. surface tension
   D. viscosity

3. The molecular weight of an *unknown* may be determined by dissolving a definite amount of *unknown* in a measured amount of solvent and determining the 3.____

   A. conductivity
   B. freezing point depression
   C. temperature coefficient of conductivity
   D. temperature coefficient of surface tension

4. Stannous chloride is 4.____

   A. a reducing agent
   B. an oxidizing agent
   C. used for galvanizing iron
   D. very insoluble in water

5. An official compound characterized as a purine derivative is 5.____

   A. succinchlorimide
   B. sulfapyridine
   C. terpin hydrate
   D. theobromine

6. Glycine has the formula 6.____

   A. $H_2NC_6H_5CHO$
   B. H_2NCH_2COOH
   C. CH_3COONH_4
   D. CH_3CONH_2

7. Needle-shaped crystals are sometimes observed on the surface of tablets of acetylsalicylic acid that have been standing for an extended period. 7.____
   This is due to the formation of

   A. CH_3COOH
   B. $C_6H_4(OH)COOH$
   C. C_6H_5OH
   D. $C_6H_4(OH)COCH_3$

8. Of the following substances, the one employed in anticoagulant therapy is 8.____

   A. cortisone
   B. diphenylhydantoin
   C. heparin
   D. tetracycline

9. The PRINCIPAL response elicited by a barbiturate is 9.____

A. depression of the central nervous system
B. elevation of blood pressure
C. reduction in body temperature
D. tachycardia and palpitation

10. An official compound containing arsenic is 10.____

A. carbachol
B. mersalyl
C. sodium alurate
D. sodium cacodylate

Questions 11-20.

DIRECTIONS: Column I lists the names of official chemicals, each of which can be properly matched with one of the options listed in Column II. For each item in Column I, write on you answer sheet the letter in front of the option in Column II which is its synonym.

COLUMN I	COLUMN II	
11. Amylene hydrate	A. Acetic ether	11.____
	B. Crystal violet	
12. Antimony potassium tartrate	C. Diethylmalonylurea	12.____
	D. Dihydrotheelin	
13. Antipyrine	E. Ethyl carbamate	13.____
	F. Gluside	
14. Barbital	G. Methylthionine chloride	14.____
	H. N-glucose	
15. Calciferol	I. Orthohydroxybenzoic acid	15.____
	J. Phenazone	
16. Cyclopropane	K. Stilbestrol	16.____
	L. Tartar emetic	
17. Estradiol	M. Tartar emetic	17.____
	N. Tertiary amyl alcohol	
18. Methylrosaniline chloride	O. Vitamin B_1 Hydrochloride	18.____
19. Saccharin	P. Vitamin D_2	19.____
20. Urethane		20.____

21. Xerophthalmia is a symptom of 21.____

A. atropine poisoning
B. diabetes mellitus
C. paralysis agitans
D. vitamin A deficiency

22. Sulfanilamide is detoxified in the body by 22.____

A. acetylation
B. ammonolysis
C. hydrolysis
D. sulfonation

23. The administration of Atropine results in 23.____

A. dysmenorrhea
B. miosis
C. mydriasis
D. rhinitis

24. Hexachlorophene is employed as a 24.____

A. bacteriastat
B. detergent
C. insecticide
D. wetting agent

25. Syphilis is an infection caused by the organism 25.____

A. Endamoeba histolytica
B. Escherichia coli
C. Proteus vulgaris
D. Treponema pallidum

KEY (CORRECT ANSWERS)

1.	A	11.	N
2.	C	12.	M
3.	B	13.	K
4.	A	14.	C
5.	D	15.	Q
6.	B	16.	O
7.	B	17.	D
8.	C	18.	B
9.	A	19.	F
10.	D	20.	E

21. D
22. A
23. C
24. A
25. D

TEST 4

DIRECTIONS: Each question or incomplete statement is followed by several suggested answers or completions. Select the one that BEST answers the question or completes the statement. *PRINT THE LETTER OF THE CORRECT ASWER IN THE SPACE AT THE RIGHT.*

1. *Negri bodies* are associated with 1.____

   A. diphtheria
   B. poliomyelitis
   C. rabies
   D. yellow fever

2. Ammonium chloride prescribed in doses of 0.3 grams every four hours would be expected to act as a(n) 2.____

   A. alkalinizer
   B. antispasmodic
   C. expectorant
   D. systemic anti-infective

3. The main actions of papaverine are exerted on the 3.____

   A. cardiac and smooth muscle
   B. central nervous system
   C. cranial nerves
   D. haematopoietic system

4. A calcium compound MOST suitable for intravenous administration is the 4.____

   A. acetate
   B. glycerophosphate
   C. levulinate
   D. phosphate

5. Diphenhydramine Eydrochloride is used as an 5.____

   A. amebicide
   B. anhydrotic
   C. antihistamine
   D. expectorant

6. Benzyl Benzoate is characterized as an 6.____

   A. antibacterial
   B. antiperspirant
   C. antipsoriatic
   D. antiscabietic

7. Zinc Undecylenate is generally employed as a(n) 7.____

   A. astringent
   B. deodorant
   C. fungistat
   D. germicide

8. An official product obtained from Liquidambar orientalis is 8.____

   A. benzoin
   B. peru balsam
   C. storax
   D. tolu balsam

9. An official glycoside obtained from Digitalis Lanata is 9.____

   A. digitalin
   B. digitogenin
   C. digitonin
   D. digoxin

10. Cinnamic Aldehyde is the active constituent of ______ oil. 10.____

    A. cassia
    B. clove
    C. myrcia
    D. nutmeg

11. Ouabain is obtained from 11.____

A. Claviceps purpurea
B. Eriodictyon californicum
C. Strophanthus gratus
D. Urginea maritima

12. Tyrothricin is an anti-bacterial substance produced by the growth of 12.____

A. Bacillus brevis
B. Bacillus polymyxa
C. Streptomyces aureofaciens
D. Streptomyces griseus

13. Urginea maritima is the source of 13.____

A. carmine
B. ichthammol
C. squill
D. tragacanth

14. Calabar Bean is the source of 14.____

A. aloin
B. eserine
C. procaine
D. theophylline

15. Gum Karaya is the official synonym for 15.____

A. ghatti gum
B. gum kino
C. gum thus
D. sterculia gum

16. Rhamnus Purshiana is the source of 16.____

A. bachu
B. cascara sagrada
C. cubeb
D. podophyllum

17. The volume of 9 lb. (avoirdupois) of Sulfuric Acid having a specific gravity of 1.83 is 17.____

A. 4.73
B. 4.91
C. 5.00
D. none of these answers

18. From the following formula, calculate the quantity of arsenic trioxide required to make one gallon of Potassium Arsenite Solution: 18.____

Arsenic Trioxide	10.0 grams
Potassium Bicarbonate	7.6 grams
Alcohol	30.0 c.c.

Distilled water–a sufficient quantity to make 1000 c.c. of

A. 26.29 gm.
B. 33.71 gm.
C. 37.85 gm.
D. 47.23 gm.

19. The number of 1/40 grain doses that can be prepared, from 3/5 grams of Strychnine Sulfate is 19.____

A. 24
B. 28
C. 44
D. 72

20. The molecular weight of acetic acid is 60.05. The weight of acetic acid present in 500 milliliters of a 0.2 N solution of $HC_2E_3O_2$ is ______ grams. 20.____

A. 2.009
B. 6.005
C. 14.327
D. 79.406

21. The maximum number of tablets, each containing 1/4 grain of codeine sulfate, that can be prepared from one avoirdupois ounce of Codeine Sulfate is 21.____

A. 327 B. 639 C. 1142 D. 1750

22. A liniment preparation has the formula: 22.____
Methyl Salicylate 8%
Rubbing Alcohol to make 3 fluid ounces
The volume of Methyl Salicylate required is ______ minims.

A. 47 B. 86 C. 115 D. 221

23. A prescription calls for 1% of pilocarpine nitrate in four fluid drains of solution. The weight of pilocarpine nitrate required to prepare this solution is ______ grains. 23.____

A. 2.40 B. 3.39 C. 4.83 D. 4.92

24. The USP Rectal dose of Tribromoethanol is 60 mg for each kilogram of body weight. The quantity of Tribromoethanol to be administered to a 150-lb. adult is ______ grams. 24.____

A. 0.210
B. 0.370
C. 0.420
D. none of these answers

25. A stock solution of potassium permanganate contains 2.50 grams of the salt in 100 milliliters of solution. The volume of this stock solution required to prepare two liters of a 1:2500 potassium permanganate solution is ______ milliliters. 25.____

A. 32 B. 38 C. 56 D. 72

KEY (CORRECT ANSWERS)

1. C
2. C
3. A
4. C
5. C

6. D
7. C
8. C
9. D
10. A

11. C
12. A
13. C
14. B
15. D

16. B
17. D
18. C
19. A
20. B

21. D
22. C
23. A
24. D
25. A

EXAMINATION SECTION
TEST 1

DIRECTIONS: Each question or incomplete statement is followed by several suggested answers or completions. Select the one that BEST answers the question or completes the statement. *PRINT THE LETTER OF THE CORRECT ANSWER IN THE SPACE AT THE RIGHT.*

Questions 1-2.

DIRECTIONS: Questions 1 and 2 are to be answered on the basis of the information given below.

JOAN SMITH	40yoWO+	437B
Protein Hydrolysate 5% NaCl 40mEq KCl 40mEq $MgSO_4$ 5mEq B & C		
	DR. JONES	

1. Which of the following medications has been ordered by the physician for the patient Joan Smith? 1.____

   A. 500 mg ascorbic acid
   B. Monosodium glutamate
   C. 5M magnesium sulfate
   D. 40 Milliequivalents sodium chloride

2. The above prescription may be termed ______ therapy. 2.____

   A. hyperalimentation
   B. hyperlimitation
   C. nitrogen infusion
   D. hypoalimentation

3. The effect of dimenhydrinate given in a dose of 25-50 mg, 3-4 times a day, on a patient is that it 3.____

   A. exhibits a high incidence of sedation
   B. exhibits a low incidence of sedation
   C. is contra-indicated in patients taking phenoxymethyl penicillin
   D. exhibits a negative antivertilian effect

4. A physician's order for *acetominophen USP, 10 grs Q4H prn* should be interpreted as a MAXIMUM of ______ tablets daily. 4.____

   A. 4 B. 5 C. 6 D. 12

5. Assume that you are reviewing an order for 2mg Busulfan tablets from a physician. Which of the following should be dispensed? 5.____

   A. Auralgan B. Leukeran C. Myleran D. Immuran

6. *Pro Time* refers to ______ time. 6.___

A. prothrombin determination
B. positive reactive oxygenation
C. professional rate observation
D. sedimentation

7. Which one of the following doses does NOT legally require a physician's prescription? 7.___

A. Chlorpheniramine malcate 2mg/dose
B. Nitroglycerine 0.6mg/dose
C. Chlorpromazine 10 mg/dose
D. Methyltestosterone 25mg/dose

8. Toxius, toxoids, and vaccines MUST conform to standards established by the 8.___

A. W.H.O. B. N.I.H. C. U.S.P. D. F.D.A.

9. The MINIMUM amount that may be weighed on a Class A prescription balance is 9.___

A. 120mg
B. 200mg
C. determined by the sensitivity reciprocal
D. 4 grains

10. Pyrogen testing, as outlined by acceptable standards, requires biological testing on 10.___

A. goldfish B. rabbits C. cats D. pigeons

11. A Laminar Flow Hood is used when sterile intravenous solution additives are 11.___

A. labeled
B. prepared
C. stored
D. administered

12. Which of the following gives the meaning of *HEPA* as used in *HEPA filter*? 12.___

A. High efficiency particulate air
B. High energy particle aeration
C. The name of the manufacturer
D. High energy particulate aerosol

13. Which one of the following is TRUE with regard to Phenylephrine hydrochloride, USP? It 13.___

A. is a parasympathomimetic agent
B. exhibits a vasodilatory activity in hypotensive states
C. is a useful mydriatic when used opthalmically
D. may be administered only topically

14. Which of the following drugs are placed under Controlled Substances requirements? 14.___

A. Trancycypromine
B. Trinitoin
C. Chlordiazepoxide
D. Chlorpheniramine

15. Which one of the following preparations should be kept at a temperature of 0 to -10C during storage? 15.____

A. Insulin, USP
B. Rocky mountain spotted fever vaccine
C. ACTH gel (80 U only)
D. Immunine serum globin (human)

16. *Tablet friability* refers to tablet 16.____

A. dissolution rate
B. disintegration time
C. fragility and durability when tested
D. size

17. Iodine solution, N.F., should MOST preferably be stored 17.____

A. in a frozen gel
B. below 35°C
C. at room temperature
D. above 35°C

18. Which class or classes of controlled substances require a Bureau of Narcotics and Dangerous Drugs order form? 18.____

A. II
B. I & II
C. I, II, & III
D. All classes

19. Fenfluramine, a new anorexigenic, falls into which control class? 19.____

A. II
B. III
C. IV
D. V

20. Secobarbital falls into which control class? 20.____

A. V
B. IV
C. III
D. II

21. Which one of the following is a MAJOR disadvantage in the implementation of a unit dose system? 21.____
It

A. requires the pharmacist to increase his involvement with the nursing staff
B. requires additional equipment and labor costs to package those drugs not readily available in unit dose form from drug manufacturers
C. makes the dispensing process a monotonous task due to the standardization of doses and drugs
D. requires the pharmacist to prepare all injectable doses

22. A unit dose package can be defined as a 22.____

A. vial of 1 gram of Keflin, to be reconstituted by the nurse sent to the nursing unit (assuming the dose is 1 gram q 4h 1V)
B. package containing the exact dosage of drugs to be administered to a patient at a specific time
C. package containing enough medication for the next three doses
D. bottle containing enough medication for 24 hours

23. Which one of the following statements is an advantage of the *floor stock* system of drug distribution? 23.____
It

A. requires the increased professional involvement of the pharmacist
B. brings the drug to the patient the fastest
C. has the lowest incidence of medication errors
D. is the most efficient, from a fiscal point of view

24. Which one of the following is unaffected by unit dose dispensing? 24.____

A. Drug inventory levels
B. Medication errors
C. Drug administration to patients
D. Personnel allotment

25. Which one of the following is NOT an acceptable method of sterilization? 25.____

A. Autoclave
B. Laminar flow
C. Membrane
D. Gas

26. In pharmaceutical terms, *proof* is defined as 26.____

A. the receipt from the distiller showing proof of purchase of the alcohol
B. one-half the percent of ethyl alcohol by volume of 60° F
C. twice the percent of ethyl alcohol by volume at 60° F
D. matching records of dispensation of alcohol to actual inventory

27. A Patterson-Kelly powder blender is ALSO called a(n) 27.____

A. Waring blender
B. twin shell blender
C. Hobart mixer
D. oscillating vibrator

28. For an existing ongoing program, which one of the following is MOST desirable for the pharmacist to have in preparing an annual budget? 28.____

A. Last year's budget and this year's estimated actual expenses
B. This year's budget and this year's estimated actual expenses
C. Budgets and actual expense figures for the last five years
D. Last year's budget and actual expenses

29. Which one of the following is NOT a recommended code account for a pharmacy department budget? 29.____

A. Miscellaneous supplies and expense
B. Drugs and Pharmaceuticals
C. Salaries and wages
D. Floor stock drugs

30. Pharmacy workload reports compare workload to 30.____

A. available professional time
B. number of prescriptions filled
C. pharmacists' time devoted to it
D. pharmacy personnel budget

KEY (CORRECT ANSWERS)

1. D
2. C
3. A
4. D
5. C

6. A
7. A
8. B
9. A
10. B

11. B
12. A
13. C
14. A
15. B

16. C
17. B
18. A
19. C
20. C

21. B
22. B
23. B
24. C
25. B

26. C
27. B
28. B
29. D
30. A

TEST 2

DIRECTIONS: Each question or incomplete statement is followed by several suggested answers or completions. Select the one that BEST answers the question or completes the statement. *PRINT THE LETTER OF THE CORRECT ANSWER IN THE SPACE AT THE RIGHT.*

1. Which one of the following groups is LEAST vital for treatment in an *Emergency Box* situation? 1.____

   A. Sengstachen Blakemore tube and Xylocaine HCl
   B. Nalorphine, HCl and Epinephrine, HCl
   C. Triplennamine HCl tablets and bropheniramine maleate
   D. Heparin, USP, and Nalorphine, HCl

2. For sterility tests to be definitive, suture material must be incubated under standard conditions for a period of ______ day(s). 2.____

   A. 1 B. 4 C. 15 D. 30

3. Which one of the following sieve sizes has the SMALLEST openings? 3.____

   A. 1.0 B. 2.0 C. 20.0 D. 200.0

4. A low rate of inventory turnover is GENERALLY indicative of 4.____

   A. the presence of dead inventory on the shelves
   B. poor servicing of accounts by drug companies
   C. failure to take advantage of discounts
   D. small volume purchasing

5. Of the following, an example of an injectable unit dose is 5.____

   A. kapseal B. spansule C. tubex D. insulin

6. When dispensing tetracycline capsules to a patient in an OPD pharmacy, the pharmacist should 6.____

   A. dispense the medication without comment
   B. tell the patient to take the capsules one hour before or 2 hours after meals and to avoid milk and antacids immediately before and after his dose of the drug
   C. tell the patient not to take the capsules with milk, antacids or food
   D. tell the patient to take the capsules immediately after meals and to avoid antacids and milk

7. When conducting nursing station inspections, one need NOT look for ______ drugs. 7.____

   A. improperly stored B. expiration dates on
   C. unlabelled D. unlicensed

8. Which one of the following statements regarding the formulary system generally is TRUE? 8.____
   It does not

   A. allow the pharmacist the right of product selection
   B. deprive the physician of his right to prescribe the drug of his choice

C. save the hospital any money
D. represent the current thinking of the medical staff of the hospital

9. The one of the following factors which does NOT affect the removal of an active drug from a site of action is 9.____

A. the amount of carboxymethylcellulose present
B. excretion of the active drug
C. redistribution to other tissues
D. metabolism of an active drug to an inactive metabolite

10. Of the following types of pharmaceutical products, which is LEAST often manufactured by the hospital pharmacy? 10.____

A. Sterile irrigating solutions
B. Allergenic extracts
C. Galenicals
D. Non-commercially available products

11. Even though the purchasing agent, a non-pharmacist, may actually procure medications for a hospital, a pharmacist MUST 11.____

A. receive on-site inspection reports of the purchasing agent
B. provide price range and a list of generics
C. provide acceptable vendors and specific procurement requirements
D. provide general specifications of storage requirements

12. A non-proprietary hospital is usually eligible to purchase tax-free alcohol. In order to do so, it must meet certain criteria, among which is that it 12.____

A. add a denaturant to all stored alcohol to prevent its consumption by unauthorized personnel
B. charge patients for any medicinal product containing tax-free alcohol
C. store alcohol in containers smaller than one gallon proof
D. obtain a bond of surety

13. According to the regulations established by the State Bureau of Narcotics, a *running* inventory must be maintained by the primary source of distribution (pharmacy) in all institutions for drugs in Class(es) 13.____

A. II, III, IV, and V
B. II and III
C. II only
D. II, III, and IV

14. Pharmacy purchase records must contain all of the following information EXCEPT 14.____

A. last price
B. therapeutic class
C. usage rate
D. vendor

15. Drug inventory files must contain all of the following information EXCEPT 15.____

A. minimum order quantity
B. usage rate
C. last price
D. vendor

16. Inventory turnover rate is determined by 16.____

    A. dividing the average of opening and closing inventories by the cost of goods sold
    B. dividing the cost of goods sold by the average of opening and closing inventories
    C. dividing the opening inventory by the closing inventory
    D. multiplying the average of opening and closing inventories by one-tenth of the cost of goods sold and dividing that result by 25

17. The ratio, *cost of drugs per patient day,* compares cost of drugs with 17.____

    A. average daily census
    B. annual admissions
    C. total of all the daily censuses for the year, excluding bassinets
    D. total of all the daily censuses for the year, including bassinets

18. In order to provide accurate drug information, MOST local hospital pharmacies have developed 18.____

    A. a 24-hour drug information service
    B. computerized techniques to disseminate drug information
    C. consumer-oriented information centers
    D. monthly newsletters covering drug information highlights

19. The PRIMARY goal of a hospital formulary is to 19.____

    A. save a hospital money
    B. strictly control prescribing in a hospital
    C. insure that patients receive the best care possible
    D. influence medical staff to use approved drugs only

20. The pharmacy and therapeutics committee is NOT designed to 20.____

    A. serve an educational function
    B. advise on professional policies involving the use of drugs in the hospital
    C. save the hospital money
    D. recommend in-service programs relating to drugs

21. When a supervising pharmacist serves on the pharmacy and therapeutics committee, which of the following types of detailed information SHOULD be supplied by him for consideration and evaluation? 21.____

    A. The agenda and minutes of the meetings
    B. Information pertaining to the economic aspects of a drug only
    C. Information pertaining to the pharmaceutic and economic aspects of a drug
    D. Information pertaining to the therapeutic, pharmaceutic, and economic aspects of a drug

22. Administrative policies for a pharmacy unit are GENERALLY developed 22.____

    A. with the approval of the pharmacy and therapeutics committee
    B. with the approval of the medical and/or nursing staffs (depending upon the particular policy)
    C. with the approval of the administrative officers of the hospital
    D. by the pharmacy unit alone

23. Which one of the following does NOT have to be in the form of a written policy and procedure in the pharmacy? 23.____

A. Patient admissions
B. Handling flammable materials
C. Orienting new pharmacy employees
D. Handling of narcotics

24. Non-licensed personnel play an IMPORTANT role in the hospital pharmacy because 24.____

A. many of them aspire to be pharmacists, and working in the hospital pharmacy provides training
B. they can be trained to act in the place of a pharmacist within 3 months
C. they can perform certain functions under the supervision of a registered pharmacist and, therefore, frees other pharmacists to perform more professional duties
D. two technicians can be hired in place of each pharmacist, thereby increasing staff complement without increasing expenditure

25. The use of an investigational new drug within a particular institution requires that the 25.____

A. institution be certified by the FDA
B. licensed prescriber be approved by the manufacturer or chief investigator
C. hospital administrator, licensed prescriber, and pharmacy be certified by the FDA
D. institution and the physician be certified by the FDA

26. One requirement of the State Bureau of Narcotics for registered hospital pharmacies is that 26.____

A. they dispense all Schedule I, II, III, IV, and V medications with an orange label
B. they maintain accurate procurement and distribution records and perform a physical inventory annually
C. they maintain a *running* inventory on all Schedule II, III, and IV drugs
D. the hospitals' nursing staffs must inventory all *floor stock* every 24 hours

27. The Internal Revenue Service requires that annual inventory on all tax-free alcohol be reported in which of the following units? 27.____
_______ gallons.

A. *Alcohol* B. Proof C. Wine D. Spirit

28. The documentation and preparation of the pharmacy annual report should be based PRIMARILY on the 28.____

A. general activities of the previous fiscal year only
B. general activities to be developed during upcoming fiscal year only
C. qualifications of the director of pharmacy service
D. fiscal activities only for the previous year

29. It is suggested that in hospitals where manufacturing of any drug or dosage is being performed, the *manufacturing standards* conform to the Food, Drug and Cosmetics Act standards known as 29.____

A. GNP B. NDA C. GMP D. IND

30. A written proposal for a new project or service submitted by a supervising pharmacist should 30.____

A. contain as many technical terms as possible
B. substantiate any claims in professional literature and how it relates to the institution
C. emphasize the advantages of the project or service and minimize its shortcomings
D. contain information relative to another institution which has implemented a similar administrative proposal

---

KEY (CORRECT ANSWERS)

1.	C	16.	B
2.	C	17.	C
3.	D	18.	D
4.	A	19.	C
5.	C	20.	C
6.	B	21.	D
7.	D	22.	C
8.	B	23.	A
9.	A	24.	C
10.	B	25.	B
11.	C	26.	B
12.	D	27.	B
13.	C	28.	A
14.	B	29.	C
15.	C	30.	B

PHARMACOLOGY

EXAMINATION SECTION
TEST 1

DIRECTIONS: Each question or incomplete statement is followed by several suggested answers or completions. Select the one that BEST answers the question or completes the statement. *PRINT THE LETTER OF THE CORRECT ANSWER IN THE SPACE AT THE RIGHT.*

1. Which of the following statements regarding the occupation theory of drug-receptor interaction are TRUE? 1.____
   I. The affinity of a drug is dependent on its inherent intrinsic activity.
   II. The maximum effect of the drug occurs when all receptors are occupied.
   III. An antagonist has affinity for the receptor but less intrinsic activity than an agonist.
   IV. The effect of the drug is proportional to the number of receptors occupied.
   V. It does not follow the law of mass action.

   The CORRECT answer is:

   A. I, II, III
   B. II, III, V
   C. III, IV, V
   D. II, IV
   E. II, III

2. Which of the following contribute to the analgesic effects of morphine? 2.____
   I. Sedation
   II. Euphoria
   III. Impairment of nerve conduction
   IV. Altered threshold of nerve endings
   V. Elevation of nerve thresholds within the CNS

   The CORRECT answer is:

   A. I, II, III
   B. I, II, V
   C. II, III, IV
   D. II, IV, V
   E. III, IV, V

3. Which of the following statements regarding a schedule II prescription are TRUE? 3.____
   I. Cannot be prescribed by telephone
   II. Must contain both the generic and brand name of the drug
   III. In addition to federal statutes, individual states may have additional requirements
   IV. Cannot be refilled even with the consent of the prescriber
   V. Only valid when accompanied by a narcotic registry number

   The CORRECT answer is:

   A. I, II, III
   B. II, III, IV
   C. I, III, V
   D. I, II, III, IV
   E. I, III, IV, V

4. Which of the following compounds after metabolizing to form acetaminophen is an ACTIVE analgesic and antipyretic agent? 4.____

   A. Propoxyphene (Darvon®)
   B. Phenacetin
   C. Aminopyrine
   D. Phenylbutazone
   E. Acetylsalicylic acid

5. Which of the following statements regarding drugs are TRUE? 5.____
   I. Drugs usually have more than one generic name.
   II. Prescribing a drug by its generic name allows the pharmacist to dispense any brand name preparations.
   III. Brand name preparations are usually more expensive than the comparable generic preparation.
   IV. All narcotics by law must be prescribed by their brand names.

   The CORRECT answer is:

   A. I, II
   B. I, II, III
   C. II, III
   D. II, III, IV
   E. III, IV

6. Which of the following statements concerning ethyl is TRUE? It 6.____

   A. produces a true stimulation of the central nervous system
   B. protects individuals against exposure to cold by preventing heat loss
   C. is metabolized primarily by the lungs
   D. is partially absorbed in the stomach
   E. possesses teratogenic properties

7. A 19-year-old, well-developed, well-nourished young man reports to a dental office for the extraction of a tooth. Normal body temperature and a number of scars on the tongue are noted. Shortly after making an injection of 2 percent Carbocaine, with levonordefrin (Neo-Cobefrin) 1:20,000, using an aspirating syringe through which no blood was withdrawn, the patient has a convulsion. These facts are CONSISTENT with a diagnosis of 7.____

   A. benign syncopy
   B. epileptic seizure
   C. febrile convulsion
   D. toxic overdose of the anesthetic

8. Prolonged and continued use of which of the following antibiotics will MOST likely result in damage to the VIII cranial nerve? 8.____

   A. Streptomycin
   B. Aureomycin
   C. Penicillin
   D. Tetracyn

9. A side-effect unique with erythromycin estolate (Ilosone) is 9.____

   A. hypersensitivity response involving the liver
   B. staphylococcal enteritis
   C. bone marrow depression
   D. cranial nerve damage
   E. renal damage

10. The active metabolite of the biotransformation of phenacetin is 10.____

    A. aniline
    B. gentisic acid
    C. salicylic acid
    D. acetaminophen
    E. phenylacetylurea

11. The MOST probable cause for a serious toxic reaction to a local anesthetic is 11.____

    A. psychogenic
    B. deterioration of the anesthetic agent

C. hypersensitivity to the vasoconstrictor
D. hypersensitivity to the local anesthetic
E. excessive blood level of the local anesthetic

12. The PRIMARY effect produced by digitalis at therapeutic dose levels is to 12.____

A. slow the cardiac rate
B. increase the force of myocardial contraction
C. decrease the venous pressure
D. decrease cardiac enlargement

13. The ONLY local anesthetic which increases the pressor activity of both epinephrine and norepinephrine is 13.____

A. cocaine B. procaine C. dibucaine
D. lidocaine E. mepivacaine

14. Alkalization of tubular urine slows the rate of excretion of 14.____

A. water B. chlorides
C. weak acids D. weak bases

15. Local anesthetic agents act PRIMARILY 15.____

A. at a cortical level to decrease the patient's awareness of pain impulses
B. at the myoneural junction to decrease frequency of pain impulses reaching the CNS
C. on the axon membrane to prevent depolarizing potentials
D. at ganglionic sites to decrease central pain input
E. none of the above

16. Atropine is DESIRABLE for preanesthetic medication because it 16.____

A. prevents vomiting
B. obtunds the cough reflex
C. reduces glandular secretion in the airway
D. increases secretions of the gastrointestinal tract
E. decreases the physiologic dead space of the airway

17. Which of the following would be the drug of choice for the rapid relief of suspected coronary vasoconstriction (spasm) characterized by sharp chest pain, shortness of breath, and a history of previous attacks? 17.____

A. Morphine B. Digitalis
C. Quinidine D. Nitroglycerin
E. Pentobarbital sodium

18. A patient receiving propranolol has an acute asthmatic attack while undergoing dental treatment.
The MOST useful agent for management of the condition would be 18.____

A. morphine B. epinephrine C. phentolamine
D. aminophylline E. norepinephrine

19. For which of the following conditions would steroids be used? 19.____

A. Diabetes
B. Acromegaly
C. Tuberculosis
D. Collagen diseases

20. Iron will be absorbed from the duodenum when 20.____

A. pH in the stomach is high
B. the metal is in the ferrous form
C. high concentrations of phosphate are present in the diet
D. the level of ferritin in the mucosal cells is high
E. oxidizing agents are present in the duodenum

21. Action of the sympathetic nervous system may be blocked by which of the following types of agents? 21.____

A. Ganglionic block agents *only*
B. Curariform agents *only*
C. Adrenergic block agents *only*
D. Both ganglionic and adrenergic blocking agents

22. An excess of which of the following hormones may be associated with increased sensitivity to epinephrine? 22.____

A. Testosterone
B. Parathyroid
C. Insulin
D. Thyroid

23. Which of the following would LIKELY appear with atropine overdosage? 23.____

A. Dryness of mouth and throat
B. Pallor of face and neck
C. Constricted pupils
D. None of the above

24. Which is NOT an estrogenic substance? 24.____

A. Premarin
B. Theelin
C. Estradiol
D. Stilbesterol
E. Follicle-stimulating hormones

25. Which of the following statements describes in part the cardiovascular effects of a pressor dose of epinephrine? 25.____

A. An increase in blood pressure is followed by a decrease, i.e., a biphasic pressure response.
B. Total peripheral resistance is never decreased.
C. The myocardium is stimulated by exogenous epinephrine only at the sympathetic accelerator nerve endings.
D. All blood vessels are constricted.

KEY (CORRECT ANSWERS)

1.	D	11.	E
2.	B	12.	B
3.	E	13.	A
4.	B	14.	D
5.	C	15.	C
6.	D	16.	C
7.	B	17.	D
8.	A	18.	D
9.	A	19.	D
10.	D	20.	B

21. D
22. D
23. A
24. E
25. A

TEST 2

DIRECTIONS: Each question or incomplete statement is followed by several suggested answers or completions. Select the one that BEST answers the question or completes the statement. *PRINT THE LETTER OF THE CORRECT ANSWER IN THE SPACE AT THE RIGHT.*

1. The side effects associated with the Rauwolfia derivatives (such as reserpine) are 1.____
   I. tachycardia
   II. nasal stuffiness
   III. postural hypotension
   IV. potentiation of barbituate and narcotic agents

   The CORRECT answer is:

   A. I, II, IV
   B. I, III, IV
   C. II, III, IV
   D. All of the above

2. The concentration of a volatile anesthetic agent in the blood depends upon the 2.____
   I. partial pressure of the anesthetic agent in alveolar space
   II. permeability of the alveolar membrane
   III. respiratory minute volume
   IV. hemoglobin content of the blood

   The CORRECT answer is:

   A. I, II
   B. I, IV
   C. I, II, III
   D. II, III, IV
   E. All of the above

3. Some general anesthetic agents predispose the patient to epinephrine-induced cardiac irregularities, even when the patient receives adequate amounts of oxygen. Examples of such agents include: 3.____
   I. ethylene
   II. chloroform
   III. diethyl ether
   IV. ethyl chloride
   V. nitrous oxide
   VI. trichloroethylene

   The CORRECT answer is:

   A. I, II, III
   B. I, III, IV
   C. I, V, VI
   D. II, IV, V
   E. II, IV, VI
   F. III, V, VI

4. A hypnotic LIKELY to be suitable for use in an individual allergic to secobarbital is 4.____

   A. thiopental
   B. pentobarbital
   C. chloral hydrate
   D. phenobarbital
   E. propoxyphene

5. Currently available local disinfectants act by 5.____
   I. selective and specific metabolic interference in
   II. the growth of only gram-positive organisms
   III. precipitation of bacterial protein
   IV. oxidizing bacterial protoplasmic constituents
   V. increasing the membrane permeability of the bacterium

   The CORRECT answer is:

A. I, III
B. I, IV
C. II, IV
D. II, III, IV
E. All of the above

6. The OUTSTANDING advantage of diphenylhydantoin over phenobarbital in the treatment of grand mal epilepsy is that diphenylhydantoin 6.____

A. exerts less sedation for a given degree of motor cortex depression
B. is effective in a greater percent of cases
C. needs to be given much less frequently
D. does not bring about addiction

7. Both reserpine and chlorpromazine have which of the following effects? 7.____

I. Antiemetic
II. Tranquilizing
III. Muscle relaxation
IV. Cause Parkinson-like syndrome

The CORRECT answer is:

A. I, II
B. I, III
C. I, IV
D. II, III
E. II, IV
F. III, IV

8. Some antidepressant drugs are known to inhibit the enzyme 8.____

A. cholinesterase
B. choline-acetylase
C. monomine oxidase
D. O-methyltransferase

9. Which of the following clinical situations are indications for the use of the phenothiazines? 9.____

I. Neuroses
II. LSD overdosage
III. Nausea due to motion sickness
IV. Psychoses
V. Analgesic potentiation

The CORRECT answer is:

A. I, II, III
B. I, III, V
C. II,III, IV
D. II, IV, V
E. III, IV, V

10. If a patient requiring an extraction reports that he is on bishydroxycoumarin therapy, the laboratory test that would be MOST valuable in evaluating the surgical risk is 10.____

A. clotting time
B. bleeding time
C. sedimentation rate
D. complete blood count
E. plasma prothrombin time

11. Prolonged use of which of the following drugs may predispose to postoperative bleeding? 11.____

I. Acetylsalicylic acid
II. Diphenylhydantoin
III. Chlorpromazine
IV. Bishydroxycoumarin
V. Phenobarbital
VI. Tripelennamine

The CORRECT answer is:

A. I, IV B. I, V C. II, III
D. II, IV E. III, VI

12. Which of the following clinically useful agents is active against fungi but NOT bacteria? 12.____
I. Nystatin
II. Neomycin
III. Cephalothin
IV. Griseofulvin
V. Amphotericin B
The CORRECT answer is:

A. I, II, III B. I, II, V C. I, IV, V
D. II, III, IV E. II, III, V

13. Dilantin is the drug of choice for 13.____

A. Jacksonian epilepsy
B. relief of visceral pain
C. relief of peripheral pain
D. grand mal epilepsy
E. petit mal epilepsy

14. Which of the following agents should be available for treatment of emergencies in the dental office? 14.____
I. Oxygen
II. Epinephrine
III. Isoproterenol
IV. A long-acting vasopressor
V. Aromatic spirit of ammonia
VI. An injectable antihistaminic
VII. Hydrocortisone sodium succinate
The CORRECT answer is:

A. I, II, IV B. I, III, IV C. I, IV, V
D. II, III, VI E. II, VI, VII F. IV, VI, VII
G. V, VI, VII H. All of the above

15. Which is NOT a general anesthetic? 15.____

A. Benzylalcohol B. Cyclopropane C. Ethylene
D. Vinyl ether E. Trichlorethylene

16. Which of the following are IMPORTANT criteria for an adequate clinical evaluation of the efficacy of a new drug? 16.____
I. Control groups
II. Placebo indication
III. Double blind experimental design
IV. Comparison with a standard drug
V. Evaluation of toxicity
The CORRECT answer is:

A. I, II, III B. II, III, IV C. III, IV, V
D. I, III E. All of the above

17. Which of the following should NOT be administered to a patient with myasthenia gravis? 17.____

A. Atropine
B. Curare
C. Insulin
D. Digitalis
E. Prostigmine

Questions 18-25.

DIRECTIONS: The sentences in Questions 18 through 25 consist of two main parts: a statement and a reason for the statement. Which of the following describes each item?

A. Both statement and reason are correct and related.
B. Both statement and reason are correct but NOT related.
C. The statement is correct but the reason is NOT.
D. The statement is NOT correct but the reason is an accurate statement.
E. NEITHER statement nor reason is correct.

18. Procaine may cause cardiovascular collapse *because* procaine blocks autonomic ganglia. 18.____

19. In clinical testing of a new drug, the double blind design is not usually necessary *because* few drugs possess a true placebo effect. 19.____

20. Dimercaprol (BAL) is effective in early poisoning by mercuric salts *because* it successfully competes with essential sulfhydryl groups in the body for the binding and subsequent excretion of mercuric ions. 20.____

21. Acid medium will increase the local anesthetic potency of procaine HCl *because* the undissociated form of procaine can penetrate easily the nerve membrane. 21.____

22. Nitroglycerin can increase the coronary blood flow *because* it blocks the sympathetic nervous system. 22.____

23. Epinephrine is contraindicated in asthmatic patients *because* epinephrine exerts a beta adrenergic effect on bronchial smooth muscle. 23.____

24. The available evidence suggests that drugs penetrate or enter into cell membranes at the most rapid rate when they are in the unionized form *because* unionized drugs possess maximal water solubility. 24.____

25. The plasma level of weak organic acids may be reduced by sodium bicarbonate *because* this alkalizing agent promotes the renal elimination of such acids. 25.____

KEY (CORRECT ANSWERS)

1. C
2. C
3. E
4. C
5. D

6. A
7. E
8. C
9. D
10. E

11. A
12. C
13. D
14. H
15. A

16. E
17. B
18. C
19. E
20. A

21. D
22. C
23. D
24. C
25. A

PHARMACOLOGY

EXAMINATION SECTION
TEST 1

DIRECTIONS: Each question or incomplete statement is followed by several suggested answers or completions. Select the one that BEST answers the question or completes the statement. *PRINT THE LETTER OF THE CORRECT ANSWER IN THE SPACE AT THE RIGHT.*

1. What is the BASIC chemical moiety of the dilantin molecule which is responsible for dilantin's action? 1.____
_______ nucleus.

   A. Acetylurea
   B. Barbiturate
   C. Hydantoin
   D. Oxazolidine
   E. Isoquinoline

2. Which of the following has the LEAST anti-inflammatory activity? 2.____

   A. Prednisone
   B. Aldosterone
   C. Prednisolone
   D. Hydrocortisone

3. Which of the following statements is NOT true regarding procainamide? 3.____
It(s)

   A. differs substantially from quinidine in its anti-arrhythmic effect
   B. is less susceptible to serum cholinesterases than is procaine
   C. actions are qualitatively the same, but quantitatively different from those of procaine
   D. can be administered orally
   E. has a more favorable ratio of cardiac to CNS effects than does procaine

4. Which of the following antibiotics is NOT considered to be a broad spectrum antibiotic? 4.____

   A. Chlortetracycline
   B. Oxytetracycline
   C. Chloramphenicol
   D. Penicillin

5. Which of the following statements is NOT true regarding the adrenal corticosteroids? 5.____

   A. Therapeutically beneficial when administered orally, parenterally or topically
   B. High blood levels can produce a diabetes-like syndrome
   C. Decrease activity in lymphoid tissue
   D. Prevent antibody-antigen union in the allergic reaction
   E. Can produce mental disturbances

6. The sulfonylurea hypoglycemic drugs are usually NOT useful in childhood diabetes because 6.____

   A. they are antagonized by ACTH
   B. they have a low therapeutic index
   C. they inhibit the physiologic production of insulin
   D. few pancreatic islet cells are active

7. When a laryngospasm occurs during general anesthesia, the specific drug of choice is 7.___

A. dilantin
B. mephenesin
C. methantheline
D. succinylcholine

8. Curare may be used in oral surgery when thiopental sodium is used alone or in combination with nitrous oxide or cyclopropane and oxygen for the express purpose of 8.___

A. relaxing muscles
B. preventing hypoxia
C. elevating blood pressure
D. stimulating the respiratory center

9. The secretion of parathyroid hormone is controlled by the blood level of 9.___

A. protein bound calcium
B. complexed calcium
C. ionic calcium
D. calcium-mobilizing hormone
E. calcium gluconate

10. Propylthiouracil is a drug used in the treatment of 10.___

A. diabetes
B. hyperthyroidism
C. sodium retention
D. intestinal parasites
E. allergic manifestations

11. Cetyl dimethyl ethyl ammonium bromide, a quaternary base, is MOST likely to be used as a 11.___

A. sedative
B. ganglionic blocking agent
C. stimulant to myeloid tissue
D. mild acting hypnotic for children
E. cold disinfecting solution for instruments

12. Of the following substances, the MOST effective agent against mild fungus infections of the skin is 12.___

A. hexachlorophene
B. undecylenic acid
C. polymyxin ointments
D. saturated magnesium sulfate
E. 10 percent aluminum chloride solution

13. The antibiotic well known to induce an occasional case of aplastic anemia is 13.___

A. penicillin
B. streptomycin
C. tetracycline
D. erythromycin
E. chloramphenicol

14. Which of the following statements are TRUE regarding the halogenated hydrocarbon anesthetic agents? 14.____

    I. Potential for liver toxicity
    II. Cause fall in blood pressure
    III. Progressive respiratory depressants
    IV. Explosive
    V. Little tendency to produce cardiac arrhythmias

    The CORRECT answer is:

    A. I, II, III
    B. II, IV, V
    C. III, IV, V
    D. I, III
    E. IV, V

15. Which of the following statements are TRUE regarding the general anesthetics? 15.____

    I. Selectively depress the reticular activating system
    II. Potency may be related to degree of lipid solubility
    III. Transported through tissues by active transport mechanisms
    IV. Effects dependent on partial pressure of gas in brain
    V. High therapeutic index

    The CORRECT answer is:

    A. I, II, III
    B. I, III, IV
    C. II, III, IV
    D. III, IV, V
    E. II, IV

16. Which of the following drugs are considered to be direct-acting catecholamines? 16.____

    I. Epinephrine
    II. Amphetamine
    III. Tyramine
    IV. Isoproterenol
    V. Norepinephrine

    The CORRECT answer is:

    A. I, II, III
    B. I, IV, V
    C. II, IV, V
    D. I, III, V
    E. III, IV, V

17. The antibiotic of choice to protect a patient with a history of rheumatic heart disease prior to oral surgical procedures is 17.____

    A. penicillin
    B. novobiocin
    C. erythromycin
    D. streptomycin

18. The penicillin nucleus necessary for biologic activity is 18.____

    A. penicillamine
    B. penicilloic acid
    C. penaldic acid
    D. 6-aminopenicillanic acid
    E. none of the above

19. Permanent auditory nerve deafness is FREQUENTLY associated with use of 19.____

    A. polymyxin B
    B. chloramphenicol
    C. the penicillins
    D. the tetracyclines
    E. the streptomycins

20. Toxic systemic effects of procaine hydrochloride are USUALLY associated with 20.____

    A. overdosage
    B. use of a hypotonic solution

C. use of a solution having an incorrect pH
D. use with a vasoconstrictor

21. The penetration of a local anesthetic into nervous tissue is a function of 21.____

A. length of central alkyl chain
B. lipid solubility of unionized form
C. lipid solubility of the ionized form
D. ester linkage between aromatic nucleus and alkyl chain
E. amide linkage between aromatic nucleus and alkyl chain

22. From the behavior of the patient under ether anesthesia, the MOST resistant part of the central nervous system is the 22.____

A. spinal cord
B. medulla oblongata
C. cerebral cortex (motor area)
D. cerebral cortex (sensory area)

23. In edema related to congestive heart failure, the MOST effective and reliable diuretics are the 23.____

A. chlorothiazide
B. spironolactone
C. osmotic diuretics
D. xanthine diuretics

24. Which of the following drugs belong to the xanthine group of CNS stimulants? 24.____

I. Strychnine
II. Aminophylline
III. Pentylenetetrazol
IV. Cocaine
V. Caffeine

The CORRECT answer is:

A. I, II, III
B. I, III, IV
C. II, III, IV
D. II, V
E. III, IV, V

25. Which of the following situations are examples of bio-transformation? 25.____
A drug

I. is excreted by the kidney
II. is made less toxic or nontoxic in the body
III. changes the functioning of an organ in the body
IV. is made more or less therapeutically active in the body

The CORRECT answer is:

A. I, II
B. I, III
C. I, IV
D. II, III
E. II, IV
F. III, IV

KEY (CORRECT ANSWERS)

1. C
2. B
3. A
4. D
5. D
6. D
7. D
8. A
9. C
10. B
11. E
12. B
13. E
14. A
15. E
16. B
17. A
18. D
19. E
20. A
21. B
22. B
23. A
24. D
25. E

TEST 2

DIRECTIONS: Each question or incomplete statement is followed by several suggested answers or completions. Select the one that BEST answers the question or completes the statement. *PRINT THE LETTER OF THE CORRECT ANSWER IN THE SPACE AT THE RIGHT.*

1. A consideration in the therapeutic choice of trimethadione (U.S.P.) as an anticonvulsant is that the compound is 1.____

   A. useful in petit mal, especially in children
   B. recommended for control of grand mal in adults
   C. contraindicated for the treatment of psychomotor seizures
   D. an anticonvulsant without any hypnotic or analgesic action
   E. devoid of toxic effects so needs no precautions in its use

2. The barbiturate which MOST readily penetrates the blood-brain barrier is 2.____

   A. barbital B. thiopental C. secobarbital
   D. phenobarbital E. pentobarbital

3. Many highly ionized drugs are more poorly absorbed, less generally distributed, and more rapidly excreted than less ionized drugs because highly polar drugs are 3.____

   A. less lipid-soluble
   B. less water-soluble
   C. more rapidly metabolized
   D. more extensively bound to tissues

4. Penicillin activity is made ineffective by penicillinase-producing bacteria. This action is related to 4.____

   A. splitting of the beta-lactam ring
   B. splitting of the thiazolidine ring
   C. formation of penicilloic acid
   D. formation of 6-aminopenicillanic acid

5. Lidocaine is a(n) 5.____

   A. amide B. ester C. lipid
   D. hydrocarbon E. carbohydrate

6. The systemic manifestations of a serious toxic reaction to a local anesthetic agent include some combination of the following: hypotension, respiratory depression and/or convulsions. 6.____
   The MOST probable cause is

   A. psychogenic
   B. deterioration of the anesthetic agent
   C. patient hypersensitivity to the vasoconstrictor
   D. excessive blood level of the anesthetic agent
   E. patient hypersensitivity to the anesthetic agent

7. Which of the following general anesthetics belong to the group termed the halogenated hydrocarbons? 7.____

   I. Nitrous oxide
   II. Halothane
   III. Chloroform
   IV. Cyclopropane
   V. Methoxyflurane

   The CORRECT answer is:

   A. I, II, III
   B. II, III, IV
   C. II, III, V
   D. II, IV, V
   E. III, IV, V

8. Which of the following agents would affect coagulation time of blood when added to a sample in vitro? 8.____

   I. Heparin
   II. Thrombin
   III. Menadione
   IV. Dicumarol

   The CORRECT answer is:

   A. I, II
   B. I, II, III
   C. I, III
   D. II, III, IV
   E. III, IV

9. An action of the nitrite ion is to 9.____

   A. decrease heart rate
   B. increase blood pressure
   C. dilate blood vessels
   D. decrease coronary blood flow

10. Quinidine is used to treat 10.____

    A. hypertension
    B. angina pectoris
    C. ventricular tachycardia
    D. congestive heart failure

11. A ganglionic blocking agent such as mecamylamine will block 11.____

    A. sympathetic ganglia *only*
    B. parasympathetic ganglia *only*
    C. both sympathetic and parasympathetic ganglia
    D. none of the above

12. To suppress excessive salivation in an adult, atropine sulfate may be used in a dosage of _______ mg. 12.____

    A. 0.05
    B. 0.5
    C. 5
    D. 50
    E. 100

13. The following drug produces inhibition of sympathetic adrenergic nerve activity by causing a depletion of the sympathetic mediator: 13.____

    A. Ergotamine
    B. Tolazoline
    C. Reserpine
    D. Phentolamine
    E. Phenoxybenzamine

14. Alcoholic euphoria results from 14.___

A. increased activity of the cerebrum
B. increased activity of cerebral areas
C. increased activity of spinal synapses
D. decreased activity of medullary centers
E. removal of inhibitory activity of the cortex

15. When an attempt is made to distinguish between habituation and addiction, GREATEST importance is usually given to the presence or absence of 15.___

A. the development of tolerance to the drug
B. psychic dependence upon the drug
C. acceptability of the drug in our society
D. harmfulness of the drug
E. physical dependence upon the drug

16. Which of the following drugs produce an effect comparable to stimulation of the parasympathetic nervous system? 16.___

I. Pilocarpine
II. Physostigmine
III. Acetylcholine
IV. Muscarine
V. Amphetamine
VI. Phenylephrine
VII. Ergotamine

The CORRECT answer is:

A. I, II, III, IV
B. I, II, III, V
C. I, II, IV, VI
D. II, IV, VI, VII

17. Which of the following is the drug of choice for the treatment of a severe, immediate allergic reaction? 17.___

A. Oxygen
B. Caffeine
C. Cortisone
D. Epinephrine
E. Diphenhydramine

18. Which of the following types of drug dependence probably produces the GREATEST amount of tissue damage in the individual? 18.___

A. Alcohol
B. Marijuana
C. Barbiturate
D. LSD
E. Cocaine

19. Of the choices listed below, which BEST conforms to the following facts? 19.___
It is readily reabsorbed from glomerular filtrates.
If allowed to accumulate in the body, it tends to produce edema.
It may cause diuresis when high concentrations are in the bloodstream.
The CORRECT answer is:

A. Insulin
B. Na^+
C. K^+
D. NH_4^+

20. Following the administration of lidocaine 1 percent, the patient feels faint and lightheaded and begins to wheeze. The injection of 0.5 cc of 1:1000 epinephrine s.c. will produce all of the following effects EXCEPT 20.____

A. sedation
B. bronchodilation
C. cardiac acceleration
D. increased systolic blood pressure

21. A patient suffers an accidental wound of the oral cavity. The dentist should 21.____

A. prescribe tetanus toxoid
B. suture wound and prescribe tetanous toxoid
C. suture wound to control bleeding
D. control hemorrhage and refer to physician for necessary tetanus toxoid therapy

22. Patient has uncontrolled diabetes. The offending tooth requiring extraction is causing severe pain. 22.____
The dentist should proceed by

A. referring to physician for treatment of diabetes
B. removing the offending tooth and prescribing appropriate antibiotics
C. prescribing analgesics
D. prescribing analgesics, consultation with physician, and appointment for extraction

23. A 35-year-old woman with acute suppurative pulpitis is scheduled for tooth extraction. Because of a history of rheumatic heart disease, 600,000 units of procaine penicillin G and 300,000 units of aqueous penicillin are administered one hour prior to an anesthetic of 2 percent lidocaine with 1:100,000 epinephrine. Fifteen minutes later, it is noted that periorbital tissue and lips of the patient are edematous. 23.____
These facts are CONSISTENT with a diagnosis of

A. hematoma formation
B. angioneurotic edema
C. congestive heart failure
D. an acute anaphylactoid reaction

24. Streptokinase activity may result in 24.____

A. dissolution of blood clots
B. fibrinolysin activation
C. neither A nor B above
D. both A and B above

25. The absorption of dietary calcium is an active process which is 25.____

A. facilitated by vitamin D
B. facilitated by vitamin E
C. dependent upon dietary fluoride
D. dependent upon the presence of dietary phosphate

KEY (CORRECT ANSWERS)

1. A
2. B
3. A
4. A
5. A
6. D
7. C
8. A
9. C
10. C
11. C
12. B
13. C
14. E
15. E
16. A
17. D
18. A
19. B
20. A
21. D
22. D
23. B
24. D
25. A

PHARMACOLOGY EXAMINATION SECTION TEST 1

DIRECTIONS: Each question or incomplete statement is followed by several suggested answers or completions. Select the one that BEST answers the question or completes the statement. *PRINT THE LETTER OF THE CORRECT ANSWER IN THE SPACE AT THE RIGHT.*

1. The PROPER antibiotic to be employed prophylactically in a patient with rheumatic heart disease (RHD) not receiving prophylactic penicillin is 1.____

   A. erythromycin
   B. lincomycin
   C. cephalosporin
   D. penicillin G
   E. penicillin V or phenethicillin

2. MOST life-threatening adverse drug reactions affect the 2.____

   A. central nervous system
   B. liver and kidney systems
   C. bronchial smooth muscle
   D. cardiovascular and respiratory systems
   E. none of the above

3. Drugs which are either synergistic with or potentiate the effects of acetylcholine include: 3.____

   I. Methacholine (Mecholyl®)
   II. Scopolamine
   III. Pralidoxime (2-PAM)
   IV. Neostigmine
   V. Pilocarpine

   The CORRECT answer is:

   A. I, II, III
   B. I, III, IV
   C. I, IV, V
   D. II, IV, V
   E. III, IV, V
   F. All of the above

4. Drugs which are commonly used in the control of excessive salivation include: 4.____

   I. Meprobamate
   II. Atropine sulfate
   III. Methantheline bromide
   IV. Codeine phosphate
   V. Chlorpromazine HCl

   The CORRECT answer is:

   A. I, II
   B. I, II, III
   C. II, III
   D. III, IV, V
   E. III, IV
   F. IV, V

5. Local anesthetics are COMMONLY chemical derivatives of 5.____
   I. Barbituric acid
   II. Aniline
   III. Ethanol
   IV. Para-aminobenzoic acid
   V. Acetic acid

   The CORRECT answer is:

   A. I, II, III
   B. I, III
   C. II, III, IV
   D. II, IV
   E. III, IV, V

6. The blood-alcohol level is determined PRIMARILY by 6.____
   I. rate of metabolism
   II. body weight
   III. mind-set
   IV. presence of food in stomach
   V. rate of urinary excretion

   The CORRECT answer is:

   A. I, II, III
   B. I, II, IV
   C. I, IV, V
   D. II, III, IV
   E. III, IV, V

7. The FIRST sensations usually lost after local anesthetic administration are 7.____
   I. touch
   II. pressure
   III. pain
   IV. temperature
   V. skeletal muscle movement

   The CORRECT answer is:

   A. I, II
   B. I, III
   C. II, III
   D. III, IV
   E. None of the above

8. Place in proper order the following events occurring during transmission of nerve impulses at synapses: 8.____
   I. Release of chemical mediator by nerve action potential
   II. Binding of chemical mediator to vesicles
   III. Depolarization of postsynaptic membrane
   IV. Diffusion of chemical mediator across synaptic cleft
   V. Enzymatic destruction or re-uptake of chemical mediator

   The CORRECT answer is:

   A. I, II, III, IV, V
   B. I, IV, V, III, II
   C. II, I, IV, III, V
   D. II, III, I, IV, V
   E. IV, I, II, III, V

9. Gastrointestinal activity may be modified by which of the following types of compounds? 9.____
   I. Ganglionic blocking drugs
   II. Cathartics
   III. Opiates
   IV. Parasympathomimetics

   The CORRECT answer is:

A. I, IV
B. I, II, IV
C. II, III, IV
D. All of the above
E. None of the above

10. Which of the following regarding the oral hypoglycemic agent tolbutamide (Orinase) are TRUE? 10.____

I. Blocks the destruction of insulin
II. Stimulates the beta cells of the pancreas
III. Used primarily in maturity-onset diabetics
IV. Increases glucose utilization by activating hexokinase
V. Decreases activity of insulin antagonists

The CORRECT answer is:

A. I, II, III, V
B. I, II, III
C. II, III, IV
D. II, III
E. III, IV, V

11. Which of the following drugs can cause depletion of norepinephrine from the sympathetic nerve terminals? 11.____

I. Meprobamate
II. Reserpine
III. Chlorpromazine
IV. Benactyzine
V. Guanethidine

The CORRECT answer is:

A. I, II
B. I, IV
C. I, V
D. II, III
E. II,V
F. III, IV
G. IV, V

12. Which of the following properties apply to procainamide? 12.____

I. Depresses cardiac automaticity
II. Delays conduction in bundle of His
III. Increases atrial refractory period
IV. Decreases incidence and severity of arrhythmias following cardiac infarction
V. Causes tachycardia by direct cardio-accelerator action on SA node

The CORRECT answer is:

A. I, II, III, IV
B. I, II
C. II, IV
D. III *only*
E. All of the above

Questions 13-25.

DIRECTIONS: The sentences in Questions 13 through 25 consist of two main parts: a statement and a reason for the statement. Which of the following describes each item?
Mark your answer:

A. If both statement and reason are correct and related
B. If both statement and reason are correct but NOT related
C. If the statement is correct but the reason is NOT
D. If the statement is not correct but the reason is an accurate statement
E. If NEITHER statement nor reason is correct.

13. In clinical testing of a new drug, the double blind design is not usually necessary *because* few drugs possess a true placebo effect. 13.____

14. Epinephrine is contraindicated in asthmatic patients *because* epinephrine exerts a beta-adrenergic effect on bronchial smooth muscle. 14.____

15. Hypertension caused by a phenochromocytoma may be reduced by phentolamine *because* sympatholytic agents destroy catecholamines as they are secreted. 15.____

16. Pentylenetetrazol is occasionally used as an antidote in acute barbiturate poisoning *because* it may stimulate vital medullary centers. 16.____

17. The immediate use of pentylenetetrazol (Metrazol) is contraindicated for barbiturate over-dosage *because* barbiturates with a short duration of action are metabolized more slowly than are those with a long duration of action. 17.____

18. Cumulation can occur upon repeated administration of any drug *because* cumulation of a drug will occur any time the rate of administration exceeds the rate of elimination. 18.____

19. Aspirin is contraindicated in patients receiving the coumarin anticoagulants *because* high doses of aspirin may induce a hypoprothrombinemia. 19.____

20. Energy expenditure via active transport mechanisms is usually required to move a drug across a membrane *because* drugs move from a higher to a lower concentration according to the law of passive diffusion. 20.____

21. Many nonprescription *sleeping tablets* contain an anti-histamine *because* some antihistamines are effective against motion sickness. 21.____

22. Caution must be exercised in using glucosteroids to reduce inflammation in the face of bacterial infection *because* glucosteroids have masculinizing as well as salt and water retention properties. 22.____

23. A local anesthetic which is x times as potent as procaine never offers any therapeutic advantage over procaine *because* a local anesthetic which is x times as potent as procaine will also be x times as toxic. 23.____

24. Neostigmine is useful in the treatment of an overdose of d-tubocurarine *because* neostigmine increases the amount of acetylcholine released from the motor nerve terminal. 24.____

25. Pretreatment with phenobarbital accelerates the oxidation of a subsequently injected dose of pentobarbital *because* phenobarbital induces an increase in the activity of drug-metabolizing enzymes of the liver microsomes. 25.____

KEY (CORRECT ANSWERS)

1. E
2. D
3. C
4. C
5. D
6. B
7. D
8. C
9. D
10. D
11. E
12. A
13. E
14. D
15. C
16. A
17. C
18. A
19. B
20. D
21. B
22. B
23. E
24. C
25. A

TEST 2

DIRECTIONS: Each question or incomplete statement is followed by several suggested answers or completions. Select the one that BEST answers the question or completes the statement. *PRINT THE LETTER OF THE CORRECT ANSWER IN THE SPACE AT THE RIGHT.*

1. Which of the following are TRUE regarding marijuana (cannabis) dependence? 1._____
   I. Active ingredient is tetrahydrocannabinol
   II. Botanical source is Indian help plant
   III. Not absorbed from the G-I tract
   IV. Proven teratogen
   V. May induce severe physical dependence and tolerance

   The CORRECT answer is:

   A. I, II, III B. I, II C. II, III, IV
   D. III, IV, V E. III, V

2. Which of the following are TRUE regarding the major tranquilizers? 2._____
   I. Principally used in the treatment of neurotic behavior
   II. May induce extrapyrmidal syndrome
   III. Alpha-adrenergic blocking effects may induce hypotension
   IV. May induce severe drug dependencies
   V. LSD antagonists

   The CORRECT answer is:

   A. I, II, III B. I, III, V C. II,III, IV
   D. II, III, V E. III, IV, V

3. Which of the following are TRUE regarding drug bio-transformation? 3._____
   I. Primarily occurs in the liver microsomal enzyme system
   II. Generally involves complex chemical processes
   III. Rate may be influenced by certain drugs
   IV. Usually converts a drug to its lipid-soluble, ionized form
   V. Rate may differ significantly in various animal species

   The CORRECT answer is:

   A. I, II, III B. I, III, V C. II, III, IV
   D. II, III E. III, IV, V

4. Which of the following are halogenated hydrocarbon general anesthetics? 4._____
   I. Cyclopropane
   II. Halothane (Fluothane®)
   III. Nitrous oxide
   IV. Methoxyflurane (Penthrane®)
   V. Diethyl ether
   VI. Chloroform

   The CORRECT answer is:

   A. I, II, III B. I, III, V, VI
   C. II, III, IV D. II, IV, VI
   E. III, IV, V, VI

5. Which of the following are TRUE regarding belladonna alkaloids? 5.____
   I. Competitive antagonists of acetylcholine at muscarinic receptor sites
   II. Usually first systems affected are those for secretions (salivary, etc.)
   III. Produce tachycardia due to blockage of vagus nerve
   IV. Produce miosis
   V. Contraindicated in presence of glaucoma

   The CORRECT answer is:

   A. I, II, III, V
   B. I, II, III
   C. I, III, V
   D. I, V
   E. II, IV, V

6. Which of the following penicillins are well absorbed orally? 6.____
   I. Methicillin (Staphcillin®)
   II. Penicillin V
   III. Ampicillin (Polycillin®)
   IV. Phenoxymethyl penicillin
   V. Penicillin G

   The CORRECT answer is:

   A. I, II, III
   B. I, IV, V
   C. II, III, IV
   D. II, III
   E. III, IV, V

7. Which of the following statements are TRUE regarding drug dependence and abuse? 7.____
   I. Only CNS depressants produce significant physical dependence.
   II. All victims of drug abuse have in common a desire to escape reality.
   III. Definition depends upon accepted medical practice and social custom.
   IV. Physical dependence is characterized by the abstinence or withdrawal syndrome.
   V. All forms of drug abuse produce psychic dependence.

   The CORRECT answer is:

   A. I, II, III
   B. I, IV, V
   C. II, V
   D. III, IV, V
   E. All of the above

8. Which of the following are TRUE regarding the Controlled Substances Act of 1970? 8.____
   I. Replaces the Harrison Narcotic Act classification of narcotic and addicting drugs
   II. Requires that accurate records of the receipt and dispensation of Schedule drugs be kept in the dental office
   III. Prohibits Schedule II drugs from being prescribed orally to the pharmacist unless under extreme emergency
   IV. Prohibits the dentist from prescribing any drug not directly related to dental practice
   V. Prohibits the dentist from dispensing any Schedule II drugs in the dental office

   The CORRECT answer is:

   A. I, II, III
   B. I, III
   C. II, III, IV
   D. III, IV, V
   E. III, V

9. Which of the following are TRUE regarding barbiturates? 9.____
   I. Suppress REM sleep
   II. Cause of death in overdosage is respiratory depressior
   III. Metabolized primarily in the liver
   IV. Severe myocardial depressants in sedative doses
   V. Significant alpha-adrenergic blocking effects in therapeutic doses

   The CORRECT answer is:

   A. I, II, III B. I, III, V C. II, III, IV
   D. III, IV, V E. IV, V

10. Which of the following treatments would likely be instituted on the first visit of the patient with temporo-mandibular joint pain? 10.____
   I. Immobilization of the mandible
   II. Application of moist heat
   III. Prescribing of pain-relieving systemic drugs
   IV. Removal of gross occlusal interferences
   V. Alcohol injection in painful area

   The CORRECT answer is:

   A. I, II, III B. I, V C. I *only*
   D. II, III E. II, III, IV F. II, IV

11. Which of the following local disinfectants is inactivated by the presence of soap? 11.____
   A. Iodine tincture
   B. Thimerosal tincture
   C. Nitromersol tincture
   D. Compound cresol solution
   E. Benzalkonium chloride solution

12. Fluoride exchanges with what components of teeth? 12.____
   A. Amino groups B. Hydroxyl groups
   C. Carboxyl groups D. Sulfhydryl groups
   E. None of the above

13. Chlorpromazine belongs to which of the following groups of chemical compounds? 13.____
   A. Catecholamine B. Phenothiazine C. Sulfonamide
   D. Pyridine E. Quinoline

14. An epileptic (grand mal) patient MOST likely would be under treatment with which of the following drugs? 14.____
   A. Meprobamate B. Pentobarbital
   C. Trimethadione D. Chlorpromazine
   E. Diphenylhydantoin

15. Which of the following statements regarding local anesthesia is TRUE? 15.____
   A. Onset and duration are independent of the tissue pH.
   B. Recovery time is usually shorter than the onset time.
   C. The smaller the concentration, the shorter the latency of onset of action.
   D. Degree and duration depend upon the intrinsic potency of the anesthetic.
   E. The larger the nerve fiber, the shorter the onset and the greater the duration.

16. Aplastic anemia is a serious toxic effect which particularly occurs after a course of treatment with which of the following antibiotics? 16.____

A. Penicillin
B. Tetracycline
C. Chloramphenicol
D. Chlortetracycline
E. Lincomycin

17. Which of the following is considered a broad-spectrum penicillin? 17.____

A. Penicillin G
B. Phenoxymethyl penicillin
C. Ampicillin
D. Methicillin

18. What does ED_{50} mean? 18.____

A. Lethal dose
B. Therapeutic ratio
C. Median lethal dose
D. Median effective dose

19. Which of the following types of drug responses is LEAST predictable in occurrence? 19.____

A. Side effect
B. Idiosyncrasy
C. Tachyphylaxis
D. Therapeutic action
E. Overdosage toxicity

20. Which of the following is NOT true of diazepam (Valium)? 20.____

A. Structurally related to chlordiazepoxide (Librium)
B. A minor tranquilizer
C. May be habit-forming
D. Anti-anxiety agent
E. Potent diuretic

21. Which of the following effects is NOT obtained by administration of sodium bicarbonate? 21.____

A. Increase in intestinal absorption of acetylsalicylic acid
B. Increase in renal excretion of Na phenobarbital
C. Decrease in renal toxicity of sulfadiazine
D. Decrease in gastric acidity
E. Acid rebound

22. Which of the following is NOT true regarding acetaminophen (Tylenol®)? 22.____

A. Antipyretic properties
B. Not cross-allergenic with aspirin
C. Anti-inflammatory properties
D. Can be combined with codeine
E. May induce methemoglobinemia

23. Which of the following is NOT true regarding ethyl alcohol? 23.____

A. Induces cutaneous vasodilation
B. Initial CNS stimulant effect followed by CNS depression
C. Limited tolerance development
D. No proven chromosomal damage
E. None of the above

24. All of the following vasodilators are useful as anti-hypertensive agents EXCEPT 24.____

A. reserpine
B. amyl nitrite
C. guanethidine
D. mecamylamine
E. alpha-methyldopa

25. Excessive doses of acetylsalicylic acid can produce each of the following EXCEPT 25.____

A. hypothermia
B. hyperventilation
C. metabolic acidosis
D. central nervous system stimulation

KEY (CORRECT ANSWERS)

1. B
2. D
3. B
4. D
5. A
6. C
7. E
8. A
9. A
10. E
11. E
12. B
13. B
14. E
15. D
16. C
17. C
18. D
19. B
20. E
21. A
22. C
23. B
24. B
25. A

PHARMACOLOGY

EXAMINATION SECTION
TEST 1

DIRECTIONS: Each question or incomplete statement is followed by several suggested answers or completions. Select the one that *BEST* answers the question or completes the statement. *PRINT THE LETTER OF THE CORRECT ANSWER IN THE SPACE AT THE RIGHT.*

1. Which of the following drugs does *NOT* possess an action common to the other four? 1.____

   A. Caffeine B. Ephedrine C. Strychnine
   D. Amphetamine E. Scopolamine

2. Generally, each of the following factors is important in assuring maximum effeetive absorption of a drug from the gastrointestinal tract *EXCEPT* 2.____

   A. high degree of ionization of the drug
   B. high lipid solubility of the drug
   C. particle size of the drug administered
   D. size of the drug molecule
   E. None of the above

3. All of the following pairs of drugs are opposite in their pharmacological action on smooth muscle of intestine *EXCEPT* 3.____

   A. morphine and papaverine
   B. neostigmine and atropine
   C. amphetamine and ephedrine
   D. acetylcholine and epinephrine
   E. None of the above

4. Hydrochlorothiazide has all of the following actions in man *EXCEPT* 4.____

   A. a hypotensive effect
   B. mobilization of edema fluid
   C. increased excretion of potassium
   D. increased excretion of uric acid
   E. increased excretion of sodium

5. Each of the following is useful as an antihypertensive agent *EXCEPT* 5.____

   A. reserpine B. amyl nitrite
   C. hydralazine D. chlorothiazide
   E. alpha-methyldopa

6. Each of the following local anesthetics is a benzoic acid ester *EXCEPT* 6.____

   A. procaine B. tetracaine C. piperocaine
   D. mepivacaine E. ethyl aminobenzoate

7. Which of the following statements *BEST* describes the toxicity of most drugs? 7.___

   A. Toxicity is unpredictable and random.
   B. Toxicity and therapeutic effect always arise from different mechanisms.
   C. Toxicity is not produced by the average dose listed in the U. S. PHARMACOPEIA.
   D. Toxicity is often an extension of the desired drug effect.
   E. Toxicity is predictable and consistent.

8. Organophosphate insecticides and nerve gases inhibit the action of which of the following enzymes? 8.___

   A. Adenylate cyclase
   B. Monoamine oxidase
   C. Phosphodieterase
   D. Acetylcholinesterase
   E. None of the above

9. Which of the following forms of drug toxicity is particularly associated with the halogenated hydrocarbon general anesthetics? 9.___

   A. Liver damage
   B. Myocardial atrophy
   C. Peripheral neuritis
   D. Severe hypertension
   E. None of the above

10. Which of the following statements is *TRUE* regarding the use of the barbiturates in treating convulsions due to local anesthesia? 10.___

   A. Barbiturates are incapable of terminating local anesthetic convulsions.
   B. Barbiturates may delay return to consciousness and are synergistic with respiratory and cardiovascular depressant effects of local anesthetics.
   C. Premedication with the barbiturates may prevent the convulsions due to local anesthetics.
   D. All of the above
   E. None of the above

11. How is the therapeutic index of a drug calculated? 11.___

   A. The therapeutic dose is divided by the toxic base
   B. Half the toxic dose is divided by half the therapeutic dose
   C. The maximum tolerated dose is divided by the minimum therapeutic dose
   D. The lethal dose for 50 percent of animals is divided by the therapeutic dose for 50% of animals
   E. The toxic base is divided by the therapeutic dose

12. The systemic activity of the ester (procaine) types of local anesthetics is terminated *PRIMARILY* by 12.___

   A. elimination by the kidney
   B. storage in adipose tissue
   C. metabolism in the liver only
   D. metabolism in the liver and by pseudocholinesterase in the plasma
   E. all of the above

13. A patient receiving propranolol has an acute asthmatic attack while undergoing treatment. The *MOST* useful agent for management of the condition is 13.____

A. morphine
B. epinephrine
C. phentolamine
D. aminophylline
E. norepinephrine

14. Anithistaminic compounds exert their effect by 14.____

A. chemically neutralizing histamine
B. competing with histamine for peripheral receptor sites
C. preventing the release of histamine in injured tissues
D. preventing the antigen-antibody reaction upon exposure to an allergen
E. chemically freeing histamine

15. A patient states that he has been taking mecamylamine regularly for the past year. Oral examination is *most likely* to reveal 15.____

A. ptyalism
B. xerostomia
C. palatal petechiae
D. gingival hypertrophy
E. bullous lesions on the buccal mucosa

16. Prolonged therapeutic administration of cortisone induces 16.____

A. hypoglycemia
B. hypofunction of the adrenal cortex
C. hypofunction of the adrenal medulla
D. hyperfunction of the pituitary gland
E. hyperfunction of the thyroid gland

17. Which of the following statements are *TRUE* regarding general anesthetics? 17.____

A. All are gases at room temperature.
B. Speed of induction is inversely related to blood solubility.
C. Effects are dependent upon attaining a critical partial pressure in the CNS.
D. All are associated with a decrease in central synaptic activity.
E. All are explosive.

The *CORRECT* answer is:

A. I, II, III
B. I, IV, V
C. II, III, IV
D. III, IV
E. III, IV, V

18. Which of the following are side-effects of anti-anxiety drugs such as diazepam? 18.____

I. Drug dependence similar to the barbiturates
II. Ataxia
III. Impaired mechanical abilities
IV. Drowsiness
V. Hypnosis

The *CORRECT* answer is:

A. I, II, V
B. I, III, IV
C. II, III, IV
D. III, IV, V
E. All ofthe above

19. Which of the following drugs may cause adverse reactions when administered in the presence of the monoamine oxidase inhibitors? 19.____

I. Epinephrine
II. Amphetamine
III. Tyramine
IV. Penicillin
V. Aspirin

A. I, II, III, IV
B. I, II, III
C. II, IV, V
D. III, IV, V
E. All of the above

20. Scopolamine is often used for premedication prior to administration of a general anesthetic because it 20.____

A. *increases* heart rate
B. *decreases* heart rate
C. *decreases* blood pressure
D. *decreases* the possibility of laryngospasm by inhibiting salivation
E. *retards* liver metabolism of the general anesthetic agent

21. The activity of benzalkonium chloride is markedly antagonized by 21.____

A. soap
B. sodium nitrite
C. sodium chloride
D. cetylpyridinium chloride
E. alkylbenzyldimethyl ammonium chloride

22. Inadvertently, an overdose of morphine is administered to a patient. To treat this condition, it is appropriate to administer 22.____

A. oxygen and inject naloxone hydrochloride
B. caffeine sodium benzoate intravenously
C. doxapram intramuscularly
D. nalorphine and epinephrine intramuscularly
E. none of the above

23. The *single MOST* useful agent in resuscitation is 23.____

A. oxygen
B. an endotracheal tube
C. a respiratory stimulant
D. aromatic spirits of ammonia
E. 1:1000 epinephrine for injection

24. The advantages of nitrous oxide sedation over intravenous sedation include: 24.____

I. Shorter recovery time
II. Less respiratory depression
III. The ability to discharge the patient without an escort
IV. The ability to alter the depth of sedation from moment to moment
V. Lack of toxicity and allergenicity of the agent

The *CORRECT* answer is:

A. I, II, III
B. I, IV
C. II, III, IV
D. III, IV, V
E. All of the above

25. Which of the following is *NOT* true regarding combined oral contraceptives? 25.____

A. Inhibit ovulation
B. Stimulate pituitary secretion of FSH and LH
C. Chemically contain an estrogen and a progestin
D. Produce endometrial changes resembling pregnancy
E. Are contraindicated in the presence of estrogen-dependent cancers

---

KEY (CORRECT ANSWERS)

1.	E	11.	D
2.	A	12.	D
3.	C	13.	D
4.	D	14.	B
5.	B	15.	B
6.	D	16.	B
7.	D	17.	C
8.	D	18.	E
9.	A	19.	B
10.	B	20.	D

21. A
22. A
23. A
24. E
25. B

TEST 2

DIRECTIONS: Each question or incomplete statement is followed by several suggested answers or completions. Select the one that *BEST* answers the question or completes the statement. *PRINT THE LETTER OF THE CORRECTANSWER IN THE SPACE AT THE RIGHT.*

1. Tolerance is *LEAST* likely to develop with use of 1.___

   A. LSD B. heroin C. marihuana
   D. methadone E. amphetamines

2. The *MOST* important pharmacologic action of drugs which suppress cardiac arrhythmias is 2.___

   A. blockade of the vagus nerve
   B. stimulation of cardiac ATP-ase activity
   C. blockade of the beta-adrenergic receptor
   D. stimulation of the alpha-adrenergic receptor
   E. increased refractory period of cardiac muscle

3. Adrenergic neuron blocking drugs, such as guanethidine, are useful *PRIMARILY* in the treatment of 3.___

   A. mental disease B. cardiac arrest
   C. cholinergic crisis D. paroxysmal tachycardia
   E. essential (primary) hypertension

4. A patient on anticonvulsant therapy exhibits marked gingival hypertrophy. This patient, *MOST* likely, is regularly taking 4.___

   A. primidone B. mephobarbital
   C. phenacemide D. phenobarbital
   E. diphenylhydantoin

5. When methohexital is used to induce general anesthesia, the initial effect wears off within a short time and the patient awakens. This occurs because the drug is 5.___

   A. detoxified B. biotransformed
   C. eliminated from the body D. redistributed from the brain
   E. None of the above

6. At a pH of 7.8, lidocaine (pKa = 7.8) will exist in 6.___

   A. the ionized form
   B. the unionized form
   C. an equal mixture of ionized and unionized forms
   D. all of the above
   E. none of the above

7. The blood level of a drug is determined by its: 7.___

   I. Rate of absorption
   II. Rate of excretion
   III. Dose
   IV. Rate of metabolism
   V. Route of administration

The *CORRECT* answer is:

A. I, II, III
B. I, II, V
C. I, IV
D. II, III, IV
E. All of the above

8. The inhalation of amyl nitrite may result in: 8.____
   I. Coronary artery dilation
   II. Peripheral arteriolar dilation
   III. Bradycardia
   IV. Increased motility of the small bowe
   V. A decrease in arterial blood pressure

The *CORRECT* answer is:

A. I, II, IV
B. I, II, V
C. I, III, IV
D. II, III, V
E. III, IV, V

9. An intravenous injection of epinephrine will cause: 9.____
   I. A constriction of cutaneous vascular beds
   II. An increase in cardiac rate
   III. An increase in the activity of the intestinal musculature
   IV. A depression of the central nervous system
   V. An increased blood sugar level

The *CORRECT* answer is:

A. I, II, III
B. I, II, V
C. I, IV, V
D. II, III, IV
E. III, IV, V
F. All of the above

10. Which of the following drugs are categorized as "controlled" drugs under the Controlled Substances Act? 10.____
   I. Codeine
   II. Pentobarbital
   III. Meprobamate
   IV. Oxycodone

The *CORRECT* answer is:

A. I, II, III
B. I, III, IV
C. I, IV
D. II, III, IV
E. All of the above

11. The cholinergic effect of pilocarpine is due to 11.____

A. reversible inactivation of acetylcholinesterase at the postganglionic synapse
B. irreversible inactivation of acetylcholinesterase at the postganglionic synapse
C. direct action upon the cholinergic receptor site
D. stimulation of release of acetylcholine from the nerve terminal
E. none of the above

12. An enzyme involved in the inactivation of epinephrine in the body is 12.____

A. cholinesterase
B. choline acetylase
C. carbonic anhydrase
D. cytochrome oxidase
E. catechol-o-methyltransferase

13. The *first* clinically useful and systemically effective anti-infective agent was 13.___

A. penicillin B. sulfanilamide C. tetracycline
D. streptomycin E. bacitracin

14. The drugs phenformin, tolbutamide, and acetohexamide have in common the fact that they 14.___

A. prevent symptoms of metaphase
B. are anti-inflmmatory
C. reduce blood pressure in the hypertensive patient
D. are antithyroid drugs generally used before thyroid surgery
E. are hypoglycemic agents which may induce cardiovascular disease

15. If a patient requiring an extraction reports that he is on bishydroxyeoumarin therapy, the laboratory test *MOST* valuable in evaluating the surgical risk is 15.___

A. clotting time B. bleeding time
C. sedimentation rate D. complete blood count
E. plasma prothrombin time

16. Which of the following drugs is *MOST* commonly employed in an attack of angina pectoris? 16.___

A. Sodium nitrate B. Epinephrine
C. Theophylline D. Nitroglycerin
E. Isosorbide dinitrate

17. Which of the following antibiotics may cause discoloration of the teeth of the newborn if administered to the mother in the third trimester of pregnancy? 17.___

A. Penicillin B. Tetracycline C. Streptomycin
D. Clindamycin E. Erythromycin

18. Which of the following is the *BEST* substitute drug for a patient allergic to penicillin? 18.___

A. Lincomycin B. Tetracycline C. Sulfonamide
D. Erythromycin E. Ampicillin

19. Which of the following properties may be attributed to warfarin? 19.___

I. Interferes in the *in vivo* synthesis of Factor VII
II. Related structurally to vitamin K
III. Inhibits formation of prothrombin in vivo
IV. Immediate onset of anticoagulant activity
V. Hematological activity is reversed by whole blood administration

The *CORRECT* answer is:

A. I *only* B. I, II, III, V C. I, III, IV
D. II, IV, V E. All of the above

Questions 20-25.

DIRECTIONS: The information contained in Questions 20-25 consists of two main parts: a statement and a reason for the statement. *Which* of the following evaluations *BEST* describes each question?

A. Both statement and reason are correct and related
B. Both statement and reason are correct but not related
C. The statement is correct but the reason is not
D. The statement is not correct but the reason is an accurate statement
E. Neither statement nor reason is correct

20. Epinephrine is contraindicated in treating the vascular collapse of chlorpromazine toxicity *because* chlorpromazine blocks the vasoconstricting properties of epinephrine. 20.____

21. The liver affects the excretion rate of a drug *because* the liver is capable of chemically changing a drug to its lipid insoluble form. 21.____

22. Tincture of iodine is not used as a local anti-infective agent over large areas of the body *because* tincture of iodine causes many allergic reactions and is destructive of skin. 22.____

23. Neostigmine can be useful in treating an overdose of d-tubucurarine *because* neostigmine increases the release of acetylcholine from motor nerve endings. 23.____

24. Many nonprescription "sleeping tablets" contain an antihistamine because some antihistamines are effective against motion sickness. 24.____

25. Dimercaprol (BAL) is effective in early poisoning by mercuric salts *because* it forms a chelate with mercury. 25.____

KEY (CORRECT ANSWERS)

1. C
2. E
3. E
4. E
5. D

6. C
7. E
8. B
9. B
10. E

11. C
12. E
13. B
14. E
15. E

16. D
17. B
18. D
19. B
20. A

21. A
22. A
23. C
24. B
25. A

PHARMACOLOGY
EXAMINATION SECTION
TEST 1

DIRECTIONS: Each question or incomplete statement is followed by several suggested answers or completions. Select the one that BEST answers the question or completes the statement. *PRINT THE LETTER OF THE CORRECT ANSWER IN THE SPACE AT THE RIGHT.*

1. The diuresis seen after adequate digitalis therapy in a patient with congestive heart failure results from 1.____
   A. a direct action of digitalis on glomeruli of the kidney
   B. increased efficiency of the heart and increased renal blood flow
   C. decreased water reabsorption caused by a direct tubular action
   D. an inhibition of antidiuretic hormone output
   E. decreased efficiency of the heart and decreased renal blood flow

2. The action of local anesthetic drugs on nerve fibers resulting in blockage of impulse conduction is 2.____
   A. a decrease in action potential duration
   B. a decrease in magnitude of resting membrane potential
   C. prevention of the depolarization phase of the action potential
   D. a decrease in the rate of repolarization of the membrane
   E. an increase in magnitude of resting membrane potential

3. The PRINCIPAL therapeutic action of the glucocorticoids is 3.____
   A. antidiuretic B. antianabolic C. anti-infective
   D. antihypertensive E. anti-inflammatory

4. If the pH of an area is lower than normal body pH, the concepts involved for the membrane theory of local anesthetic activity would predict that the local anesthetic activity would be 4.____
   A. greater, due to an increase in the free-base form of the drug
   B. greater, due to an increase in the cationic form of the drug
   C. less, due to an increase in the free-base form of the drug
   D. less, due to a decrease in the free-base form of the drug
   E. none of the above

5. The PRIMARY effect produced by digitalis at therapeutic dose levels is a(n) 5.____
   A. slowing of the cardiac rate
   B. decrease in the venous pressure
   C. decrease in cardiac enlargement
   D. increase in the force of myocardial contraction
   E. increase in the venous pressure

6. Which of the following pertain to general anesthesia induced by thiopental? 6.____
   I. Fast induction
   II. Long duration of anesthesia
   III. Predisposition to laryngospasm
   IV. Decreased secretions
   The CORRECT answer is:
   A. I, III B. I, IV C. II, III
   D. III, IV E. All of the above

7. Which of the following therapeutic measures would be appropriate in attempting to ensure the recovery of a patient in coma (with six respiratory movements per minute) as a result of an overdose of pentobarbital? 7.____
   I. Artificial respiration
   II. Administration of oxygen
   III. Injection of nikethamide as an analeptic drug
   IV. Removal of secretions from nasopharynx and trachea
   V. Administration of neomycin by intramuscular injection
   VI. Intravenous infusion of electrolytes to maintain electrolyte balance
   The CORRECT answer is:
   A. I, II, III, V B. I, II, IV, V C. I, II, IV, VI
   D. I, III, IV, VI E. II, III, V, VI F. III, IV, V, VI

8. Which of the following are TRUE regarding the therapeutic index? 8.____
   I. Expresses the relationship between efficacy and toxicity of a drug
   II. The lower the number, the safer the drug
   III. Expresses the margin of safety of the drug
   IV. Determined by comparing ED_{30} and LD_{50} for a drug
   V. Identical for drugs belonging to the same general group (sedatives, antibiotics, etc.)
   The CORRECT answer is:
   A. I, II, III B. I, III, IV C. I, IV, V
   D. II, IV, V E. III, IV, V

9. Alpha adrenergic drugs are used in combination with local anesthetics to: 9.____
   I. Stimulate myocardial contraction
   II. Reduce vascular absorption of the local anesthetic
   III. Increase the rate of liver metabolism of the local anesthetic
   IV. Increase the concentration of the local anesthetic at its receptor site
   V. Antagonize the vasodilatory effects of the local anesthetic
   The CORRECT answer is:
   A. I, II, III B. II, III, IV C. II, IV, V
   D. III, IV, V E. IV, V

10. The side effects associated with the rauwolfia derivatives (e.g., reserpine) are: 10.____
   I. Tachycardia
   II. Nasal stuffiness
   III. Postural hypotension
   IV. Potentiation of barbiturate and narcotic agents
   V. Xerostomia

The CORRECT answer is:
A. I, II, IV
B. I, III, V
C. I, V
D. II, III, IV
E. All of the above

11. The FIRST sensations usually lost after local anesthetic administration are: 11.____
I. Touch
II. Pressure
III. Pain
IV. Temperature
V. Skeletal muscle movement
The CORRECT answer is:
A. I, II
B. I, III
C. II, III
D. III, IV
E. III, V

12. Which of the following are TRUE regarding neuroleptic analgesia? 12.____
I. Combination of an anti-psychotic agent and a Schedule II narcotic
II. May induce general anesthesia
III. Contraindicated in patients with impaired respiration
IV. Low therapeutic index
The CORRECT answer is:
A. I, II, III
B. I, IV
C. II, III, IV
D. II, IV
E. All of the above

13. Which of the following drugs of abuse produce little, if any, physical dependence? 13.____
I. Marijuana
II. Barbiturates
III. Amphetamine
IV. Cocaine
V. Heroin
The CORRECT answer is:
A. I, II, III
B. I, III, IV
C. I, IV
D. II,III, V
E. III, IV, V

14. Which of the following reduce skeletal muscle tone by action of the central nervous system? 14.____
I. Chlordiazepoxide
II. Mephenesin
III. Meprobamate
IV. Diazepam
The CORRECT answer is:
A. I, II, III
B. I, III
C. II, IV
D. III, IV
E. All of the above

15. Which of the following are TRUE regarding ethyl alcohol? 15.____
I. Diuretic
II. Respiratory depressant
III. Selectively concentrates in the brain
IV. 30% excreted by the kidney
V. No tolerance development
The CORRECT answer is:
A. I, II
B. I, II, III
C. I, IV, V
D. II, IV, V
E. II, V

Questions 16-25.

DIRECTIONS: Questions 16 through 25 are to be answered on the basis of the following case.

Mrs. Martin is scheduled in the office for minor periodontal surgery. She has a documented history of rheumatic heart disease, but is not receiving any prophylactic antibiotic therapy. Her medical history reveals narrow angle glaucoma and acute intermittent porphyria (porphyrism). She is anxious regarding her dental procedure and pharmacosedation procedures are deemed necessary. She has no known drug allergies.

16. In view of Mrs. Martin's rheumatic heart condition, the prophylactic antibiotic of choice to be administered orally is 16.____
    A. erythromycin B. penicillin V C. cephalexin
    D. lincomycin E. ampicillin

17. This prophylactic antibiotic therapy should begin _____ prior to the dental procedure. 17.____
    A. immediately B. one hour C. four hours
    D. one day E. two days

18. Due to Mrs. Martin's history of porphyrism, which of the following drug groups is contraindicated for pharmacosedation? 18.____
    A. Minor tranquilizers B. Antihistamines C. Barbiturates
    D. Narcotics E. None of the above

19. Which of the following pharmacosedation agents are contraindicated in the presence of glaucoma? 19.____
    I. Meperidine II. Scopolamine III. Diazepam
    IV. Pentobarbital V. Morphine
    The CORRECT answer is:
    A. I, II, III B. II, III, IV C. II, IV
    D. III, IV, V E. III, V

20. Considering Mrs. Martin's history of glaucoma and porphyrism, which of the following pharmacosedation techniques is PREFERRED? 20.____
    A. Intravenous secobarbital B. Intravenous diazepam
    C. Nitrous oxide-oxygen D. Intravenous thiopental
    E. None of the above

21. Because Mrs. Martin's postoperative discomfort is expected to be minimal, aspirin is advised for analgesia. Which of the following are TRUE regarding aspirin in therapeutic doses? 21.____
    I. Active form is salicylic acid
    II. Has antipyretic properties
    III. Produces central nervous system depressant effects
    IV. Produces central nervous system stimulant effects
    V Retards platelet (thrombocyte) function

The CORRECT answer is:
A. I, II, III
B. I, II, V
C. I, III
D. II, III, IV
E. III, IV, V

22. A SIGNIFICANT mechanism by which aspirin produces its analgesic and anti-inflammatory effects is 22.____
A. antagonism of histamine
B. inhibition of prostaglandin synthesis
C. local anesthetic effect on pain fibers
D. release of adrenal steroids from the adrenal cortex
E. synaptic inhibition in the dorsal column of the spinal cord

23. Mrs. Martin calls the office with complaints suggesting a diffuse cellulitis and lymphadenopathy. A superinfection with a penicillinase-producing staphylococcus is immediately suspected. 23.____
Which of the following antibiotics is the drug of choice in treating this condition?
A. Chloramphenicol
B. Cephalexin
C. Penicillin G
D. Erythromycin
E. Polymyxin B

24. If this superinfection were to be confined to the gastrointestinal tract as a staphylococcal enteritis, which of the following antibiotics would be the drug of choice to be administered topically? 24.____
A. Bacitracin
B. Polymyxin B
C. Erythromycin
D. Lincomycin
E. Benzathine penicillin

25. If Mrs. Martin developed severe gastrointestinal upset from aspirin, which of the following analgesics would be ACCEPTABLE substitutes? 25.____
I. Pentazocine
II. Empirin® Compound
III. Acetaminophen
IV. Darvon® Compound-65
V. Codeine
The CORRECT answer is:
A. I, II, III
B. I, III
C. I, III, V
D. II, IV, V
E. II, V

KEY (CORRECT ANSWERS)

1. B
2. C
3. E
4. D
5. D

6. A
7. C
8. B
9. C
10. D

11. D
12. E
13. B
14. E
15. A

16. B
17. B
18. C
19. A
20. C

21. B
22. B
23. B
24. A
25. C

TEST 2

DIRECTIONS: Each question or incomplete statement is followed by several suggested answers or completions. Select the one that BEST answers the question or completes the statement. *PRINT THE LETTER OF THE CORRECT ANSWER IN THE SPACE AT THE RIGHT.*

1. Which of the following xanthine derivatives produces the BEST bronchodilation? 1.____
   A. Caffeine B. Theobromine C. Theophylline
   D. All of the above E. None of the above

2. The cardiac glycosides will reduce the concentration of which ion in an active heart muscle? 2.____
   A. Sodium B. Bromide C. Calcium
   D. Chloride E. Potassium

3. Pre-treatment with which of the following drugs will potentiate the ability of an intravenous injection of acetylcholine to lower blood pressure? 3.____
   A. Methacholine B. Epinephrine C. Pilocarpine
   D. Physostigmine E. Pralidoxime

4. Which of the following drugs might act by biotransformation into a FALSES adrenergic neurotransmitter? 4.____
   A. Alpha-methyldopa B. Hydralazine C. Phentolamine
   D. Dibenamine® E. Reserpine

5. An excess of which of the following hormones may be associated with increased sensitivity to epinephrine? 5.____
   A. Testosterone B. Parathyroid C. Insulin
   D. Thyroid E. None of the above

6. Which of the following procedures would be expected to increase the incidence and the severity of reactions to local anesthetic agents? 6.____
   A. Aspiration prior to injection
   B. Premedication with a barbiturate
   C. Rapid injection of the anesthetic solution
   D. Use of a vasoconstrictor agent along with the local anesthetic agent
   E. Aspiration after injection

7. Potassium is one of the most important and prevalent ions in the mammalian species. Which of the following statements about this ion are TRUE? 7.____
   I. It is the principal intracellular cation.
   II. High concentrations of the chloride salt can be safely injected intravenously.
   III. It is necessary for normal function of nerve and muscle.
   IV. It is the principal ion responsible for edema.

   The CORRECT answer is:
   A. I, II, III B. I, III C. I, III, IV
   D. II, III E. II, IV

8. Which of the following factors should be considered in adjusting the dose of a drug administered to a specific patient? 8.____
I. Age
II. Sex
III. Weight
IV. Disease state
V. Emotional state
The CORRECT answer is:
A. I, II, III
B. I, II, V
C. I, III, V
D. III, IV, V
E. All of the above

9. Which of the following statements is TRUE regarding prescriptions? 9.____
A. A dentist may legally prescribe only those drugs useful in a dental office.
B. Federal law prohibits the doctor's prescribing a drug over the phone to a pharmacist.
C. Drugs must be prescribed in dosage unit amounts greater than ten.
D. It is ethical and legal to prescribe a placebo.
E. Prescriptions may be signed by a dental assistant as long as the dentist initials the prescription.

10. Which of the following drug groups is currently the mainstay of treatment in depressive psychoneurotic disease? 10.____
A. Amphetamines
B. Phenothiazines
C. Benzodiazepines
D. Monoamine oxidase inhibitors
E. Tricylic (imipramine-like) antidepressants

11. The mechanism of action by which the fluoride ion when taken orally reduces dental caries is 11.____
A. inhibition of bacterial enzymes located in dental plaque
B. alteration in developing tooth morphology
C. alteration in developing tooth collagen matrix
D. alteration in tooth eruption pattern
E. production of less soluble fluorohydroxyapatite

12. The sulfonamides act by 12.____
A. suppressing bacterial protein synthesis
B. inhibiting cytoplasmic bacterial membrane formation
C. inducing the formation of "lethal" bacterial proteins
D. inducing folic acid deficiency by competition with para-aminobenzoic acid
E. releasing bacterial protein synthesis

13. The MOST serious and life-threatening blood dyscrasia associated with drug toxicity is 13.____
A. aplastic anemia
B. agranulocytosis
C. thrombocytopenia
D. hemolytic anemia
E. megaloblastic anemia

14. "Epinephrine reversal" of blood pressure can BEST be demonstrated by injecting epinephrine intravenously following pretreatment with 14.____
   A. atropine
   B. neostigmine
   C. guanethidine
   D. phenoxybenzamine
   E. dichloroisoproterenol

15. During a visit, a patient develops a severe, acute bronchial asthmatic attack. He should IMMEDIATELY receive 15.____
   A. cortisone
   B. epinephrine
   C. tripelennamine
   D. 90 percent oxygen, 10 percent CO_2
   E. none of the above

16. Derivatives of 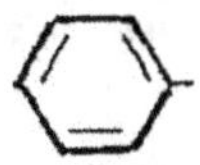 CH_2 CH_2 NH_2 are 16.____
   A. adrenergic drugs
   B. cholinergic drugs
   C. anticholinesterases
   D. cholinergic blocking agents
   E. synaptic transmitters in sympathetic ganglia

17. Which of the following statements are TRUE regarding the occupation theory of drug-receptor interaction? 17.____
   I. The affinity of a drug is dependent on its intrinsic activity.
   II. The maximum effect of the drug occurs when all receptors are occupied.
   III. An antagonist has affinity for the receptor but less intrinsic activity than its agonist.
   IV. The effect of the drug is proportional to the number of receptors occupied.
   V. It does not follow the law of mass action.
   The CORRECT answer is:
   A. I, II, III
   B. II, III
   C. II, III, IV
   D. II, IV
   E. III, IV, V

18. Concomitant administration of which of the following drugs tends to increase the depressant actions of morphine? 18.____
   I. Phenothiazines
   II. Barbiturates
   III. Alcohol
   IV. Monoamine oxidase inhibitors
   V. Tranquilizers
   The CORRECT answer is:
   A. I, II
   B. I, II, III
   C. II, IV, V
   D. III, IV, V
   E. All of the above

Questions 19-25.

DIRECTIONS: The information contained in Questions 19 through 25 consists of two main parts: A STATEMENT and a REASON FOR THE STATEMENT. Which of the following evaluations BEST describes each question?

A. Both statement and reason are correct and related.
B. Both statement and reason are correct but not related.
C. The statement is correct but the reason is not.
D. The statement is not correct but the reason is an accurate statement.

19. Atropine is a competitive inhibitor of acetylcholine at parasympathetic postganglionic autonomic sites because atropine and acetylcholine have the same affinity for all cholinergic receptor sites. 19.____

20. Penicillin is bactericidal because it inhibits the enzymatic processes responsible for determining the final three-dimensional structure of the bacterial cell wall. 20.____

21. Guanethidine can result in an initial sympathomimetic effect when administered intravenously because guanethidine, by rapidly inhibiting monoamine oxidase, produces an increase in intraneuronal norepinephrine. 21.____

22. Some patients are abnormally sensitive to succinylcholine because these individuals are congenitally deficient in pseudocholinesterase. 22.____

23. Hydrogen peroxide is useful in the management of necrotizing ulcerative gingivitis because hydrogen peroxide can result in the hypertrophy of the filiform papillae of the tongue. 23.____

24. Adenylate cyclase and cyclic AMP are thought to be intimately involved with the β-adrenergic receptor because increased tissue levels of cyclic AMP are seen in almost all cases of β-adrenergic stimulation. 24.____

25. Atropine in therapeutic doses can produce tachycardia because atropine has a depressant action on the myocardium. 25.____

KEY (CORRECT ANSWERS)

1. C
2. E
3. D
4. A
5. D

6. C
7. B
8. E
9. D
10. E

11. E
12. D
13. A
14. D
15. B

16. A
17. C
18. E
19. A
20. A

21. C
22. A
23. B
24. A
25. C

PHARMACOLOGY

EXAMINATION SECTION
TEST 1

DIRECTIONS: Each question or incomplete statement is followed by several suggested answers or completions. Select the one that BEST answers the question or completes the statement. *PRINT THE LETTER OF THE CORRECT ANSWER IN THE SPACE AT THE RIGHT.*

1. The drug of choice for prophylaxis against subacute bacterial endocarditis for the patient sensitive to penicillin is 1.____

   A. lincomycin
   B. ampicillin
   C. tetracycline
   D. streptomycin
   E. erythromycin

2. The mechanism by which 70 percent ethyl alcohol may act as a disinfectant is attributed to 2.____

   A. a metabolic degradation product of ethyl alcohol
   B. the lack of alcohol dehydrogenase in bacterial cells
   C. the interference of ethyl alcohol with carbohydrate metabolism
   D. the inebriating effect of ethyl alcohol on cells
   E. the ability of ethyl alcohol to denature proteins

3. d-tubocurarine is used in conjunction with general anesthesia to 3.____

   A. relax skeletal muscles
   B. prevent respiratory failure
   C. prevent a fall in blood pressure
   D. hasten the emergence from anesthesia
   E. increase the duration of anesthesia

4. When a laryngospasm occurs during general anesthesia, the drug of choice is 4.____

   A. atropine
   B. phenytoin
   C. meprobamate
   D. methantheline
   E. succinylcholine

5. Alcoholic euphoria results from 5.____

   A. *increased* activity of the cerebrum
   B. *increased* activity of thalamic areas
   C. *increased* activity of limbic synapses
   D. *decreased* activity of medullary centers
   E. *removal* of inhibitory effect of the cortex

6. Chlorothiazide administration results in a(n) 6.____

   A. *increased* urinary output of sodium
   B. *decreased* urinary output of chloride
   C. *increased* urinary output of glucose
   D. *decreased* urinary output of potassium
   E. *increased* urinary output of uric acid

7. Increasing the dose of a drug by a factor of 10 will INCREASE the response by a factor of 7.____

A. 10 B. 20 C. 100 D. 1,000 E. x

8. Symptoms which may be characterized as allergic manifestations during penicillin therapy are 8.____

A. deafness, dizziness, and acute anemia
B. crystalluria, nausea and vomiting, and anaphylactic shock
C. oliguria, hematuria, bronchoconstriction, and cardiovascular collapse
D. dermatitis, stomatitis, bronchoconstriction, and cardiovascular collapse
E. none of the above

9. Alpha or beta adrenergic blocking drugs, such as phentolamine and propranolol, act by 9.____

A. inhibiting synthesis of norepinephrine
B. increasing the metabolism of norepinephrine
C. competitive inhibition of postjunctional adrenergic receptors
D. a local anesthetic effect on the adrenergic nerve terminal
E. depleting norepinephrine from adrenergic nerve terminals

10. The analgesic effect of aspirin may be related to its suppression of the synthesis of 10.____

A. histamine
B. serotonin
C. bradykinin
D. prostaglandin
E. gamma-aminobutyric acid

11. The pressor action of epinephrine is reversed by 11.____

A. atropine
B. papaverine
C. neostigmine
D. phentolamine
E. propranolol

12. Drug-metabolizing enzymes are present *mainly* in liver 12.____

A. nuclei
B. lysosomes
C. microsomes
D. mitochondria
E. cell membranes

13. Termination of the action of procaine is accomplished *primarily* by 13.____

A. conjugation of the liver
B. the action of plasma amidase
C. hydroxylation in the liver
D. the action of plasma pseudocholinesterase
E. excretion in unchanged form by the kidney

14. The phenomenon in which two drugs produce opposite effects on a physiologic system but do NOT act at the same receptor site is 14.____

A. potentiation
B. chemical antagonism
C. competitive antagonism
D. physiologic antagonism
E. noncompetitive antagonism

15. When digitalis is used in atrial fibrillation, the therapeutic objective is to 15.____

A. inhibit vagal impulses to the heart
B. decrease the rate of A-V conduction
C. abolish cardiac decompensation
D. produce a decrease in the rate of atrial contraction
E. convert fibrillation to a normal sinus rhythm

16. An adrenergic drug, such as epinephrine, can be expected to 16.____

A. constrict bronchioles, systemic arterioles and cerebral arterioles
B. increase heart rate, blood pressure and myocardial contractile force
C. increase G.I. peristalsis and skeletal muscle tone, and dilate the bronchiolar smooth muscle
D. shunt blood from viscera and skin to muscles, and produce miosis without cycloplegia
E. increase body temperature, BMR and glucogenesis

17. The action of the ultra-short acting barbiturates is terminated *primarily* by the process of 17.____

A. oxidation
B. redistribution
C. renal excretion
D. plasma protein binding
E. conjugation with sulfate

18. The MAJOR therapeutic indication for the use of sulfonarnides is 18.____

A. tuberculosis
B. typhoid fever
C. urinary tract infections
D. fungal infections of the foot
E. fungal infections of the oral cavity

19. The antipsychotics are currently believed to produce their effect on the CNS by blocking the receptor for 19.____

A. dopamine
B. serotonin
C. epinephrine
D. aspartic acid
E. norepinephrine

20. A sudden INCREASE in the blood level of drug A after administration of drug B could result from 20.____

A. binding of drug A by drug B
B. chelation of drug A by drug B
C. competition for the same receptor sites
D. induction of hepatic microsomal enzymes
E. displacement of drug A by drug B from protein-binding sites

21. Spironolactone diuresis is the result of 21.____

A. increased potassium excretion
B. direct aldosterone antagonism
C. inhibition of carbonic anhydrase
D. inhibition of antidiuretic hormone release
E. increase in glomerular filtration rate

22. Oral contraceptives prevent conception *primarily* by 22.____

A. inducing abortion
B. preventing ovulation
C. a spermatocidal effect
D. causing a cessation of menses
E. preventing implantation of the fertilized ovum in the endometrial wall

23. The MOST important organ system involved in the excretion of a drug and its metabolites is the 23.____

A. lung
B. liver
C. kidney
D. gallbladder
E. gastrointestinal tract

24. Prilocaine hydrochloride four percent is supplied in a 1.8 ml. cartridge. It is recommended that 600 mg. NOT be exceeded in a two-hour period. 24.____
This amount is contained in *approximately* ______ cartridges.

A. 4 B. 8 C. 12 D. 16 E. 20

25. The current drug of choice for the treatment of the manic phase of manic-depressive psychosis is 25.____

A. amphetamine
B. imipramine
C. pargyline
D. reserpine
E. lithium

KEY (CORRECT ANSWERS)

1. E
2. E
3. A
4. E
5. E

6. A
7. E
8. D
9. C
10. D

11. D
12. C
13. D
14. D
15. B

16. B
17. B
18. C
19. A
20. E

21. B
22. B
23. C
24. B
25. E

TEST 2

DIRECTIONS: Each question or incomplete statement is followed by several suggested answers or completions. Select the one that BEST answers the question or completes the Statement. *PRINT THE LETTER OF THE CORRECT ANSWER IN THE SPACE AT THE RIGHT.*

1. When given together, the ability of two drugs to produce a response greater than either administered alone is termed 1.____

   A. synergism
   B. induction
   C. cumulation
   D. antagonism
   E. tachyphylaxis

2. Local anesthetics induce convulsions by effects on the 2.____
   I. cerebellum
   II. limbic system
   III. basal ganglia
   IV. cerebral cortex
   V. reticular activating system

   The CORRECT answer is:

   A. I, II, III B. I, V C. II, III, IV D. II, IV E. III, IV, V

3. Onset and duration of action of a drug is determined by its 3.____
   I. ability to cross membranes
   II. rate of liver metabolism
   III. degree of ionization at the urinary pH
   IV. route of administration
   V. affinity for the receptor site

   The CORRECT answer is:

   A. I, II, III, V B. I, IV C. II, III, IV D. III, IV, V
   E. all of the above

4. The adrenal steroids may be used to treat 4.____
   I. rheumatoid arthritis
   II. leukemia tuberculosis
   III. collagen diseases
   IV. Gushing disease

   The CORRECT answer is:

   A. I, II, III B. I, II, IV C. II, III, IV D. III, IV, V E. IV, V

5. The likelihood of adverse reactions to local anesthetics will be DECREASED by 5.____
   I. using an aspirating syringe
   II. injecting the anesthetic slowly
   III. taking a careful patient history
   IV. using less potent, less toxic local anesthetics
   V. limiting the amount of local anesthetics used

   The CORRECT answer is:

   A. I, II B. I, II, III C. I, II, IV D. IV, V
   E. all of the above

6. The various penicillins DIFFER in 6.____
   I. mechanism of action
   II. degree of oral absorption
   III. resistance to enzymatic degradation by penicillinase
   IV. antibacterial spectrum
   V. structural formula

   The CORRECT answer is:

   A. I, II, IV
   B. I, III, V
   C. II, III, IV
   D. II, III, IV, V
   E. III, IV, V

7. The ability of a given drug to pass through membranes is determined by the 7.____
   I. pka of the drug
   II. pH of the membrane surface
   III. lipid solubility of the drug
   IV. relative amounts of ATP in the membrane
   V. level of activity of pinocytosis in the membrane

   The CORRECT answer is:

   A. I, II
   B. I, II, III
   C. II, III, IV
   D. III, IV, V
   E. IV, V

8. Reserpine acts to 8.____
   I. block the passage of the nerve action potential in the postganglionic nerve fibers
   II. inhibit monoamine oxidase
   III. inhibit catechol-O-methyltransferase
   IV. deplete norepinephrine from the adrenergic neuron
   V. prevent re-uptake of norepinephrine by storage granules in the nerve terminal

   The CORRECT answer is:

   A. I, II
   B. I, II, III
   C. II, III, IV
   D. III, IV, V
   E. IV, V

9. Which of the following statements regarding anaphylaxis caused by drugs are TRUE? 9.____
   I. Administering drugs by the oral route diminishes the likelihood of anaphylaxis.
   II. Many, but not all, symptoms of anaphylaxis can be mimicked by injection of histamine.
   III. Anaphylaxis can appear within minutes after drug administration.
   IV. Immediate manifestations of anaphylaxis are effectively treated with epinephrine.
   V. Delayed manifestations of anaphylaxis are effectively treated with adrenal corticosteroids.

   The CORRECT answer is:

   A. I, II, III, IV
   B. I, II, IV
   C. I, III, V
   D. II, IV, V
   E. All of the above

10. Which of the following are contraindications to the use of oral contraceptives? 10.____

    I. History of thromboembolic disease
    II. Hyperthyroidism
    III. History of breast cancer
    IV. Peptic ulcer
    V. Undiagnosed genital bleeding

    The CORRECT answer is:

    A. I, II, III
    B. I, III, V
    C. I, IV
    D. II, III, IV
    E. III, IV, V

11. Which of the following drugs produce an effect comparable to stimulation of the parasympathetic nervous system? 11.____

    I. Pilocarpine
    II. Physostigmine
    III. Muscarine
    IV. Amphetamine
    V. Ergotamine

    The CORRECT answer is:

    A. I, II
    B. I, II, III
    C. II, IV, V
    D. III, IV, V
    E. IV, V

12. Which of the following statements are TRUE of the barbiturates? 12.____

    I. They suppress REM sleep.
    II. The cause of death in overdosage is respiratory depression.
    III. They are metabolized primarily in the liver.
    IV. In sedative doses, they are myocardial depressants.
    V. In sedative doses, they have significant alpha-adrenergic blocking effects.

    The CORRECT answer is:

    A. I, II, III
    B. I, III, V
    C. II, III, IV
    D. III, IV, V
    E. IV, V

13. Which of the following statements are TRUE regarding the generic form of a drug? 13.____

    I. A drug usually has more than one generic name.
    II. Prescribing a drug by its generic name allows the pharmacist to dispense any comparable brand name preparation.
    III. The generic preparation is generally less expensive than comparable brand name preparations.
    IV. A narcotic, by law, must be prescribed by its generic name.
    V. A generic preparation generally contains less of the pharmacologically active agent than comparable brand name preparations.

    The CORRECT answer is:

    A. I, II
    B. I, II, III, V
    C. II, III
    D. II, III, IV
    E. III, V

14. Which of the following are TRUE regarding the intravenous agent ketamine? It 14.____

    I. produces hypnosis and true anesthesia
    II. produces "dissociative anesthesia"
    III. may produce tonic and clonic convulsions
    IV. is now used primarily in children
    V. may produce delirium, hallucinations, and schizoid reactions

    The CORRECT answer is:

    A. I, II, III
    B. I, III, V
    C. I, IV, V
    D. II, III, IV, V
    E. II, V

15. Which of the following are *absolute* or *relative* contraindications to the use of morphine? 15.____

    I. Bronchial asthma
    II. Myocardial infarction
    III. Head injury
    IV. Patient history of drug abuse
    V. Chronic pain from terminal cancer

    The CORRECT answer is:

    A. I, II, III
    B. I, III, IV
    C. I, III, IV, V
    D. I, IV, V
    E. II, IV, V

16. Which of the following statements are TRUE regarding the cholinergic receptor? 16.____

    I. The muscarinic receptor is located in the effector organs which receive postganglionic parasympathetic fibers.
    II. No muscarinic receptors are found in the CNS.
    III. Muscarinic receptors are preferentially blocked by atropine.
    IV. Nicotinic receptors are located only at autonomic ganglia.
    V. The cholinergic receptor is closely related in structure to acetylcholinesterase.

    A. I, II, III
    B. I, III, V
    C. II, III, IV
    D. II, V
    E. III, IV, V

17. Which of the following drugs may cause miosis? 17.____

    I. Morphine
    II. Pilocarpine
    III. Physostigmine
    IV. Reserpine
    V. Phenoxybenzamine

    The CORRECT answer is:

    A. I *only*
    B. I, II, III
    C. II, III
    D. IV, V
    E. All of the above

18. Which of the following are TRUE regarding the effects of digitalis on congestive heart failure? It 18.___
    I. *decreases* heart rate through vagal and extravagal mechanisms
    II. *increases* the efficiency of the failing myocardium
    III. *increases* the force of myocardial contraction
    IV. *increases* residual diastolic volume
    V. *reduces* renal blood flow

    The CORRECT answer is:

    A. I, II, III
    B. I, IV
    C. II, III
    D. III, IV
    E. III, IV, V

19. Which of the following statements regarding drugs of abuse are TRUE? 19.___
    I. All act on the CNS to produce depression, stimulation or mood-alteration.
    II. All produce some degree of psychologic dependence.
    III. All produce some degree of physiologic dependence.
    IV. All produce drug disposition tolerance but not pharmacodynamic tolerance.
    V. None of the drugs of abuse possesses any therapeutic pharmacologic properties.

    The CORRECT answer is:

    A. I, II
    B. I, II, III
    C. I, IV, V
    D. II, III, IV
    E. II, IV, V

20. Which of the following are endogenous catecholamines? 20.___
    I. Epinephrine
    II. Isoproterenol
    III. Ephedrine
    IV. Phenylephrine
    V. Norepinephrine

    The CORRECT answer is:

    A. I, II, III, IV
    B. I, II, V
    C. I, V
    D. II, V
    E. IV, V

21. Which of the following are TRUE regarding pentazocine? 21.___
    I. Requires DEA registration to prescribe
    II. Prepared only as a parenteral analgesic
    III. Partial agonist of the opioid receptor
    IV. Equianalgesic with codeine
    V. May induce dysphoria and mental aberrations

    The CORRECT answer is:

    A. I, II, IV B. I, III, V C. I, V D. II, III, IV E. III, IV, V

22. Which of the following statements are TRUE regarding the barbiturates? They 22.____
    I. significantly elevate pain thresholds
    II. are metabolized by the liver
    III. are classified according to duration of action.
    IV. depress all levels of the CNS
    V. produce death by cardiovascular depression

The CORRECT answer is:

A. I, II, III
B. I, IV
C. II, III, IV
D. II, V
E. III, IV, V

23. Which of the following drugs possess additive depressant effects on the central nervous system when given with another depressant? 23.____
    I. Antianxiety drugs
    II. Alcohol Barbiturates
    III. Narcotics
    IV. Antipsychotics

The CORRECT answer is:

A. I, II, III, V
B. II, III
C. II, III, IV
D. IV, V
E. All of the above

24. Which of the following penicillins are readily INACTIVATED by stomach acids? 24.____
    I. Penicillin G
    II. Phenoxymethyl penicillin
    III. Methicillin
    IV. Ampicillin
    V. Cloxacillin

The CORRECT answer is:

A. I, II
B. I, III
C. II, IV
D. II, V
E. III, IV

25. Which of the following drugs are useful in the treatment of hypertension? 25.____
    I. Sodium chloride
    II. Ephedrine
    III. Thiazide diuretics
    IV. Reserpine
    V. Alpha-methyldopa

The CORRECT answer is:

A. I, II, III
B. I, III, V
C. II, III, IV
D. II, IV
E. III, IV, V

KEY (CORRECT ANSWERS)

1. A
2. D
3. E
4. B
5. E

6. D
7. B
8. E
9. E
10. B

11. B
12. A
13. C
14. D
15. B

16. B
17. E
18. A
19. A
20. C

21. E
22. C
23. E
24. B
25. E

PHARMACOLOGY

EXAMINATION SECTION
TEST 1

DIRECTIONS: Each question or incomplete statement is followed by several suggested answers or completions. Select the one that BEST answers the question or completes the statement. *PRINT THE LETTER OF THE CORRECT ANSWER IN THE SPACE AT THE RIGHT.*

1. Which of the following are often seen in patients receiving chemotherapy for cancer? 1.____
   I. Oral ulcerations
   II. Delayed wound healing
   III. Increased susceptibility to infection
   IV. Increased salivation
   V. Elevated white cell count

   The CORRECT answer is:

   A. I, II, III
   B. I, III, V
   C. II, III, IV
   D. II, IV
   E. III, IV, V

2. Therapeutic effectiveness of which of the following drugs will be DECREASED by concomitant ingestion of antacids? 2.____

   A. Penicillin V
   B. Cephalexin
   C. Tetracycline
   D. Erythromycin
   E. Sulfisoxazole

3. Which of the following barbiturates is useful in therapy of grand mal epilepsy? 3.____

   A. Thiopental
   B. Amobarbital
   C. Secobarbital
   D. Pentobarbital
   E. Phenobarbital

4. Which of the following anesthetics could be a fire hazard? 4.____

   A. Ether
   B. Halothane
   C. Nitrous oxide
   D. Methoxyflurane
   E. Xylocaine

5. Which of the following drugs is MOST frequently employed in the treatment of grand mal epilepsy? 5.____

   A. Diazepam
   B. Phenytoin
   C. Ethosuximide
   D. Methobarbital
   E. Trimethadione

6. Chlorpromazine belongs to which of the following groups of chemical compounds? 6.____

   A. Pyridine
   B. Quinoline
   C. Sulfonamide
   D. Catecholamine
   E. Phenothiazine

7. Inadequate function of which of the following organs would be *most likely* to INCREASE the toxicity of prilocaine? 7.____

A. Liver
B. Heart
C. Lung
D. Kidney
E. Spleen

8. Abuse of which of the following drugs produces the greatest physiological and psychological damage? 8.____

A. LSD
B. Cocaine
C. Alcohol
D. Marihuana
E. Barbiturate

9. Which of the following statements regarding local anesthesia is TRUE? 9.____

A. Onset and duration are independent of the tissue pH.
B. Recovery time is usually shorter than onset time.
C. The smaller the concentration, the shorter the latency of onset of action.
D. Degree and duration depend upon the intrinsic potency of the anesthetic.
E. The larger the nerve fiber, the shorter the onset and the greater the duration.

10. Which of the following is classified as an antianxiety drug? 10.____

A. Promazine
B. Haloperidol
C. Glutethimide
D. Ethchlorvynol
E. Chlordiazepoxide

11. Which of the following anesthetic agents is *most likely* to cause serious cardiac irregularities in the presence of epinephrine? 11.____

A. Ether
B. Halothane
C. Thiopental
D. Nitrous oxide
E. Pentothal

12. Which of the following drugs is a mild CNS stimulant useful in treating hyperkinetic children? 12.____

A. Caffeine
B. Doxapram
C. Nikethamide
D. Theophylline
E. Methylphenidate

13. If a patient exhibits signs and symptoms of angina pectoris, which of the following drugs acts MOST quickly to relieve this condition? 13.____

A. Morphine
B. Digitalis
C. Quinidine
D. Propranolol
E. Nitroglycerin

14. Which of the following penicillins has the BEST gram-negative spectrum? 14.____

A. Nafcillin
B. Ampicillin
C. Methicillin
D. Penicillin V
E. Phenethicillin

15. Administration of which of the following drugs would be contraindicated in patients with allergic bronchial asthma? 15.____

A. Atropine
B. Propranolol
C. Methacholine
D. Phentolamine
E. d-tubocurarine

16. Which of the following antibiotics is *most likely* to cause depression of the bone marrow? 16.____

A. Streptomycin
B. Penicillin G
C. Tetracycline
D. Chloramphenicol
E. Amphotericin B

17. Which of the following statements MOST accurately describes the effectiveness of action of alpha-methyldopa? It 17.____

A. causes marked cardiac slowing
B. directly relaxes vascular smooth muscle
C. causes rapid depletion of norepinephrine from adrenergic nerve terminals
D. causes formation of a false transmitter which is released at vascular smooth muscle
E. produces a false transmitter, the effect of which is primarily at central nuclei

18. Which of the following drugs would be useful in treating the dermatologic manifestations of an allergic response? 18.____

A. Diazepam
B. Atropine
C. Chlorpheniramine
D. Hexylresorcinol
E. Phenoxybenzamine

19. Which of the following drugs would provide the MOST IMMEDIATE relief for a patient suffering an attack of angina pectoris? 19.____

A. Digitalis
B. Phenytoin
C. Epinephrine
D. Glyceryl trinitrate
E. Isosorbide dinitrate

20. Which of the following drug groups is a classic *antagonist* for curare overdosage? 20.____

A. Anticholinesterases
B. Ganglionic stimulants
C. Ganglionic blocking agents
D. Alpha-adrenergic blocking agents
E. Adrenergic neuron blocking agents

21. Which of the following is an H_2 receptor antagonist? 21.____

A. Cimetidine
B. Promethazine
C. Tripelennamine
D. Diphenhydramine
E. Chlorpheniramine

22. Which of the following drug classes has been definitely established to be teratogenic in humans? 22.____

A. Salicylates
B. Barbiturates
C. Antianginals
D. Anticancer drugs
E. Local anesthetics

23. A drug with which of the following actions on the autonomic nervous system would be contraindicated in patients with glaucoma? 23.____

A. Nicotinic
B. Adrenergic
C. Cholinergic
D. Anticholinergic
E. Adrenergic blocking

24. Which of the following adverse effects is MOST commonly associated with administration of an intravenous barbiturate? 24.____

A. Hypotension
B. Renal failure
C. Hepatic necrosis
D. Nausea and vomiting
E. Respiratory depression

25. Which of the following classes of drugs undergoes the LEAST change in the body? 25.____

A. Alcohols
B. Barbiturates
C. Salicylates
D. Volatile anesthetics
E. Local anesthetics

KEY (CORRECT ANSWERS)

1.	A	11.	B
2.	C	12.	E
3.	E	13.	E
4.	A	14.	B
5.	B	15.	B
6.	E	16.	D
7.	A	17.	E
8.	C	18.	C
9.	D	19.	D
10.	E	20.	A

21. A
22. D
23. D
24. E
25. D

TEST 2

DIRECTIONS: Each question or incomplete statement is followed by several suggested answers or completions. Select the one that BEST answers the question or completes the statement. *PRINT THE LETTER OF THE CORRECT ANSWER IN THE SPACE AT THE RIGHT.*

1. Symptoms of atropine poisoning in man include 1.____
   I. decreased intraocular pressure
   II. burning, dry mouth
   III. nausea, vomiting and diarrhea
   IV. hyperthermia
   V. orthostatic hypotension

   The CORRECT answer is:

   A. I, III
   B. II, IV
   C. II, IV, V
   D. IV, V
   E. All of the above

2. Bioavailability of orally administered drugs may be influenced by the 2.____
   I. formulation of the drug
   II. gastrointestinal perfusion
   III. pH of the gastrointestinal tract
   IV. genetic phenotype
   V. presence of other substances in the gastrointestinal tract

   The CORRECT answer is:

   A. I *only*
   B. I, II, III, V
   C. II, III, V
   D. IV *only*
   E. I, II, III, IV, V

3. Which of the following statements are TRUE regarding onset, degree and duration of action of local anesthetics? 3.____
   I. The greater the drug concentration, the faster the onset and the greater the degree of effect.
   II. Local anesthetics block only myelinated nerve fibers at the nodes of Ranvier.
   III. The larger the diameter of the nerve fiber, the faster the onset of effect.
   IV. The faster the penetrance of the drug, the faster the onset of effect.

   The CORRECT answer is:

   A. I, II, III
   B. I, II, IV
   C. I, III
   D. II, III, IV
   E. I, II, III, IV, V

4. Which of the following are pharmacologic properties of antipsychotic drugs? They 4.____
   I. block the dopamine receptor
   II. affect the hypothalamic temperature regulation system
   III. cause emesis
   IV. are synergistic with LSD
   V. cause hypertension

   The CORRECT answer is:

   A. I, II
   B. I, II, III
   C. II, III, IV
   D. III, IV, V
   E. IV, V

5. Which of the following are TRUE regarding drug biotransformation? 5.___
   I. It primarily occurs in the liver microsomal enzyme system.
   II. It generally involves complex chemical processes.
   III. Its rate may be influenced by certain drugs.
   IV. It usually converts a drug to its lipid-soluble, ionized form.
   V. Its rate may differ significantly in various animal species.

   The CORRECT answer is:

   A. I, II, III
   B. I, III, V
   C. II, III, IV
   D. II, IV
   E. IV, V

6. Which of the following situations must prevail if pre-operative administration of vitamin K is to improve the clotting of blood? A 6.___
   I. low calcium level
   II. low prothrombin level
   III. low platelet count
   IV. normal flow of bile
   V. functioning liver

   The CORRECT answer is:

   A. I, II
   B. I, III
   C. I, IV
   D. II, III
   E. II, V

7. Which of the following local anesthetics would be expected to produce a sensitization reaction in a patient allergic to lidocaine? 7.___
   I. Mepivacaine
   II. Tetracaine
   III. Procaine
   IV. Prilocaine
   V. Dibucaine

   The CORRECT answer is:

   A. I, II, III
   B. I, IV, V
   C. II, III
   D. II, III, IV
   E. II, IV, V

8. In which of the following pairs of drugs is the pharmacologic activity of the first drug diminished or antagonized by the second drug? 8.___
   I. Histamine-epinephrine
   II. Penicillin-erythromycin
   III. Morphine-naloxone
   IV. Procaine-sulfanilamide
   V. Aspirin-phenylbutazone

   The CORRECT answer is:

   A. I, III, IV
   B. I, III, V
   C. II, IV
   D. III *only*
   E. IV *only*

9. Which of the following changes produced by intravenous administration of epinephrine result from stimulation of beta-adrenergic receptors? 9.____
   I. Respiratory inhibition
   II. Cardiac acceleration
   III. Dilation of the pupil
   IV. Increased systolic pressure
   V. Decreased diastolic pressure

   The CORRECT answer is:

   A. I, II, III
   B. I, II, IV
   C. II, V
   D. III, IV, V
   E. III, V

10. Which of the following regarding clindamycin are TRUE? It 10.____
    I. has a low incidence of diarrhea
    II. is well-absorbed orally
    III. is a broad-spectrum drug
    IV. is chemically similar to lincomycin
    V. suppresses protein synthesis

    The CORRECT answer is:

    A. I, II, III
    B. I, II, IV
    C. I, III, V
    D. II, IV, V
    E. III, IV, V

11. Which of the following occur when equilibrium conditions exist during administration of a gaseous anesthetic agent? 11.____
    I. There is no net transfer of anesthetic agent among tissues.
    II. The partial pressure of the gas at the site of action can be determined.
    III. The partial pressure of the gas is the same in all tissues.
    IV. The concentration of the anesthetic is the same in all tissues.
    V. There is no net transfer of anesthetic agent across the alveolar membrane.

    The CORRECT answer is:

    A. I, III, V
    B. I, IV
    C. I, V
    D. II, III
    E. All of the above

12. Which of the following regarding the cephalosporin antibiotics are TRUE? They 12.____
    I. are available for oral or parenteral administration
    II. may be cross-allergenic with penicillin
    III. may cause cholestatic hepatitis
    IV. have a gram-positive spectrum only
    V. have a mechanism of action similar to that of penicillin

    The CORRECT answer is:

    A. I, II, V
    B. I, IV, V
    C. II, III
    D. II, III, IV
    E. II, IV, V

13. A patient has no difficulty going to sleep at night, but awakens after a couple of hours and cannot get back to sleep. 13.____
Which of the following drug groups would be MOST appropriate to treat this condition?

A. Nitrous oxide
B. Phenothiazine compounds
C. Sympathomimetic agents
D. Tricyclic antidepressants
E. Benzodiazepine compounds

14. An excess of which of the following hormones may be associated with increased sensitivity to epinephrine? 14.____

A. Testosterone
B. Parathyroid
C. Insulin
D. Thyroid
E. Estrogen

15. Which of the following drugs is currently widely used in treating opioid-dependent individuals? 15.____

A. Codeine
B. Methadone
C. Alphaprodine
D. Pentazocine
E. Meperidine

16. A patient, without prior medication, breathes a gas mixture consisting of 50 percent nitrous oxide and 50 percent oxygen by volume. 16.____
Which of the following effects would be expected?

A. Analgesia
B. Excitation
C. Surgical anesthesia
D. Respiratory arrest
E. Damage to the brain from anoxia

17. Which of the following is TRUE of absorption from the stomach of weak acid drugs, such as salicylates? It 17.____

A. occurs most rapidly when the drugs are largely in unionized form
B. occurs most rapidly when the drugs are largely in ionized form
C. depends upon a specialized transport mechanism in the stomach
D. depends upon biotransformation in the stomach
E. is enhanced by rapid gastric emptying

18. Which of the following would be the BEST initial treatment for a person showing early signs of an anaphylactic response following a penicillin injection? 18.____

A. Intravenous cortisone
B. Sublingual isoproterenol
C. Subcutaneous epinephrine
D. Intravenous norepinephrine
E. Intravenous diphenhydramine

19. Which of the following cardiac depressants is contraindicated in a patient with cardiac arrhythmia? 19.____

A. Lidocaine
B. Quinidine
C. Phenytoin
D. Propranolol
E. Procainamide

20. Overdosage with certain steroids leads to manifestations of Cushing syndrome: hypertension, rounding of the face, hirsutism, glycosuria and sodium retention.
Which of the following steroids produces MOST of the above effects? 20.____

A. Estradiol
B. Testosterone
C. Prednisolone
D. Progesterone
E. Diethylstilbestrol

21. Abuse of which of the following drugs is associated with extreme violence and paranoid behavior? 21.____

A. LSD
B. Opioid
C. Alcohol
D. Cannabis
E. Amphetamine

22. The action of which of the following drugs will *most likely* be impaired by concurrent administration of tetracycline? 22.____

A. Chloramphenicol
B. Erythromycin
C. Sulfonamide
D. Penicillin
E. Lincomycin

23. Neuroleptanalgesia is *usually* attained by intravenous administration of 23.____

A. ketamine
B. chlorpromazine
C. droperidol and fentanyl
D. scopolamine and morphine
E. succinylcholine and thiopental

24. Which of the following barbiturates is useful in treating grand mal epilepsy? 24.____

A. Thiopental
B. Amobarbital
C. Secobarbital
D. Pentobarbital
E. Phenobarbital

25. Which of the following substances is the MOST effective agent against fungus infections of the mucous membrane? 25.____

A. Nystatin ointment
B. Undecylenic acid
C. Polymyxin ointment
D. Saturated magnesium sulfate
E. 10 percent aluminum chloride solution

KEY (CORRECT ANSWERS)

1. B
2. E
3. B
4. A
5. B
6. E
7. B
8. A
9. C
10. D
11. A
12. A
13. E
14. D
15. B
16. A
17. A
18. C
19. D
20. C
21. E
22. D
23. C
24. E
25. A

PHARMACOLOGY

EXAMINATION SECTION
TEST 1

DIRECTIONS: Each question or incomplete statement is followed by several suggested answers or completions. Select the one that BEST answers the question or completes the statement. *PRINT THE LETTER OF THE CORRECT ANSWER IN THE SPACE AT THE RIGHT.*

1. Of the following, drugs are INCAPABLE of 1.____

   A. inhibiting enzymes
   B. releasing stored chemicals
   C. altering neurohormone levels
   D. altering enzyme substrate levels
   E. initiating new cellular functions

2. When the combined action of two drugs is GREATER than the sum of their individual actions, this is 2.____

   A. induction
   B. synergism
   C. idiosyncrasy
   D. hypersensitivity
   E. cumulative action

3. Oxidized cellulose sponge aids in blood coagulation by 3.____

   A. producing vasoconstriction of the vessels
   B. aiding in the conversion of fibrinogen to fibrin
   C. increasing the amount of fibrinogen in circulating blood
   D. forming an artificial absorbable bridge for clot formation
   E. forming an artificial nonabsorbable bridge for clot formation

4. Following drug injection, a patient has difficulty breathing, loses consciousness and goes into general circulatory collapse. 4.____
   The MOST probable diagnosis is

   A. benign syncope
   B. angina pectoris
   C. coronary occlusion
   D. anaphylactic shock
   E. coronary thrombosis

5. A drug's usefulness as a therapeutic agent for man is MOST reliably assessed by 5.____

   A. determining the ratio of LD_5 to ED_{95}
   B. determining the dose at which adverse effects develop
   C. determining the dose that produces the desired therapeutic effect in man
   D. constructing a dose-response curve from the testing of a large population of animals
   E. relating the dose that produces adverse effects in man to the dose that produces the desired therapeutic effect

6. Amyl nitrate is MOST commonly administered 6.____

A. orally
B. sublingually
C. by inhalation
D. subcutaneously
E. intravenously

7. The outstanding advantage of phenytoin over phenobarbital in the treatment of grand mal epilepsy is that phenytoin 7.____

A. does not bring about addiction
B. needs to be given much less frequently
C. is effective in a greater percentage of cases
D. produces less sedation for a given degree of motor cortex depression
E. costs less

8. MOST diuretic drugs act *primarily* by 8.____

A. inhibiting the antidiuretic hormone
B. promoting renal chloride excretion
C. altering renal osmotic pressure balance
D. increasing glomerular filtration rate
E. retarding renal tubular sodium reabsorption

9. Mixtures of sulfonamides have an advantage over single sulfonamides in that mixtures 9.____

A. *decrease* renal toxicity
B. *increase* therapeutic effectiveness
C. *decrease* acetylation, plasma binding and acidity of the urine
D. convert usual bacteriostatic action to a bactericidal action
E. none of the above

10. The cause of death in poisoning from an irreversible anticholinesterase, such as diisopropylfluorophosphate, is 10.____

A. starvation, resulting from inability to swallow
B. dehydration, resulting from hypermotility of the gastrointestinal tract
C. pneumonia, resulting from excessive secretions of respiratory tract glands
D. respiratory failure, resulting from paralysis of the intercostals and the diaphragm
E. central nervous system depression, following prolonged excitation

11. The presence of a digitalis preparation in the current drug profile of a patient should alert the dentist to the possibility that this patient has 11.____

A. angina pectoris
B. atrial fibrillation
C. congestive heart failure
D. ventricular tachycardia
E. either B or C

12. The hydrolysis of procaine occurs *mainly* in the 12.____

A. liver
B. lungs
C. plasma
D. mucosa
E. kidneys

13. Succinylcholine acts to block neuromuscular transmission by 13.____

A. *inhibiting* cholinesterase
B. *inhibiting* the central nervous system
C. *depolarizing* the motor endplate of skeletal muscle
D. *inducing* the formation of cholinesterase at the endplate
E. *blocking* the release of acetylcholine at the endplate

14. Propylthiouracil is a drug used in the treatment of 14.____

A. cancer
B. hyperthyroidism
C. sodium retention
D. pheochromocytoma
E. allergic manifestations

15. Current evidence indicates that endorphins are 15.____

A. large polypeptides that regulate renal activity
B. endogenous molecules having morphine-like properties
C. central nervous system transmitters implicated in depressive psychoses
D. receptors located in the periaqueductal gray area of the brain which are sensitive to opiates
E. none of the above

16. The antianxiety drugs produce skeletal muscle relaxation by 16.____

A. depleting the neuron terminal of the mediator
B. blocking transmission at autonomic ganglia
C. depressing polysynaptic pathways in the spinal cord and higher centers
D. depressing conduction at the neuromuscular junction
E. none of the above

17. Drug-mediated inhibition of H_2-histamine receptors is MOST useful in treating 17.____

A. asthma
B. anaphylaxis
C. hypertension
D. gastric hyperacidity
E. localized allergic reactions

18. Of the following, diffusion hypoxia is *most likely* to occur with 18.____

A. ether
B. halothane
C. thiopental
D. enflurane
E. nitrous oxide

19. A drug that produces an antithrombin action in blood that is in part responsible for its anticoagulant effect is 19.____

A. heparin
B. vitamin K
C. dicumarol
D. folic acid
E. thromboplastin

20. The MOST recent data indicate that the *primary* mechanism of aspirin and other related anti-inflammatory analgesics is 20.____

A. a local anesthetic effect on peripheral nerve endings
B. inhibition of prostaglandin synthetase at the site of injury
C. prevention of histamine release from the mast cells at the site of injury
D. release of centrally active endorphins from the periaqueductal gray area of the brain
E. none of the above

21. The MOST commonly employed drugs in the treatment of simple anxiety states are the 21.____

A. benzodiazepines
B. phenothiazines
C. sedative-hypnotics
D. tricyclic antidepressants
E. monoamine oxidase inhibitors

22. Nonsteroidal anti-inflammatory agents have a tendency to produce 22.____

A. xerostomia
B. drowsiness
C. constipation
D. gastric irritation
E. metabolic alkalosis

23. During general anesthesia, the factor MOST responsible for the depth of anesthesia is 23.____

A. respiratory rate
B. oxygen concentration
C. drug concentration in the blood
D. drug concentration in inspired air
E. patient weight

24. A procaine-like local anesthetic theoretically could be LESS effective in acutely inflamed tissue because 24.____

A. high pH would inactivate the anesthetic too rapidly
B. high pH would decrease solubility of the anesthetic
C. extracellular fluid would dilute the anesthetic significantly
D. low pH would decrease available free base (transport form)
E. none of the above

25. Drug interaction in the periphery may be exemplified by the dimercaprol treatment of mercury poisoning. This interaction represents 25.____

A. chemical antagonism
B. physiologic antagonism *only*
C. pharmacologic antagonism *only*
D. physiologic and pharmacologic antagonisms
E. none of the above

KEY (CORRECT ANSWERS)

1. E
2. B
3. D
4. D
5. E
6. C
7. D
8. E
9. A
10. D
11. E
12. C
13. C
14. B
15. B
16. C
17. D
18. E
19. A
20. B
21. A
22. D
23. C
24. D
25. A

TEST 2

DIRECTIONS: Each question or incomplete statement is followed by several suggested answers or completions. Select the one that BEST answers the question or completes the statement. *PRINT THE LETTER OF THE CORRECT ANSWER IN THE SPACE AT THE RIGHT.*

1. The IMMEDIATE precursor of epinephrine is 1.____

   A. dopa
   B. tyrosine
   C. tyramine
   D. dopamine
   E. norepinephrine

2. Local anesthetics act on nerve membranes to 2.____

   A. displace Ca^{++}
   B. stimulate ATPase activity
   C. increase channel formation
   D. inhibit cyclic AMP activity
   E. increase membrane permeability

3. The LAST central nervous system function to disappear in general anesthesia is that of the 3.____

   A. medullary centers
   B. motor cortical areas
   C. spinal motor pathways
   D. spinal sensory pathways
   E. reticular activating system

4. Neostigmine produces its effect by 4.____

   A. depressing acetylcholinesterase release
   B. inhibiting acetylcholinesterase activity
   C. increasing the rate of acetylcholine synthesis
   D. acting like acetylcholine at cholinergic receptor sites
   E. increasing the amount of acetylcholine released from nerve terminals

5. The thiobarbiturates are characterized by 5.____

   A. a rapid onset and very short duration of action
   B. a rapid redistribution from the brain into body tissues
   C. a high percentage excreted as unchanged drugs
   D. all of the above
   E. A and B *only*

6. Carbidopa, a dopa-decarboxylase inhibitor, is often used in the treatment of parkinsonism because its 6.____

   A. central action potentiates the action of dopamine
   B. central action potentiates the action of norepinephrine
   C. peripheral action decreases the metabolism of levodopa
   D. peripheral action inhibits stimulatory fibers from the central nervous system
   E. none of the above

7. MOST toxic reactions to local anesthetics can be successfully treated by administering a(n) 7.____

A. corticosteroid
B. antihistamine
C. analeptic agent
D. anticonvulsant
E. none of the above

8. The MOST important drug in emergency treatment of anaphylaxis is 8.____

A. oxygen
B. naloxone
C. prednisone
D. epinephrine
E. tripelennamine

9. Salt retention, euphoria, androgenic effects and adrenal atrophy are *most likely* to be produced by 9.____

A. thyroxin
B. estrogen
C. progesterone
D. testosterone
E. hydrocortisone

10. One of the proposed mechanisms of the antihypertensive effect of B-adrenergic blockers is related to 10.____

A. sedation
B. an antirenin effect
C. a vagal blocking effect
D. a direct vasodilator action
E. an increase in cardiac output

11. Morphine causes vomiting by 11.____

A. a direct irritant action on the gastric mucosa
B. stimulation of the nodose ganglion of the vagus
C. stimulation of the medullary chemoreceptor trigger zone
D. direct stimulation of the gastrointestinal musculature
E. none of the above

12. The *primary* cause of death from overdosage with a central nervous system depressant is 12.____

A. cardiac arrest
B. autonomic blockade
C. respiratory depression
D. cardiovascular collapse
E. none of the above

13. A pharmacologic agonist is a chemical substance that 13.____

A. binds to a specific receptor and initiates a response
B. possesses the property of affinity but not intrinsic activity
C. elicits a pharmacologic response without binding to a receptor
D. exhibits no activity except to oppose the effect of an antagonist
E. none of the above

14. Administering diazepam is preferred to administering a barbiturate for emergency treatment of excessive stimulation of the central nervous system because diazepam 14.____

A. has anticonvulsive properties
B. has a shorter duration of action

C. can interrupt a seizure that is already in progress
D. is less likely to precipitate out of solution when administered intravenously
E. can produce equal protection against a seizure with less profound behavioral and cardiovascular depression

15. Current evidence indicates that the use of marihuana is associated with 15.____

A. physical deterioration
B. impairment of some skills, such as motor coordination
C. development of a marked degree of physical dependence
D. impairment of appetite leading to a decrease in caloric intake
E. serious adverse effects on peripheral nerves and the liver

16. Lidocaine produces its antiarrhythmic effects *primarily* by 16.____
I. *increasing* the refractory period of cardiac muscle
II. *increasing* cardiac conduction velocity
III. *decreasing* cardiac excitability
IV. *increasing* spontaneous pacemaker activity
V. *increasing* A-V conduction
The CORRECT answer is:

A. I, II, III
B. I, III
C. II, III, IV
D. II, V
E. III, IV, V

17. Digitalis glycoside preparations vary in 17.____
I. mechanism of action
II. route of administration
III. biologic half-life
IV. gastrointestinal absorption
V. toxic symptoms
The CORRECT answer is:

A. I, II, III
B. I, IV, V
C. II, III, IV
D. II, IV, V
E. All of the above

18. Pharmacologic effects of phenothiazines include 18.____
I. sedation
II. an antiemetic effect
III. a-adrenergic blockade
IV. potentiation of the action of narcotics
V. an antihistaminic effect
The CORRECT answer is:

A. I, II, IV
B. I, III, V
C. II, III, IV
D. III, IV, V
E. All of the above

19. Toxic effects of local anesthetics include 19.____
    I. CNS depression
    II. convulsions
    III. myocardial depression
    IV. allergic reactions

    The CORRECT answer is:

    A. I, II, III
    B. I, III
    C. II, IV
    D. IV *only*
    E. All of the above

20. General anesthetics are agents which can 20.____
    I. reduce perception of painful stimuli
    II. stimulate medullary centers
    III. produce a state of unconsciousness
    IV. decrease excitability of the motor cortex

    The CORRECT answer is:

    A. I, II, III
    B. I, II, IV
    C. I, III, IV
    D. II, III
    E. II, III, IV

21. The use of oral contraceptives has been associated with 21.____
    I. thrombophlebitis
    II. migraines
    III. nausea and vomiting
    IV. disturbances in liver function
    V. abnormal patterns of skin pigmentation

    The CORRECT answer is:

    A. I, II, III
    B. I, III, IV
    C. I, IV, V
    D. II, III, IV
    E. All of the above

22. Which of the following agents are active against fungi but NOT bacteria? 22.____
    I. Nystatin
    II. Neomycin
    III. Cephalothin
    IV. Griseofulvin
    V. Amphotericin B

    The CORRECT answer is:

    A. I, II, III
    B. I, II, V
    C. I, IV, V
    D. II, III, IV
    E. II, III, V

23. Which of the following are often seen in patients receiving chemotherapy for cancer? 23.____
    I. Oral ulcerations
    II. Delayed wound healing
    III. Increased susceptibility to infections
    IV. Increased salivation
    V. Elevated white cell count

    The CORRECT answer is:

A. I, II, III
B. I, III, V
C. II, III, IV
D. II, IV
E. III, IV, V

24. Which of the following are TRUE regarding the physical dependence associated with drug abuse? 24.____
   I. Characterized by abstinence or withdrawal syndrome
   II. Primarily associated with dependence on central nervous system depressant drugs
   III. Development unrelated to drug dosage and length of time of drug ingestion
   IV. Promotes drug-seeking behavior
   V. Constitutes a positive reinforcement to psychic dependence

   The CORRECT answer is:

   A. I, II, III
   B. I, II, IV, V
   C. I, IV
   D. II, III, IV
   E. III, IV, V

25. Allergic reactions and gastrointestinal upset may be seen as toxic effects with 25.____
   I. penicillin (G, V)
   II. erythromycins
   III. tetracyclines
   IV. ampicillin

   The CORRECT answer is:

   A. I, II, IV
   B. I, III
   C. II, III, IV
   D. III, IV
   E. All of the above

KEY (CORRECT ANSWERS)

1. E
2. A
3. A
4. B
5. E
6. C
7. E
8. D
9. E
10. B
11. C
12. C
13. A
14. E
15. B
16. B
17. C
18. E
19. E
20. C
21. E
22. C
23. A
24. B
25. E

PHARMACOLOGY

EXAMINATION SECTION
TEST 1

DIRECTIONS: Each question or incomplete statement is followed by several suggested answers or completions. Select the one that BEST answers the question or completes the statement. *PRINT THE LETTER OF THE CORRECT ANSWER IN THE SPACE AT THE RIGHT.*

1. According to the American Heart Association, the antibiotic to be used prophylactically for a penicillin-allergic patient with a replaced heart valve is 1.____

   A. vancomycin
   B. cephalexin
   C. penicillin V
   D. tetracycline
   E. clindamycin

2. A SUDDEN INCREASE in the blood level of drug A after the administration of drug B could result from 2.____

   A. binding of drug A by drug B
   B. chelation of drug A by drug B
   C. competition for the same receptor sites
   D. induction of hepatic microsomal enzymes
   E. displacement of drug A by drug B from protein-binding sites

3. The therapeutic index of a drug is the ratio of 3.____

   A. the effective dose to the toxic dose
   B. half the toxic dose to half the effective dose
   C. the maximum tolerated dose to the minimum effective dose
   D. the lethal dose for 50% of animals to the effective dose for 50% of animals
   E. none of the above

4. The appearance of a rash, itching, bronchoconstriction and fever some time after the administration of a drug is *most likely* the result of 4.____

   A. allergy
   B. tolerance
   C. idiosyncrasy
   D. teratogenicity
   E. cumulative effects

5. The MOST important therapeutic measure to be taken in a case of barbiturate poisoning is to 5.____

   A. alkalinize the urine
   B. aspirate stomach contents
   C. administer a CNS stimulant
   D. assure adequate respiration
   E. administer osmotic diuretics

6. The MOST important pharmacologic action of drugs that suppress cardiac arrhythmias is 6.____

   A. blockade of the vagus nerve
   B. stimulation of cardiac ATP-ase activity

C. blockade of the B-adrenergic receptor
D. stimulation of the a-adrenergic receptor
E. increased refractory period of cardiac muscle

7. If the pH of an area is LOWER than normal body pH, the membrane theory of local anesthetic action predicts that the local anesthetic activity would be 7.____

A. *greater,* owing to an increase in the free-base form of the drug
B. *greater,* owing to an increase in the cationic form of the drug
C. *less,* owing to an increase in the free-base form of the drug
D. *less,* owing to a decrease in the free-base form of the drug
E. none of the above

8. The sulfonamides act by 8.____

A. suppressing bacterial protein synthesis
B. inhibiting the formation of the cytoplasmic bacterial membrane
C. inducing the formation of "lethal" bacterial proteins
D. inducing a deficiency of folic acid by competition with p-aminobenzoic acid
E. all of the above

9. The MOST useful diuretic drugs act by 9.____

A. *increasing* the glomerular filtration rate
B. *decreasing* the renal reabsorption of sodium
C. *decreasing* the renal excretion of chloride
D. *increasing* the renal reabsorption of potassium
E. *increasing* the secretion of antidiuretic hormone

10. The outstanding advantage of phenytoin rather than pheno-barbital in the drug therapy of epilepsy is 10.____

A. fewer adverse side effects
B. less depression of bone marrow
C. less frequent dosage intervals
D. less sedative effects for a given degree of suppression of seizure activity
E. none of the above

11. One of the FIRST sensations usually lost after administration of a local anesthetic is 11.____

A. pain
B. touch
C. pressure
D. proprioception
E. thought

12. Administration of diazepam is preferred to administration of a barbiturate for emergency treatment of excessive CNS stimulation because diazepam 12.____

A. has anticonvulsive properties
B. has a shorter duration of action
C. is less likely to precipitate out of solution when administered intravenously
D. is the only agent that can interrupt a seizure that is already in progress
E. can produce equal protection against a seizure with less profound CNS depression

13. The action of the ultrashort-acting barbiturates is terminated *primarily* by the process of 13.____

A. oxidation
B. redistribution
C. renal excretion
D. plasma protein binding
E. conjugation with sulfate

14. Administration of angiotensin results in 14.____

A. anti-inflammatory effects
B. antihistaminic effects
C. increased blood pressure
D. increased heart rate
E. a sedative effect

15. Symptoms that may be characterized as allergic manifestations during penicillin therapy are 15.____

A. deafness, dizziness and acute anemia
B. crystalluria, nausea, vomiting and anaphylactic shock
C. oliguria, hematuria, bronchoconstriction and cardiovascular collapse
D. dermatitis, stomatitis, bronchoconstriction and cardiovascular collapse
E. none of the above

16. Biotransformation of epinephrine when administered to an intact animal occurs by 16.____

A. decarboxylation
B. conversion to acetylcholine
C. synthesis in part to norepinephrine
D. metabolism by dopamine B-hydroxylase
E. metabolism by monoamine oxidase and catechol-o-methyltransferase enzyme systems

17. Corticosteroids may be used to treat 17.____

A. asthma
B. arthritis
C. allergies
D. Addison's disease
E. any of the above

18. The MOST controllable route for administration of a general anesthetic is 18.____

A. rectal
B. inhalation
C. intramuscular
D. intravenous
E. subcutaneous

19. Morphine causes vomiting by 19.____

A. a direct irritant action on the gastric mucosa
B. stimulation of the nodose ganglion of the vagus nerve
C. stimulation of the medullary chemoreceptor trigger zone
D. direct stimulation of the gastrointestinal musculature
E. none of the above

20. Opioids have been shown to bind *specifically* with the receptor for 20.____

A. serotonin
B. histamine
C. enkephalIns
D. acetylcholine
E. y-aminobutyric acid

21. The *most likely* signs or symptoms of overdosage with atropine are 21.____

A. CNS excitation and tachycardia
B. intestinal cramps and diarrhea
C. skin rash and cutaneous itching
D. ptyalism and increased sweating
E. constriction of the pupils and blurring of vision

22. Bleeding from the oral mucosa can be REDUCED by topical use of 22.____

A. dicumarol
B. lidocaine
C. epinephrine
D. methacholine
E. hydrocortisone

23. The MOST commonly employed drugs in the treatment of simple anxiety states are the 23.____

A. benzodiazepines
B. phenothiazines
C. sedative-hypnotics
D. tricyclic antidepressants
E. monoamine oxidase inhibitors

24. Administration of succinylcholine to a patient deficient in serum cholinesterase would *most likely* result in 24.____

A. convulsions
B. hypertensions
C. prolonged apnea
D. acute asthmatic attack
E. myocardial infarction

25. A mechanism for the antiadrenergic action of guanethidine is 25.____

A. inhibition of dopa decarboxylase
B. increase rate of metabolism of norepinephrine
C. depletion of norepinephrine from the nerve terminals
D. substitution for norepinephrine and subsequent action as a false transmitter
E. uncoupling of the action potential from the norepinephrine release mechanism

KEY (CORRECT ANSWERS)

1. A
2. E
3. D
4. A
5. D

6. E
7. D
8. D
9. B
10. D

11. A
12. E
13. B
14. C
15. D

16. E
17. E
18. B
19. C
20. C

21. A
22. C
23. A
24. C
25. C

TEST 2

DIRECTIONS: Each question or incomplete statement is followed by several suggested answers or completions. Select the one that BEST answers the question or completes the statement. *PRINT THE LETTER OF THE CORRECT ANSWER IN THE SPACE AT THE RIGHT.*

1. The IMMEDIATE precursor of norepinephrine is 1.____

   A. dopa
   B. tyrosine
   C. tyramine
   D. dopamine
   E. epinephrine

2. If drug A has a GREATER efficacy than drug B, then drug A 2.____

   A. is more toxic than drug B
   B. has a greater affinity for the receptor than drug B
   C. has a greater margin of safety than drug B
   D. is capable of producing a greater maximum effect than drug B
   E. is stronger

3. A MAJOR secondary therapeutic use of the phenothiazines is as a(n) 3.____

   A. antiemetic
   B. antidepressant
   C. anticonvulsant
   D. antihypertensive
   E. CNS stimulant

4. Drug-mediated inhibition of H_2-histamine receptors is MOST useful in treating 4.____

   A. asthma
   B. anaphylaxis
   C. contact dermatitis
   D. gastric hyperacidity
   E. localized allergic reactions

5. The action of heparin may be antagonized by 5.____

   A. vitamin K
   B. menadione
   C. protamine sulfate
   D. ferrous sulfate
   E. E-aminocaproic acid

6. Carbidopa, a dopa-decarboxylase inhibitor, is often used in the treatment of parkinsonism because it 6.____

   A. *potentiates* the central action of dopamine
   B. *potentiates* the central action of norepinephrine
   C. *decreases* the peripheral metabolism of levodopa
   D. *inhibits* the peripheral stimulatory fibers from the central nervous system
   E. *increases* the permeability of the blood-brain barrier to levodopa

7. High plasma levels of local anesthetics may cause 7.____

   A. *inhibition* of peristalsis
   B. *stimulation* of baroreceptors resulting in severe hypotension
   C. *inhibition* of the vagus nerve to the heart

D. *depression* of inhibitory neurons in the CNS
E. heart failure

8. One of the proposed mechanisms of the antihypertensive effect of B-adrenergic receptor blocking agents is 8.____

A. sedation
B. a diuretic effect
C. an antirenin effect
D. a vagal blocking effect
E. an increase in cardiac output

9. Disulfiram is used in the treatment of 9.____

A. alcoholism
B. hypertension
C. agranulocytosis
D. petit mal epilepsy
E. generalized seizures of the tonic-clonic type

10. The antipyretic action of salicylates is explained in part by 10.____

A. analgesia leading to sedation
B. increased blood flow through the hypothalamus
C. cutaneous vasodilation leading to increased heat loss
D. depression of oxidative processes leading to decreased heat production
E. none of the above

11. Ethoheptazine is a chemical derivative of 11.____

A. morphine
B. methadone
C. codeine
D. papaverine
E. meperidine

12. The PRINCIPAL difference among potassium, procaine and benzathine salts of penicillin G is their 12.____

A. potency
B. toxicity
C. duration of action
D. antibacterial spectrum
E. diffusion into the cerebrospinal fluid

13. When neostigmine is administered before acetylcholine, the action of acetylcholine will be 13.____

A. blocked
B. enhanced and prolonged
C. less intense and of shorter duration
D. unaffected
E. none of the above

14. Tricyclic antidepressants have a prominent side effect that *most nearly* resembles the usual pharmacological action of 14.____

A. codeine
B. atropine
C. ephedrine
D. propranolol
E. methacholine

15. The concurrent administration of penicillin G and probenecid results in 15.____

A. *inereased* metabolism of penicillin G
B. *increased* renal excretion of probenecid
C. *decreased* renal excretion of penicillin G
D. *decreased* bactericidal effect of penicillin G
E. *increased* excretion of probenecid in the feces

16. Excretion of an acidic drug will be enhanced if the patient is given 16.____

A. sodium bicarbonate
B. ammonium chloride
C. sodium chloride
D. a high lipid diet
E. cholesterol oleate

17. Which of the following adverse effects is MOST commonly associated with administration of an intravenous barbiturate? 17.____

A. Hypotension
B. Renal failure
C. Hepatic necrosis
D. Nausea and vomiting
E. Respiratory depression

18. Which of the following forms of drug toxicity is associated with the halogenated hydrocarbon general anesthetics? 18.____

A. Liver damage
B. Myocardial atrophy
C. Peripheral neuritis
D. Severe hypertension
E. Coma

19. Which of the following is CONTRAINDICATED for a patient who had an allergic reaction to procaine six months ago? 19.____

A. Nerve block with lidocaine
B. Topical application of lidocaine
C. Topical application of tetracaine
D. Infiltration with an antihistamine
E. None of the above

20. A patient has been given a large volume of a certain local anesthetic solution and subsequently develops cyanosis with methemoglobinemia.
Which of the following drugs most *likely* was administered? 20.____

A. Procaine
B. Prilocaine
C. Dibucaine
D. Lidocaine
E. Mepivacaine

21. Which of the following is a local anesthetic subject to inactivation by plasma esterases? 21.____

A. Procaine
B. Lidocaine
C. Prilocaine
D. Mepivacaine
E. Bupivacaine

22. Which of the following B-adrenergic receptor blocking agents is thought to be cardioselective? 22.____

A. Nadolol
B. Timolol
C. Metoprolol
D. Propranolol
E. Chloramphenicol

23. The therapeutic effectiveness of which of the following drugs will be MOST affected by concomitant ingestion of antacids? 23.____

A. Cephalexin
B. Erythromycin
C. Tetracycline
D. Sulfisoxazole
E. Penicillin V

24. Which of the following barbiturates is useful in the therapy of generalized seizures of the tonic-clonic type? 24.____

A. Thiopental
B. Amobarbital
C. Secobarbital
D. Pentobarbital
E. Phenobarbital

25. Which of the following antihistamines is MOST commonly used as preoperative medication? 25.____

A. Meclizine
B. Cyclizine
C. Promethazine
D. Dimenhydrinate
E. Chlorpheniramine

KEY(CORRECT ANSWERS)

1. D
2. D
3. A
4. D
5. C
6. C
7. D
8. C
9. A
10. C
11. E
12. C
13. B
14. B
15. C
16. A
17. E
18. A
19. C
20. B
21. A
22. C
23. C
24. E
25. C

PHARMACOLOGY

EXAMINATION SECTION
TEST 1

DIRECTIONS: Each question or incomplete statement is followed by several suggested answers or completions. Select the one that BEST answers the question or completes the statement. *PRINT THE LETTER OF THE COERECT ANSWER IN THE SPACE AT THE RIGHT.*

1. Which of the following is a bactericidal antibiotic used specifically in the treatment of infections caused by Pseudomonas species and indole-positive Proteus species? 1.____

   A. Ampicillin B. Penicillin V C. Tetracycline
   D. Dicloxacillin E. Carbenicillin

2. Which of the following characterizes the mechanism of action of levodopa? It 2.____

   A. acts through a direct anticholinergic action
   B. stimulates specific L-dopa receptors in basal ganglia
   C. replenishes the otherwise deficient dopamine in patients with parkinsonism
   D. increases concentrations of norepinephrine in the brain to counterbalance an otherwise overactive cholinergic system
   E. none of the above

3. Three ml. of a local anesthetic solution consisting of 2% lidocaine with 1:100,000 epinephrine contains how many milligrams of each? ______ mg. lidocaine, ______ mg. epinephrine. 3.____

   A. 6; 0.3 B. 6; 0.03 C. 60; 0.3
   D. 60; 0.03 E. 600; 0.3

4. Inhaled ammonia acts against syncope by 4.____

   A. directly stimulating the vasomotor center
   B. directly stimulating the respiratory center
   C. releasing prostaglandins that modulate pain fibers
   D. stimulating sensory nerve endings of the nasal mucosa
   E. none of the above

5. Administration of a single 1 gm. dose of aspirin INSTEAD of the usual 650 mg. will increase 5.____

   A. bleeding time
   B. degree of analgesia
   C. anti-inflammatory response to the drug
   D. all of the above
   E. none of the above

6. Verapamil is MOST efficacious in the treatment of 6.____

   A. atrial fibrillation
   B. atrial tachycardia

C. ventricular tachycardia
D. ventricular extrasystoles
E. catecholamine-induced arrhythmias

7. The current drug of choice for treatment of the manic phase of manic-depressive psychosis is 7.____

A. lithium B. caffeine C. reserpine
D. imipramine E. amphetamine

8. The MOST useful drug to induce salivation is one which has properties that are 8.____

A. adrenergic B. cholinergic
C. ganglionic blocking D. adrenergic blocking
E. cholinergic blocking

9. Compared with the parent compound, biotransformation USUALLY results in drugs that are 9.____

A. more active B. more ionized
C. less ionized D. more lipid soluble
E. less water soluble

10. Chlortetracycline acts by interfering with 10.____

A. cell wall synthesis
B. nucleic acid synthesis
C. protein synthesis on bacterial but not mammalian ribosomes
D. protein synthesis on mammalian but not bacterial ribosomes
E. none of the above

11. Alpha- or beta-adrenergic blocking agents act by 11.____

A. inhibiting synthesis of norepinephrine
B. increasing metabolism of norepinephrine
C. competitive inhibition of postjunctional adrenergic receptors
D. a local anesthetic effect on adrenergic nerve terminals
E. depleting norepinephrine from adrenergic nerve terminals

12. Which of the following anesthetic drugs produces powerful stimulation of the cerebral cortex? 12.____

A. Cocaine B. Procaine C. Lidocaine
D. Tetracaine E. Mepivacaine

13. Which of the following is a FREQUENT side effect of anti-histamine therapy? 13.____

A. Anemia
B. Anuria
C. Diuresis
D. Drowsiness
E. Autonomic nervous system overactivity

14. Which of the following antihypertensive agents is MOST likely to cause an exaggerated response to an injected catecholamine? 14.____

A. Propranolol
B. Hydralazine
C. Guanethidine
D. A thiazide diuretic
E. All of the above

15. Tetracycline reduces the effectiveness of concomitantly administered penicillin by 15.____

A. reducing absorption of penicillin
B. increasing metabolism of penicillin
C. increasing renal excretion of penicillin
D. increasing binding of penicillin to serum proteins
E. none of the above

16. The rapidity of onset of anesthesia with an inhalation anesthetic agent is PRIMARILY related to its 16.____

A. molecular weight
B. degree of blood solubility
C. temperature in the gas phase
D. interaction with preoperative drugs
E. all of the above

17. Hepatic *first-pass* metabolism of drugs is MOST significant after which route of administration? 17.____

A. Oral
B. Rectal
C. Sublingual
D. Intravenous
E. Subcutaneous

18. The MOST serious consequence of systemic local anesthetic toxicity is 18.____

A. vertigo
B. hypertension
C. hyperventilation
D. postdepressive central nervous system convulsions
E. postconvulsive central nervous system depression

19. Local anesthetic drugs suitable for use as topical anes-thetic agents in dentistry include 19.____

A. procaine and lidocaine
B. benzocaine and procaine
C. benzocaine and lidocaine
D. benzocaine and mepivacaine
E. procaine and mepivacaine

20. The antipsychotic effects of phenothiazines result from 20.____

A. release of serotonin in the brain
B. release of norepinephrine in the brain
C. blockade of dopaminergic sites in the brain
D. an increase in the dopamine content of the cerebral cortex
E. prevention of the release of norepinephrine from brain neuron terminals

21. The PRIMARY action of therapeutic doses of digitalis on cardiac muscle is an increase in 21.____

A. force of contraction
B. ventricular excitability

C. refractory period of the atrial muscle
D. refractory period of the ventricular muscle
E. rate of conduction of impulses to the muscle

22. The maximum allowable adult dose of mepivacaine is 300 mg. How many milliliters of 2% mepivacaine should be injected to attain the maximal dosage in an adult patient? 22.____

A. 5 B. 10 C. 15 D. 20 E. 25

23. Oral contraceptives exert their PRIMARY effect by 23.____

A. blocking implantation
B. inhibiting ovulation
C. increasing LH secretion
D. inhibiting estrogen release
E. stimulating FSH release from the pituitary

24. Which of the following drugs produces *dissociative anesthesia* with little respiratory or cardiovascular depression? 24.____

A. Ketamine
B. Diazepam
C. Fentanyl
D. Pentazocine
E. Methohexital

25. Which of the following does NOT reduce skeletal muscle tone by an effect on the central nervous system? 25.____

A. Diazepam
B. Pancuronium
C. Meprobamate
D. Chlordiazepoxide
E. All of the above

KEY (CORRECT ANSWERS)

1. E
2. C
3. D
4. D
5. C
6. B
7. A
8. B
9. B
10. C
11. C
12. A
13. D
14. C
15. E
16. B
17. A
18. E
19. C
20. C
21. A
22. C
23. B
24. A
25. B

TEST 2

DIRECTIONS: Each question or incomplete statement is followed by several suggested answers or completions. Select the one that BEST answers the question or completes the statement. *PRINT THE LETTER OF THE CORRECT ANSWER IN THE SPACE AT THE RIGHT.*

1. Benzodiazepines produce their antianxiety effects by modulating which of the following neurohumors? 1.____

   A. GABA
   B. Glycine
   C. Dopamine
   D. Acetylcholine
   E. Norepinephrine

2. The agent of choice to reverse status epilepticus induced by local anesthetic overdose is 2.____

   A. oxygen
   B. diazepam
   C. epinephrine
   D. phenobarbital
   E. diphenhydramine

3. Which of the following is an IRREVERSIBLE side-effect resulting from long-term administration of phenothiazines? 3.____

   A. Sedation
   B. Xerostomia
   C. Infertility
   D. Parkinsonism
   E. Tardive dyskinesia

4. A pharmacologic agonist is a chemical substance that 4.____

   A. binds to a specific receptor and initiates a response
   B. elicits a pharmacologic response without binding to a receptor
   C. possesses the property of affinity but not of intrinsic activity
   D. exhibits no activity except to oppose the effect of an antagonist
   E. binds to any receptor but initiates no response

5. Digitalis is useful in the treatment of which of the following conditions? 5.____

   A. Atrial fibrillation
   B. Congestive heart failure
   C. Paroxysmal atrial tachycardia
   D. All of the above
   E. None of the above

6. Treatment with sulfonamides is LESS likely to be accompanied by crystalluria if 6.____

   A. a mixture of sulfonamides is used
   B. cortisone is administered concurrently
   C. probenecid is administered concurrently
   D. the urine is acidified with ammonium chloride
   E. para-aminosalicylic acid is administered concurrently

7. Which of the following is a complete antagonist of the opioid receptor and the agent of choice in the treatment of narcotic overdose? 7.____

   A. Naloxone
   B. Nalorphine
   C. Cyclazocine
   D. Levallorphan
   E. None of the above

8. Which of the following statements BEST describes the toxicity of most drugs? Toxicity 8.____

A. is unrelated to dose
B. is unpredictable and random
C. and therapeutic effect always arise from different mechanisms
D. is not produced by the average dose listed in the U.S. PHARMACOPEIA
E. is often an extension of the desired drug effect

9. Atropine and scopolamine exert their effects on peripheral structures by 9.____

A. preventing release of acetylcholine
B. preventing synthesis of acetylcholine
C. enhancing destruction of acetylcholine
D. competing with acetylcholine for receptor sites
E. producing physiologic effects opposite to those of acetylcholine

10. A patient, while not currently taking drugs, has a history (6 months ago) of narcotic dependence. 10.____
Which of the following analgesics should be avoided in this patient?

A. Aspirin
B. Pentazocine
C. Propoxyphene
D. Indomethacin
E. Acetaminophen

11. Which of the following exerts its MAJOR systemic pharmacologic action when administered orally? 11.____

A. Insulin
B. Procaine
C. Epinephrine
D. Streptomycin
E. Chloral hydrate

12. Which of the following penicillins has a broader gram-negative spectrum than penicillin G? 12.____

A. Nafcillin
B. Ampicillin
C. Cephalexin
D. Methicillin
E. Penicillin V

13. Which of the following are pathognomonic symptoms of narcotic overdose? 13.____

A. Miosis, coma, and depressed respiration
B. Mydriasis, coma, and smooth muscle spasms
C. Mydriasis, coma, and depressed respiration
D. Miosis, convulsions, and depressed respiration
E. Mydriasis, convulsions, and depressed respiration

14. Nitroglycerin dilates coronary arteries in angina pectoris by 14.____

A. decreasing the heart rate reflexly
B. blocking beta-adrenergic receptors
C. direct action on vascular smooth muscle
D. increasing metabolic work of the myocardium
E. increasing the effective refractory period in the atrium

15. Which of the following groups of antibiotics is related both structurally and by mode of action to the penicillins? 15.____

A. Polymyxins
B. Cycloserines
C. Cephalosporins
D. Chloramphenicols
E. None of the above

16. The sulfonylurea-type of oral hypoglycemic agent produces its effect by 16.____

A. promoting synthesis of insulin
B. preventing excretion of insulin
C. preventing metabolic breakdown of insulin
D. stimulating pancreatic secretion of insulin
E. increasing renal tubular threshold for glucose

17. Which of the following drugs is useful in treating dermatologic manifestations of an allergic response? 17.____

A. Diazepam
B. Atropine
C. Hexylresorcinol
D. Chlorpheniramine
E. Phenoxybenzamine

18. A substance used clinically and experimentally to decrease clotting tendency without alteration of prothrombin level is 18.____

A. heparin
B. vitamin K
C. protamine
D. purified thrombin
E. all of the above

19. Pretreatment with reserpine prevents a response to which of the following agents? 19.____

A. Amphetamine
B. Epinephrine
C. Phenylephrine
D. Isoproterenol
E. Norepinephrine

20. Administration of which of the following drugs increases the likelihood of a toxic response to digitalis? 20.____

A. Diazepam
B. Lidocaine
C. Spironolactone
D. Chlorothiazide
E. Acetylsalicylic acid

21. Which of the following drugs can cause both premature closure of the epiphysis of long bones in children and hirsutism in women? 21.____

A. Vitamin D
B. Dexamethasone
C. Growth hormone
D. Diethylstilbestrol
E. Methyltestosterone

22. A drug that produces sufficient central nervous system depression to cause a state of sleep from which one may be wakened by slapping, prodding, or pain is a(n) 22.____

A. hypnotic
B. analeptic
C. sialagogue
D. anticholinergic
E. sympathomimetic

23. A procaine-like local anesthetic theoretically should be less effective in acutely inflamed tissue than in normal tissue because, in inflamed tissue, 23.____

A. the high pH rapidly inactivates the anesthetic
B. the high pH decreases available free base
C. the low pH decreases available free base
D. the low pH increases available free base
E. extracellular fluid dilutes the anesthetic

24. Which of the following is NOT produced by excessive doses of acetylsalicylic acid? 24.____

A. Delirium
B. Tinnitus
C. Hypothermia
D. Hyperventilation
E. Metabolic acidosis

25. Of the following agents, ventricular fibrillation is LEAST likely to occur during anesthesia with 25.____

A. halothane
B. isoflurane
C. cyclopropane
D. nitrous oxide
E. any of the above

KEY (CORRECT ANSWERS)

1. A
2. B
3. E
4. A
5. D

6. A
7. A
8. E
9. D
10. B

11. E
12. B
13. A
14. C
15. C

16. D
17. D
18. A
19. A
20. D

21. E
22. A
23. C
24. C
25. D

TEST 3

DIRECTIONS: Each question or incomplete statement is followed by several suggested answers or completions. Select the one that BEST answers the question or completes the statement. *PRINT THE LETTER OF THE CORRECT ANSWER IN THE SPACE AT THE RIGHT.*

1. Interaction between penicillin and probenecid is BEST described by which of the following mechanisms? 1.____

   A. Acceleration of drug metabolism
   B. Competition at the receptor site
   C. Alteration in the acid-base balance
   D. Alteration in the rate of renal clearance
   E. None of the above

2. Which of the following is an endogenous catecholamine? 2.____

   A. Dopamine B. Ephedrine C. Amphetamine
   D. Isoproterenol E. Phenylephrine

3. Which of the following drugs acts to suppress the cough reflex? 3.____

   A. ASA B. Codeine C. Meperidine
   D. Acetaminophen E. Phenylbutazone

4. Administration of a ganglionic blocking agent results in 4.____

   A. miosis
   B. diarrhea
   C. copious salivation
   D. orthostatic hypotension
   E. enhanced activity of the parasympathetic nervous system

5. Which of the following erythromycins is associated with an allergic cholestatic hepatitis? 5.____

   A. Erythromycin base B. Erythromycin stearate
   C. Erythromycin estolate D. Erythromycin succinate
   E. All of the above

6. MOST drugs useful in the treatment of cardiac arrhythmias act primarily by 6.____

   A. blocking Purkinje fibers
   B. blocking the alpha-adrenergic receptor
   C. suppressing SA node impulse formation
   D. causing a positive inotropic effect
   E. increasing the refractory period of cardiac muscle

7. Neostigmine produces its effect by 7.____

   A. depressing acetylcholinesterase release
   B. inhibiting acetylcholinesterase activity
   C. increasing the rate of acetylcholine synthesis
   D. acting like acetylcholine at ganglionic sites
   E. increasing the amount of acetylcholine released from nerve terminals

8. Gastric acid secretion has been shown to be MOST effectively reduced with the use of 8.____

A. adrenal steroids
B. anticholinergic drugs
C. serotonin antagonists
D. H_1-histamine receptor antagonists
E. H_2-histamine receptor antagonists

9. The hydrolysis of procaine occurs MAINLY in the 9.____

A. liver
B. lungs
C. plasma
D. muscles
E. kidneys

10. Prominent toxic effects of mercury include 10.____

A. gingivitis
B. speech difficulties
C. visual disturbances
D. all of the above
E. none of the above

11. Speed of recovery from short-acting anesthesia with thiopental depends CHIEFLY on the rapidity of 11.____

A. renal tubular secretion
B. hepatic degradation of the thiol group
C. redistribution from the brain to skeletal muscle
D. reverse diffusion across the blood-brain barrier
E. none of the above

12. The majority of drugs penetrate biomembranes by 12.____

A. the process of exocytosis
B. passive diffusion through protein channels
C. passive diffusion through membrane protein
D. passive diffusion through membrane phospholipid
E. active transport through membrane phospholipid

13. The cause of death from acute barbiturate poisoning is 13.____

A. convulsions
B. liver damage
C. renal failure
D. respiratory failure
E. cardiovascular depression

14. Abuse of which of the following drugs causes extreme violence and paranoid psychotic behavior? 14.____

A. Opioids
B. Alcohol
C. Cannabis
D. Barbiturates
E. Amphetamines

15. Disorientation, confusion, and hallucinations resulting from an overdose of scopolamine are MOST efficaciously treated by administering 15.____

A. levodopa
B. dantrolene
C. neostigmine
D. physostigmine
E. glycopyrrolate

16. A drug with a high LD_{50} and a low ED_{50} has a 16.____

A. high therapeutic index and is, therefore, very dangerous
B. high therapeutic index and is, therefore, relatively safe
C. low therapeutic index and is, therefore, very dangerous
D. low therapeutic index and is, therefore, relatively safe
E. none of the above

17. When an attempt is made to distinguish between habituation and addiction, the GREATEST importance is usually given to the presence or absence of 17.____

A. harmfulness of the drug
B. psychic dependence on the drug
C. physical dependence on the drug
D. development of tolerance to the drug
E. acceptability of the drug in society

18. Administration of which of the following drugs is MOST likely to prolong clotting time? 18.____

A. Diazepam
B. Vitamin K
C. Secobarbital
D. Acetaminophen
E. Acetylsalicylic acid

19. Local anesthetics block nerve conduction by 19.____

A. depolarizing the nerve membrane to neutrality
B. increasing membrane permeability to K^+
C. increasing membrane permeability to Na^+
D. preventing an increase in membrane permeability to K^+
E. preventing an increase in membrane permeability to Na^+

20. Administration of angiotensin results in 20.____

A. a sedative effect
B. increased heart rate
C. increased blood pressure
D. antihistaminic effects
E. anti-inflammatory effects

21. Which of the following antihypertensives are USUALLY reserved for treatment of severe hypertension? 21.____

A. Sedatives and reserpine
B. Thiazide diuretics and reserpine
C. Sedatives and thiazide diuretics
D. Guanethidine and ganglionic blocking agents
E. Guanethidine and reserpine

22. When broad-spectrum antibiotics are administered with coumarin anticoagulants, the anticoagulant action may be 22.____

A. reduced because of enhanced hepatic drug metabolism
B. reduced because of increased protein-binding
C. reduced because of reduction of vitamin K sources

D. increased because of reduction of vitamin K sources
E. increased because of decreased renal excretion of the anticoagulant

23. Of the following side-effects, which is COMMON to many antihypertensive drugs? 23.____

A. Constipation
B. Renal insufficiency
C. Orthostatic hypotension
D. Decreased prothrombin time
E. All of the above

24. Which of the following may be useful as an infiltrative local anesthetic in a patient allergic to both amide and ester anesthetic derivatives? 24.____

A. Bupivacaine
B. Phenylephrine
C. Nitrous oxide
D. Diphenhydramine
E. Ethylaminobenzoate

25. The presence of which of the following conditions is NOT a contraindication to the use of corticosteroids? 25.____

A. Peptic ulcer
B. Herpes simplex
C. Aphthous ulcer
D. Latent tuberculosis
E. None of the above

KEY (CORRECT ANSWERS)

1. D
2. A
3. B
4. D
5. C

6. E
7. B
8. E
9. C
10. D

11. C
12. D
13. D
14. E
15. D

16. B
17. C
18. E
19. E
20. C

21. D
22. D
23. C
24. D
25. C

TEST 4

DIRECTIONS: Each question or incomplete statement is followed by several suggested answers or completions. Select the one that BEST answers the question or completes the statement. *PRINT THE LETTER OF THE CORRECT ANSWER IN THE SPACE AT THE RIGHT.*

1. How many international units are in 125 mg. of penicillin G? 1.____

   A. 100,000
   B. 200,000
   C. 300,000
   D. 400,000
   E. 500,000

2. Signs and stages of anesthesia are MOST likely to be seen with a general anesthetic that has a 2.____

   A. low potency
   B. slow rate of induction
   C. low Ostwald coefficient
   D. high oil-water solubility coefficient
   E. high tissue-blood partition coefficient

3. A paralyzing dose of succinylcholine INITIALLY elicits 3.____

   A. CNS depression
   B. CNS stimulation
   C. decreased salivation
   D. muscle fasciculation
   E. extrapyramidal reactions

4. The disulfiram reaction produces a number of toxic symptoms that are caused by accumulation of 4.____

   A. acetic acid
   B. formic acid
   C. formaldehyde
   D. acetaldehyde
   E. glutaraldehyde

5. Which of the following drugs is often used successfully to treat trigeminal neuralgia? 5.____

   A. Clonazepam
   B. Carbamazepine
   C. Acetazolamide
   D. Carbamylcholine (carbachol)
   E. All of the above

6. Diazepam is preferred to a barbiturate as an antianxiety agent because diazepam 6.____

   A. produces no sedation
   B. has less addiction potential
   C. is a very short-acting drug
   D. is substantially less expensive
   E. does not potentiate the action of CNS depressants

7. Two drugs, A and B, have the same mechanism of action. Drug A in a dose of 5 mg. produces the same magnitude of response as drug B in a dose of 500 mg. Which of the following statements is CORRECT? Drug 7.____

   A. A is less toxic
   B. A is more efficacious

C. A is 100 times as potent
D. A has a shorter duration of action
E. A is a better drug to use when a maximal response is desired

8. Specificity of a drug is MOST commonly accomplished by altering 8.____

A. dose
B. dosage regimen
C. molecular structure
D. route of administration
E. any of the above

9. Administration of an otherwise effective pressor dose of epinephrine could cause an *epinephrine reversal* in a patient taking which of the following drugs? 9.____

A. Reserpine
B. Propranolol
C. Amphetamine
D. Chlorpromazine
E. Lithium carbonate

10. The behavior of patients under general anesthesia suggests that the MOST resistant part of the central nervous system is the 10.____

A. spinal cord
B. medulla oblongata
C. cerebral cortex (motor area)
D. cerebral cortex (sensory area)
E. none of the above

11. A 14-year-old girl with a history of absence epilepsy is being treated with sodium valproate.
During dental prophylaxis, this patient is LIKELY to exhibit 11.____

A. xerostomia
B. fetid breath
C. furred tongue
D. gingival hyperplasia
E. spontaneous gingival bleeding

12. Which of the following situations MUST prevail if pre-operative administration of vitamin K is to improve the clotting of blood? 12.____
A

I. low calcium level
II. low prothrombin level
III. low platelet count
IV. normal flow of bile
V. functioning liver

The CORRECT answer is:

A. I, II
B. I, III
C. I, IV
D. II, III
E. II, V

13. Which of the following are pharmacologic effects of morphine? 13.____

    I. Respiratory depression
    II. Euphoria
    III. Sedation
    IV. Constipation
    V. Dysphoria

    The CORRECT answer is:

    A. I, II, III
    B. I, II, IV
    C. I, V
    D. III, IV, V
    E. All of the above

14. Which of the following does NOT result from prolonged treatment with adrenal steroids? 14.____

    A. Gastric ulcer
    B. Osteoporosis
    C. Hyperglycemia
    D. Myocardial atrophy
    E. Redistribution of body fat

15. Which of the following pharmacologic actions is NOT produced by prostaglandins? 15.____

    A. Pyrexia
    B. Uterine contraction
    C. Increased gastric acid secretion
    D. Increased capillary permeability
    E. Pain when injected intradermally

16. Which of the following antibiotics is LEAST effective against penicillinase-producing microorganisms? 16.____

    A. Ampicillin
    B. Cephalexin
    C. Methicillin
    D. Clindamycin
    E. Erythromycin

17. Which of the following anti-inflammatory agents does NOT act primarily by inhibiting activity of prostaglandin synthetase? 17.____

    A. Diflunisal
    B. Ibuprofen
    C. Triamcinolone
    D. Oxyphenbutazone
    E. Acetylsalicylic acid

18. Which of the following is NOT a criterion for inclusion of a drug in one of the five schedules specified by the Controlled Substances Act of 1970? 18.____

    A. Relative potency
    B. Medical usefulness
    C. Potential for abuse
    D. Degree to which it produces psychological dependence
    E. Degree to which it produces physical dependence

19. Which of the following is NOT a characteristic side-effect of cancer chemotherapeutic agents? 19.____

    A. Loss of hair
    B. Increased blood pressure
    C. Gastrointestinal disturbance

D. Involution of lymphatic tissues
E. Increased incidence of infection

20. Which of the following is NOT an important consideration in selecting an analgesic agent for a patient? 20.____

A. Type of pain
B. Age of the patient
C. Potency of the drug
D. Concurrent medication
E. None of the above

21. Which of the following is NOT an action of epinephrine, when administered intravenously in a high dose? 21.____

A. Increases liver glycogenolysis
B. Causes bronchiolar constriction
C. Produces a rise in blood pressure
D. Evokes extrasystoles in the heart
E. Produces restlessness and anxiety

22. Which of the following prescriptions CANNOT be repeated without written authority? 22.____

A. ASA, 300 mg.
B. Diazepam, 10 mg.
C. Chloral hydrate, 500 mg.
D. Codeine phosphate, 30 mg.
E. ASA, 300 mg., with caffeine, 30 mg., and codeine, 30 mg.

23. In man, which of the following responses is NOT caused by histamine? 23.____

A. Bronchodilation
B. Dilation of arterioles
C. Intestinal constriction
D. Stimulation of gastric secretion
E. Increased capillary permeability

24. Which of the following does NOT delay metabolic transformation of a drug? 24.____

A. Tachyphylaxis
B. Liver disease
C. Storage in tissues
D. Extensive protein binding
E. Presence of other drugs that inhibit metabolism of the first drug

25. Which of the following is NOT characteristic of barbiturates? 25.____

A. Possess anticonvulsant properties
B. Possess significant analgesic properties
C. Possess serious drug dependence potential
D. Vary in degree of lipid solubility and hypnotic potency
E. All of the above

KEY (CORRECT ANSWERS)

1. B
2. B
3. D
4. D
5. B
6. B
7. C
8. C
9. D
10. B
11. E
12. E
13. E
14. D
15. C
16. A
17. C
18. A
19. B
20. C
21. B
22. D
23. A
24. A
25. B

CLINICAL CHEMISTRY

EXAMINATION SECTION
TEST 1

DIRECTIONS: Each question or incomplete statement is followed by several suggested answers or completions. Select the one that *BEST* answers the question or completes the statement. *PRINT THE LETTER OF THE CORRECT ANSWER IN THE SPACE AT THE RIGHT.*

1. *Which one* of the following solutions has the *LOWEST* pH above neutrality? 1.____

   A. Sodium bicarbonate
   B. 1N sodium hydroxide
   C. Potassium hydroxide
   D. 1N sodium carbonate

2. *Which* substance is miscible with water? 2.____

   A. Toluene
   B. Alcohol
   C. Chloroform
   D. Immersion oil

3. Assume that a urine sample was measured with a hydrometer, and the value was found to be 1.036. Of the following, the *MOST* likely explanation is that the urine sample 3.____

   A. was taken over a 24-hour period
   B. contained too many dissolved substances
   C. contained erythrocytes
   D. was too dilute

4. Thirty-seven degrees centigrade *MOST* closely approximates *which one* of the following temperatures? 4.____

   A. Temperature at which water freezes
   B. Temperature at which water boils
   C. Normal refrigerator temperature
   D. Normal body temperature

5. The weight of the container or paper used on a balance to hold the specimen is called 5.____

   A. zero weight
   B. adjustable weight
   C. tare weight
   D. vernier weight

6. An osmometer is an instrument used to measure 6.____

   A. osmosis
   B. osmolality
   C. osmotic pressure
   D. osmoles

7. *Which one* of the following methods is *MOST* appropriate for the quantitative measurement of triglyceride? 7.____

   A. Electrophoresis
   B. Gas chromatography
   C. UV spectrophotometry
   D. Atomic absorption

8. When not in immediate use, the electrodes of a pH meter should be 8.____

   A. stored in a refrigerator
   B. kept immersed in distilled water

C. kept immersed in normal saline
D. dried and the fluid emptied from inside the electrode

9. The normal pH of blood is about 7.4. This means that blood is 9.____

A. strongly acidic
B. very slightly acidic
C. strongly alkaline
D. very slightly alkaline

10. Bile is secreted by the 10.____

A. small intestine
B. pancreas
C. gallbladder
D. liver

11. *Which one* of the following solutions has the *LOWEST* pH? 11.____

A. 1N hydrochloric acid
B. 1N acetic acid
C. 1N ammonium hydroxide
D. 1N sodium hydroxide

12. *What* is the molecular weight of oxygen? 12.____

A. 1 B. 8 C. 16 D. 40

13. *Which one* of the following chemicals is *NOT* flammable, and can be used if there is a burning flame in the room? 13.____

A. Amyl alcohol
B. Potassium hydroxide
C. Benzene
D. Xylene

14. If 17.3 gms of copper sulfate are required to make one liter of a solution, *how much* copper sulfate would be needed to make 350 ml of solution? 14.____

A. 1.73 gms B. 6.06 gms C. 17.3 gms D. 35.0 gms

15. A biological substance that increases the rate of a chemical reaction is a(n) 15.____

A. solvent B. antigen C. enzyme D. buffer

16. *Which one* of the following is *NOT* a carbohydrate? 16.____

A. Starch B. Glucose C. Glycine D. Galactose

17. Electrophoresis measures the 17.____

A. migration of proteins
B. ionic strength of a solution
C. solubility product
D. voltage of a solution

18. The purpose of the photocell in a flame photometer is to 18.____

A. remove dust particles
B. filter out the proteins
C. convert light energy to electrical energy
D. multiply the electrical signal

19. Titration of an acid with a base yields a(n) 19.____

A. acid B. alcohol C. base D. salt

20. *What* is the pH of the commonly used buffer, phosphate buffered saline? 20.____

A. 6.5 B. 7.4 C. 8.3 D. 9.2

21. A potential explosive chemical which is used in clinical chemistry is 21.____

A. nitric acid
B. picric acid
C. potassium nitrate
D. sodium nitrate

22. In using an Autoanalyzer, the *PRIMARY* reason for dialysis is to 22.____

A. prevent coagulation
B. prepare a clear solution
C. remove salt
D. remove protein

23. Of the following materials that are commonly added to whole blood, *which one* will have the *LEAST* effect on a calcium assay? 23.____

A. Heparin B. EDTA C. Oxalate D. Fluoride

24. Isotonic saline is 24.____

A. 0.1% NaCl
B. 0.9% NaCl
C. 5% NaCl
D. 9% NaCl

25. *Which* element is used as an internal standard in clinical chemistry? 25.____

A. La B. I^{125} C. Sr D. Li

KEY (CORRECT ANSWERS)

1. A
2. B
3. B
4. D
5. C
6. B
7. C
8. B
9. D
10. D
11. A
12. C
13. B
14. B
15. C
16. C
17. A
18. C
19. D
20. B
21. B
22. D
23. A
24. B
25. D

TEST 2

DIRECTIONS: Each question or incomplete statement is followed by several suggested answers or completions. Select the one that *BEST* answers the question or completes the statement. *PRINT THE LETTER OF THE CORRECT ANSWER IN THE SPACE AT THE RIGHT.*

1. In using micropipettes, the *usual* source of measurement error is caused by 1.____

   A. dirt
   B. hanging drops
   C. poor tips
   D. contamination

2. Enzymes are reported in 2.____

   A. pH units
   B. concentration units
   C. mg/dl units
   D. activity units

3. Assume that a beaker contains 700 ml. of 0.3M NaOH. *HOW much* of a 10M NaOH solution must be added to the solution in the beaker to bring it to 0.5M NaOH? 3.____

   A. 7 ml
   B. 10 ml
   C. 14 ml
   D. 30 ml

4. If one dissolves 25 gms of a solid in a liter, *how much* is present in 100 microliters? 4.____

   A. 2.5 mgms
   B. 25 mgms
   C. 250 micrograms
   D. 250 nanograms

5. Cholesterol does *NOT* exist in the form of a(n) 5.____

   A. hormone
   B. alcohol
   C. steroid
   D. fat

6. Amylase is an enzyme that acts on starch to produce 6.____

   A. alcohol
   B. sucrose
   C. amyloid
   D. glucose

7. *Which* is *NOT* an electrolyte? 7.____

   A. Phosphate
   B. Urea nitrogen
   C. Calcium
   D. icarbonate

8. The protein component found in the greatest concentration in normal human serum is 8.____

   A. hemoglobin
   B. globulia
   C. fibrinogen
   D. albumin

9. *Which one* cannot be used as a substrate for alkaline phosphatase? 9.____

   A. Sodium phosphate
   B. Phenyl phosphate
   C. δ-napthyl phosphate
   D. p-nitrophnyl phosphate

10. Insulin is secreted by the 10.____

    A. pancreas
    B. liver
    C. thyroid
    D. spleen

11. *Which* of the following is *NOT either* a product *or* a reactant in a SGOT assay? 11.____

    A. Alanine
    B. δ-Ketoglutaric acid
    C. Glutamic acid
    D. Oxalocetic acid

12. *Which one* of the following is *MOST* alkaline? 12.____

A. 1N ammonia hydroxide
B. 1N sodium bicarbonate
C. 1N sodium carbonate
D. 1N sodium hydroxide

13. How many more hydrogen ions does a solution of pH3 have compared to a solution of pH5? ______ as many. 13.____

A. One hundred times
B. Two times
C. 1.67 times
D. 1.33 times

14. *Which one* of the following statements *BEST* describes the pH of distilled water? Freshly distilled water is 14.____

A. slightly alkaline because of the CO_2 dissolved in it
B. slightly acid because of the CO_2 dissolved in it
C. neutral
D. neither acid, alkaline, nor neutral

15. The *MOST* effective buffer consists of a 15.____

A. strong acid and a strong base
B. weak acid and a weak base
C. mixture of two salts
D. strong acid and its salt

16. A double beam colorimeter is *better* than a single beam colorimeter because 16.____

A. two measurements can be made at the same time
B. corrections for non-specific absorbances can be done
C. two substances can be determined at the same time
D. corrections for light intensity fluctuations can be made

17. The *advantage* of a bichromatic colorimeter over a monochromatic colorimeter is that 17.____

A. two measurements can be made at the same time
B. corrections for non-specific absorbances can be done
C. two substances can be determined at the same time
D. corrections for light intensity fluctuations can be made

18. If one thickness of a neutral density filter reduces the transmitted light by 50%, *how much* will two thicknesses of the same filter reduce the transmitted light? 18.____

A. 25%
B. 50%
C. 75%
D. 100%

19. If all the controls in the day's run for the assay of glucose come out proportionately high, *which* of the following would *MOST* likely be the cause? A 19.____

A. systematic error due to elevated room temperature
B. random error due to faulty pipetting
C. systematic error due to deterioration of the standards
D. systematic error due to the colorimeter not being set properly

20. *Why* is it important to have *GREATER* precision in sodium assay than for a glucose assay? 20.____

A. Sodium is a more important clinical component.
B. There is more sodium in the body.
C. There is more glucose in the body.
D. There is less percentage variation in the normal range of sodium.

21. *Which* of the following components is *NOT* found in the usual chart recorder? 21.____

A. Pen driver
B. Amplifier
C. Cathode ray
D. Chant driver

22. CPK is an enzyme *MAINLY* found in the 22.____

A. serum B. pancreas C. liver D. muscle

23. The *MOST* effective method of preserving a serum specimen for acid phosphatase assay is to 23.____

A. refrigerate it
B. add one drop of 10% Na Citrate per 2 ml
C. add 50 mg NaF per 2 ml
D. add one drop of 5% Thymol per 2 ml

24. Bilirubin is a 24.____

A. hemoglobin metabolite
B. steroid
C. bile salt
D. digestive by-product

25. Thyroxine is a 25.____

A. hormone B. steroid C. lipid D. protein

KEY (CORRECT ANSWERS)

1. B
2. D
3. C
4. A
5. A
6. D
7. B
8. D
9. A
10. A
11. A
12. C
13. A
14. C
15. B
16. D
17. B
18. C
19. C
20. D
21. C
22. D
23. B
24. A
25. A

DRUG LAWS OF THE UNITED STATES

CONTENTS

DRUG LAWS OF THE UNITED STATES

1. **Laws governing pharmacy.** There are Federal laws pertaining to pharmacy which must be followed by everyone practicing pharmacy who is associated with the U.S. Government. There are also State laws which pertain to the practice of pharmacy in a particular state. Any State law may be more stringent or strict than the Federal law, but it may not be less so. The practice of Army pharmacy is also governed by Army Regulations such as AR 40-2, AR 40-4, AR 40-7, AR 40-18, and AR 40-61. In the Army, we must abide by the Federal pharmacy laws and Army Regulations, but we do not have to abide by the State laws. It is a matter of local policy whether a particular installation will also abide by the pharmacy laws of the state in which the installation is located.

2. **The Federal Food, Drug, and Cosmetic Act.** The Federal Food, Drug, and Cosmetic Act first became law in 1906, followed by revision, amendment, and final emergence as our present law in 1965. This act is intended to protect the consumer from adulterated and misbranded food, drugs, devices, and cosmetics, and for other purposes. It directly prohibits adulterated or misbranded items from movement across state lines (interstate commerce).

a. Adulterated drugs. By provision of the Federal Food, Drug, and Cosmetic Act, a drug or device is construed as being adulterated under the following conditions if:

(1) It contains any filthy, putrid, or decomposed substance, or is packed under conditions which would result in its contamination; if it is a drug and its container is composed of any poisonous or injurious substance which could be passed on to the contents; or if it contains a coal tar color not certified by regulations.

(2) It is said or advertised to be a drug of official nature and differs from or is not the same quality as the official standard.

(3) Its strength differs from or the purity and quality fall below that indicated on the label.

(4) It is a drug and any other drug has been substituted for it or mixed with it to reduce its quality or strength.

b. Misbranded drugs. A drug or device is misbranded if–

(1) The labeling is not truthful or is misleading.

(2) It is in a package and does not contain the name and address of the manufacturer, packager, or distributor, and an accurate statement of the weight, measure, or numerical count of the contents.

(3) Any word or information required by the Act to appear on the label is not prominently placed (in comparison with the rest of the label) so that it is likely to be read and understood by ordinary individuals.

(4) It is intended for human use and contains any quantity of a substance which is habit-forming, unless the label shows the name and quantity of that substance and adjacent to it, the statement "Warning: May be habit-forming."

(5) It is a drug and is not labeled by a name official in our compendia (USP and NF), unless it bears the common name, if one exists; and if it is made of two or more ingredients, the common or usual name of each active ingredient.

(6) It is a drug of one or more active ingredients and the name, quantity, and proportion of any alcohol contained is not specified on the label.

(7) It is a drug and the label does not specify the name and quantity or proportion of any bromides, ether, chloroform, acetanilid, acetophenetidin, aminopyrine, antipyrine, atropine, hyoscine, hyoscyamus, arsenic, digitalis, digitalis glucosides, mercury, ouabain, strophanthin, strychnine, thyroid, or any derivative or preparation of any such substances. If compliance with this item or items *(5)* and *(6)* above is impracticable, exemptions may be established by regulation.

(8) The labeling does not bear adequate directions for use and appropriate warnings against use under specific circumstances (for example, laxatives where abdominal pain is present).

(9) It is stated or advertised to be an official preparation and is not packaged and labeled according to the official directions in the monograph.

(10) The packaging is such that it is misleading; it is an imitation of another drug; or it is offered under the name of another drug.

(11) It is dangerous to health when used as recommended by the label on it.

(12) It is, or is stated to be, made of or in part of insulin or antibiotic unless it be from a batch certified by this law.

c. Labeling. All drugs leaving the pharmacy must be labeled adequately.

(1) Labeling drugs dispensed on prescription. Drugs dispensed on prescription must bear the proper information on a prescription-type label–including the name and location of the facility, the name of the patient, the date of issuance, the number assigned to the prescription, the directions for use, the prescriber's name, and the initials of the person typing the label. In the Army, AR 40-2 also requires us to place the name and strength of the drug on the label, except when the prescriber directs otherwise, and also the legend "KEEP OUT OF THE REACH OF CHILDREN" in boldface type on all prescription labels. In addition, the labels for controlled substances must contain the legend, "CAUTION: FEDERAL LAW PROHIBITS THE TRANSFER OF THIS DRUG TO ANY PERSON OTHER THAN THE PATIENT FOR WHOM IT WAS PRESCRIBED" in boldface type.

(2) Labeling drugs dispensed to patients without a prescription. Drugs dispensed by the pharmacy without a prescription as provided in AR 40-2 must be properly labeled. According to law, the label must show the name of the medication; adequate directions for use; the quantity contained; the name of the facility and location; special notes or warnings; and if any habit-forming drugs are contained in any amount, the name of such drug and the amount per unit must be stated on the label as well as the statement–"Warning: May be habit-forming." Items which have an expiration date or deteriorate after mixing must bear a label stating such information. AR 40-2 also states that the legend "KEEP OUT OF THE REACH OF CHILDREN" must appear in boldface type on the label.

(3) Labels of drug stock in using activities. It is the duty of pharmacy personnel to insure that the stock in wards and in treatment rooms is labeled properly. A little bottle on the shelf in a treatment room marked "Achromycin–250 mg" is not adequate and is in direct violation of the law. When possible, drugs dispensed for ward stock should remain in their original container and with their original labeling. If labeled by pharmacy personnel, the label should contain such things as the name of the drug; trade name, if applicable; strength; quantity; date; name of manufacturer and manufacturer's lot number; and expiration date.

d. Coal tar colors. A list of certified coal tar colors for the purpose of coloring foods or drugs is set forth in this law. These coloring agents must be proved harmless and suitable for the purpose for which they are intended. A list of these coal tar colors can be found in *Remington's Practice of Pharmacy.*

e. New drugs. Before being introduced into interstate commerce, all new drugs must be first approved by the Secretary of the Department of Health, Education, and Welfare. Only "approved" drugs will be procured, prescribed, or dispensed except those unapproved drugs authorized by The Surgeon General to save life or prevent suffering. Investigational drugs may be used within the provisions of AR 40-2 (sec. 15) and AR 40-7.

3. The Durham-Humphrey Act. The Durham-Humphrey Act (Durham-Humphrey Amendment) is nothing more than a set of changes to the Food, Drug, and Cosmetic Act. This amendment groups drugs into two main classes–those which may be dispensed only on prescription, and those which may be sold over-the-counter (OTC); that is, without a prescription.

a. Prescription legend drugs. The Durham-Humphrey Act rules that drugs which by their nature are unsafe, or require medical supervision or advice with their use, must bear the legend "Caution: Federal Law Prohibits Dispensing Without a Prescription." Any drug so labeled is known as a prescription legend drug (sometimes called a legend drug) and cannot be sold without a prescription. Conversely, all drugs considered safe to use without medical supervision must not bear the caution and may be sold OTC.

b. Telephoned prescriptions. The Durham-Humphrey Amendment permits a physician to prescribe medication in the legend category by telephone. The pharmacist must reduce the prescription to writing and include the medication, strength, dose or directions for use, the name of the patient, and all other data given him by the physician. AR 40-2 states that all prescriptions will be signed by an authorized prescriber and that prescriptions for potentially harmful drugs (legend drugs) will be dispensed only upon receipt of a *written* prescription.

c. Renewing legend drug prescriptions. One of the most important stipulations of the Durham-Humphrey Act is that prescriptions for legend drugs may not be renewed (refilled), except when authorized by the prescriber. Such authorization may be made at the time of writing the prescription by stating the number of times the prescription may be refilled. The interpretation of this act, like all the others, must be in accordance with good professional judgment and good faith.

d. Enforcement of the acts. The Food, Drug, and Cosmetic Act and the Durham-Humphrey Act are enforced by the Food and Drug Administration (FDA) of the Department of Health, Education, and Welfare. Violations of the acts are misdemeanors and are punishable by "imprisonment for not more than one year, or a fine of not more than $1,000, or both."

4. The drug efficacy studies

a. As a result of the 1962 Kefauver-Harris New Drug Amendments to the Food, Drug, and Cosmetics Act of 1938, it was ruled that *drugs must not only have proof of "safety," but also proof of "effectiveness."* This was the basis for the commissioner of the Food and Drug Administration (FDA) requesting the National Academy of Sciences/National Research Council (NAS/NRC) to make a comprehensive survey of effectiveness for all drugs marketed under new drug applications (NDA) approved between 1938 and October 1962. Their findings are called the *Drug Efficacy Study.* Each drug after review is classified in one of four categories:

(1) Effective. The drug is effective for the presented indications.

(2) Probably effective. The effectiveness of the drug is probable for the indications presented but additional evidence of effectiveness is required of the manufacturer within 12 months before it can be classified *effective.*

(3) Possibly effective. There is little evidence of effectiveness for presented indications; however, the manufacturer is allowed 6 months to submit additional data to provide substantial evidence of effectiveness.

(4) Ineffective. There is no acceptable evidence to support a claim of effectiveness, and immediate administrative action by the FDA is justified in withdrawing the drug from the market or deleting the claimed indication(s) from the label. The manufacturer has 30 days to submit pertinent data bearing on this regulatory proposal.

b. As a direct result of the Drug Efficacy Study and FDA enforcement and regulatory action, the Department of Defense established the following policy regarding the procurement and prescribing of three of the above categories of drugs:

(1) Category 1A, "Ineffective" drugs.

- These drugs have definitely been determined to be ineffective by the FDA.
- No further procurement or issue is authorized for those items that have been withdrawn from the market.
- Remaining stocks of standard and nonstandard items will be destroyed or other appropriate action taken.

(2) Category 1B, "Ineffective" drugs.

- These drugs have been determined to be ineffective by the FDA; however, manufacturers have been given time to refute the FDA decision.
- Authorization for central or local procurement is suspended until final action is taken by FDA.
- These drugs will be suspended from use and issue until final status of drug is resolved.

(3) Category 2, "Possibly Effective" drugs.

- Standard and local procurement of these items are no longer authorized. Remaining stocks may be used until exhausted. Exception: continued therapeutic use of these drugs will depend upon the decision of the medical facility Therapeutic Agents Board (TAB). Local procurement is authorized if the TAB decides no alternate means of therapy are available.
- Requisitioning of "possibly effective" drugs (if approved by TAB) is minimized to no more than 60 days stock on hand in the medical facility.

(4) Category 3, "Probably Effective" drugs.

- All central and local procurement of these items

is minimized so that there is no more than 60 days stock on hand in the medical facility.

- Continued issue and use is authorized until further change in classification by FDA.

c. Information concerning the classification of a drug within these categories is not specifically included in this manual. If further information is needed, a consolidated listing of drugs classified as "Ineffective," "Possibly Effective," or "Probably Effective" was summarized in SB 8-75-4, 18 January 1972. An updating of this list and current "Drug Safety and Effectiveness Information" will be published periodically in the SB 8-75 series.

5. Controlled substances

a. General. The ordering, dispensing, and destruction of controlled substances in the United States is governed by the "Comprehensive Drug Abuse Prevention and Control Act of 1970" (also known as the Controlled Substances Act or Public Law (PL) 91-513, October 27, 1970). Essentially, this act combines the control of drugs formerly known as Class A, B, X, and M narcotics and DACA (Drug Abuse Control Amendment of 1965, which identified those drugs that have potential for high abuse) into one statute, with responsibility for enforcement placed on one agency, the Bureau of Narcotics and Dangerous Drugs (BNDD), of the U.S. Department of Justice. Most states have their own laws which supplement the Federal law. Although the practice of pharmacy on a military installation is not governed by the law of the state in which the installation is located, it is subject to the provisions of the "Comprehensive Drug Abuse Prevention and Control Act," PL 91-513. The Army does have regulations governing the handling of controlled substances which, in essence, are comparable to state laws. Army regulations are often more stringent than, or at least parallel to, the Federal law, but they are never less stringent than the Federal law. The question of which law or regulation to follow in a given situation then arises. The following rule of thumb should be followed if Army's regulations and Federal law differ, "the more stringent law or regulation is applicable." Regarding the handling of controlled substances, differences between the Federal law and Army regulation will be seen in several areas, such as labeling requirements and filing and destruction procedures. Where these differences exist, the more stringent requirements will be covered here.

b. Schedule substances. The Controlled Substances Act designated controlled drugs into five schedules based on their potential for abuse. As pharmacy specialists, it is easy for you to determine which schedule a given drug belongs to simply by examining the commercial container in which the drug is supplied. The container will bear an identification symbol indicating the schedule in which the drug belongs. The symbol can appear in either of two ways: a capital C followed by the roman numeral indicating the schedule number (for example, C-II), or a capital C with the Roman numeral inside of it (for example, ⒸII). The five schedules are defined as follows:

(1) Schedule I substances. Have no accepted medical use in the United States. Some examples are heroin, marihuana, LSD, peyote, mescaline, psilocybin, tetrahydrocannabinols, ketobemidone, levomoramide, racemoramide, benzylmorphine, dihydromorphine, morphine methylsulfonate, nicocodeine, nicomorphine, and others.

(2) Schedule II substances. Have a high abuse potential with severe psychic or physical dependence liability. Many have been known in the past as Class A Narcotic Drugs. Non-narcotic substances are currently included in this schedule. Some examples are: amphetamines, methamphetamines, methylphenidate, phenmetrazine, opium, morphine, codeine, dihydromorphinone, methadone, pantopon, meperidine, cocaine, anileridine, oxymorphone, and any other substance so designated by amendments to the Controlled Substances Act. The first difference between Federal law and Army regulations is encountered with Schedule II substances. By Army regulation, paregoric (which by Federal law is classified in Schedule III) and ethyl alcohol and alcoholic beverages (which by Federal law are not included in any schedule), must be received, dispensed, and accounted for in Army hospitals in the same manner as Schedule II substances. (However, commercial containers of paregoric, alcohol, or alcoholic beverages will *not* be imprinted with the C-II or ⒸII symbol when you receive them.) You must be aware of the fact that these substances are being controlled by the Army in this manner because the Army Regulation, which in this case is more stringent than the Federal law, has to be followed.

(3) Schedule III substances. Have an abuse potential less than those in Schedules I and II, and includes those drugs formerly known as Class B Narcotics and, in addition, non-narcotic

drugs, such as glutethimide, methyprylon, chlorhexadol, phencyclidine, sulfondiethylmethane, sulfonmethane, nalorphine, and some barbiturates, and any other items so designated by amendments to the Controlled Substances Act.

(4) Schedule IV substances. Have an abuse potential less than those listed in Schedule III and include drugs such as barbital, phenobarbital, methylphenobarbital, chloral betaine, chloral hydrate, ethchloruynol, ethinamate, meprobamate, paraldehyde, pentaetythritol chloral, methohexital, chlordiazepoxide, diazepam, and any other items so designated by amendments to the Controlled Substances Act.

(5) Schedule V substances. Have an abuse potential less than those listed in Schedule IV, and consist of those preparations formerly known as Exempt Narcotics, with the exception of paregoric. Paregoric is now listed as a Schedule III Controlled Substance but, as you have seen in *(2)* above, is received, dispensed, and accounted for in the Army as a Schedule II substance.

c. *Code R and Code K items.* Another method of classifying controlled substances is used in military medical supply channels and the Federal Supply Catalog: classification as Code R or Code K items. To be sure you are fully aware of the relationship between these items and the schedules, each term will be defined.

(1) Code R item is defined as those controlled substances classified in Schedule II, plus ethyl alcohol, alcoholic beverages, and paregoric.

(2) Code K item is defined as those controlled substances classified in Schedules III, IV, and V.

d. *Ordering.*

(1) The Controlled Substances Act outlines general guidelines which must be followed by everyone who orders and dispenses controlled substances. In the Army, the specific methods by which these guidelines are carried out are outlined in AR 40-2.

(2) While a special BNDD order form is used by medical supply to locally purchase Schedule II substances, all schedule substances are normally ordered by the pharmacy from medical supply by using a DA Form 2765-1 (Request for Issue or Turn-In). This policy may vary with installation policy, and other forms may be used.

e. *Record keeping.*

(1) When any controlled substance is received from medical supply, you will also receive a numbered voucher which shows the date and quantity of the substance you received. This voucher must be filed and will serve as your debit record when accounting for that substance. By law, Schedule II vouchers must be filed separately from Schedule III, IV, and V vouchers. The date, quantity received, and voucher number will be entered in the appropriate column of the DA Form 3862 (Controlled Substances Stock Record) which is maintained for that specific item. A separate DA Form 3862 must be maintained for each form in which the controlled substance is supplied. The metric system must be used for all entries where appropriate. When you receive controlled substances from medical supply, you will be required to sign a voucher, which is retained by medical supply, showing that these controlled substances have been delivered to you. Make sure that everything ordered is present, or deleted as appropriate, and that all items received are the exact items ordered before you sign for them.

(2) Individual prescriptions serve as your credit record for subtracting from DA Form 3862 the control substance dispensed. The manner in which specific preparations are accounted for depends on the schedule to which the preparation belongs.

(3) For Schedule II substances, ethyl alcohol, alcoholic beverages, and paregoric, each order for stock expended will be subtracted from the balance on hand shown on the DA Form 3862 maintained for that item. Each entry will show the date expended, the prescription number, and the amount expended. The *last* figure in the "Balance on Hand" column of the DA Form 3862 for that item will always reflect the *actual* amount on hand.

(4) Entries for Code R items will be made on DA Form 3862 on a daily basis with each prescription and/or voucher being recorded.

(5) For Schedule III, IV, and V controlled substances (and any other items designated by the commander), expenditures for each item will be summarized weekly and subtracted from the balance on hand shown on the DA Form 3862 maintained for that item. Concurrently, an inventory of all the stocks on hand will be conducted by pharmacy personnel and the inventory balance compared with the balance shown on DA Form 3862. An adjustment for minor overages and shortages caused by

operational handling or undiscoverable posting errors will be made by posting an inventory adjustment to the stock record since a series of small losses over an extended period of time could result in a major inventory shortage. All major inventory shortages will be investigated immediately and remedial action taken. Records of all investigations and remedial actions should be maintained in the pharmacy records.

(6) In event an error is made in posting, *one* line must be drawn through the incorrect entry and initialed and the correct entry made.

f. *Filing.*

(1) While the Controlled Substances Act provides three general methods by which persons receiving and dispensing controlled substances may maintain their prescription files, AR 40-2 provides one specific method by which prescriptions will be numbered and filed in Army pharmacies.

(2) At least three series of numbers will be used to number prescriptions filled in Army pharmacies—one for Schedule II substances, ethyl alcohol, alcholic beverages, and paregoric; one for Schedule III, IV, and V substances; and one for all other prescriptions. A corresponding file will be established for each series of numbers.

g. *Inventorying.*

(1) AR 40-2 requires that at least once each month a disinterested officer or senior noncommissioned officer be designated by the commander to inspect the stock records for controlled substances. He will conduct an inventory of each Schedule II substance, and all ethyl alcohol, alcoholic beverages, and paregoric, and verify that the amount of each drug or preparation actually in stock is the same amount show in the "Balance on Hand" column of the DA Form 3862 maintained for that item. At the same time he will verify all other entries. His findings, together with the date of the inspection and action taken, will be noted over his signature and grade immediately below the last entry on the card. Any discrepancies noted will be reported immediately in writing to the commander. Concurrently, he will inspect the stock records for at least 10 percent of the Schedule III, IV, and V items and include in his report to the commander any unusual expenditures or any major inventory discrepancies.

(2) If controlled substances are used in the manufacture of pharmaceutical preparations, a DD Form 1289 (Prescription Form) with the R_x symbol lined out will be used to account for their expenditure. Such orders will be authenticated and signed by the officer in charge of the pharmacy. The quantity expended will be subtracted from the DA Form 3862 maintained for that item, and the order will be filed in the appropriate prescription file.

h. *Security.* The Controlled Substances Act directs that Schedule II substances be stored in at least a securely locked, substantially constructed cabinet, and Schedule III, IV, and V substances be either stored in such a locked cabinet or dispersed throughout the stock of noncontrolled drugs in such a manner as to obstruct their theft or diversion. In the Army, controlled substances must be safeguarded at each storage location within a medical facility by placing stocks in appropriate security devices such as a vault, safe, locked cabinet, or locked cage. At least annually, the installation provost marshal must be requested to survey the adequacy of the security provided, and corrective action must be taken as indicated. In other words, in an Army hospital pharmacy all controlled substances must be securely locked in the pharmacy vault or stored in some other secure area.

i. *Dispensing.*

(1) The dispensing process must be examined from two aspects, inpatient dispensing and outpatient dispensing. The Controlled Substances Act sets guidelines for dispensing controlled substances which deal mostly with the outpatient situation. More specific and stringent guidance on how controlled substances are to be dispensed, labeled, and handled within an Army hospital can be found in AR 40-2.

(2) Controlled substances will be dispensed in bulk to inpatient agencies only upon receipt of a properly written and authenticated prescription (DD Form 1289) with the R_x symbol lined out. This order must be signed by an individual authorized to write prescriptions or by a registered nurse. The order will show the name of the agency receiving the controlled substance and the date. This prescription will be used as a credit voucher to deduct the quantity dispensed from the DA Form 3862 maintained for that item. Labeling requirements for controlled substances issued in bulk to wards, clinics, and other authorized agencies will be prescribed locally by the commander.

(3) While the Controlled Substances Act allows oral-prescription orders for Schedule III and IV substances (and Schedule II substances in an emergency), AR 40-2 states that all prescriptions filled in Army pharmacies will be stamped, typed, or written in ink and will be signed by the prescriber. Thus, no oral prescriptions are authorized in military pharmacies.

(4) Both the Controlled Substances Act and AR 40-2 require prescriptions for schedule drugs to contain the date of issue; name, rank, corps, organization, and address of the patient; and signature of the prescriber. The Controlled Substances Act does state that the physician's BNDD registration number has to appear on prescriptions for schedule drugs. Military physicians are exempt from the requirement to register, but by regulation they must place their service identification number, in lieu of the registration number, on all prescriptions for controlled substances. AR 40-2 also requires that the name of the prescriber be typed, handprinted, or stamped on a controlled prescription in addition to his signature.

(5) Both the Controlled Substances Act and AR 40-2 require that the label on the container of controlled substance dispensed to individual patient will contain:

(a) Prescription number.

(b) Identity of the facility dispensing the controlled substance.

(c) Name of the prescriber.

(d) Name of the patient.

(e) Date of dispensing.

(f) Directions for use and any caution or statement (such as "shake well" or "refrigerate") if needed.

(g) Transfer warning or legend "CAUTION: FEDERAL LAW PROHIBITS THE TRANSFER OF THIS DRUG TO ANY PERSON OTHER THAN THE PATIENT FOR WHOM IT WAS PRESCRIBED" in boldface type.

(6) In addition to these seven requirements, AR 40-2 also requires that all prescription labels contain the name and strength of the drug, except when the prescriber directs otherwise; the initials of the person typing the prescription label; and the legend "KEEP OUT OF REACH OF CHILDREN" in boldface type.

(7) Both by law and by regulation, prescriptions for Schedule II substances cannot be refilled. In addition, AR 40-2 extends this restriction to ethyl alcohol, alcoholic beverages, and paregoric, and prohibits personnel who are authorized to write prescriptions for Code R items from prescribing them for themselves or for members of their family.

(8) If the pharmacy does not have enough of a Schedule II item to fill a prescription order completely, partial filling of the prescription is permitted provided the balance is supplied to the patient within 72 hours. When a prescription for a Schedule II substance is partially filled, a notation of the fact must be made on the prescription and the prescriber must be notified of the action taken.

(9) Prescriptions for Schedules III through V controlled substances (and any other drug designated by the commander) cannot be refilled unless such refilling is authorized by the prescriber on the original prescription. These prescriptions cannot be refilled more than five times and cannot be refilled more than six months after the date of issue. When a prescription for any controlled substance in Schedule III or IV is refilled, the pharmacist will enter his initials, the date of refilling, and the amount of drug refilled on the back of the original prescription form or another appropriate uniformly maintained record which indicates prescription refills.

(10) The partial dispensing of Schedules III, IV, and V controlled substances is authorized provided that each partial dispensing is recorded in the same manner as a renewal, the total quantity dispensed in all partial orders does not exceed the total quantity prescribed, and no dispensing occurs six months after the issuance of the prescription order. Although authorized by law, the partial dispensing of Schedule III through V substances in Army hospitals would be a relatively rare situation such as this: the pharmacy temporarily runs out of stock of the item prescribed and dispenses only enough drug to hold the patient over until new stocks can be obtained from medical supply.

(11) While the Controlled Substances Act authorized the dispensing of Schedule V substances without a prescription provided certain conditions are met, AR 40-2 limits nonprescription dispensing to small quantities of noncontrolled pharmaceuticals suitable for relief of distress due to conditions such as simple headache and mild indigestion. Thus, as a pharmacy technician, you need not become concerned with the details of over-the-counter dispensing of Schedule V drugs.

(12) When a pharmacy does not have a controlled substance required by a patient and the patient has no alternative source of that drug reasonably available to him, the pharmacy may obtain it from a second pharmacy. In such a

situation neither pharmacy need register as a distributor. Records of the transaction must be kept, however, and the amount transferred may not exceed that necessary for immediate dispensing. The transaction is recorded as a dispensing by the pharmacy providing the drug and as a receipt by the pharmacy receiving it. Each must retain a signed receipt of the transaction which, if it involves a Schedule II drug, must be an official order form. Since the Pharmacy Service does not have official order forms for controlled substances, arrangement will have to be through medical supply for the transfer of a Schedule II substance.

j. Destruction. Under the provisions of AR 40-2, whenever controlled substances have deteriorated to the point where they are not usable for the purpose originally intended, are of questionable potency, or have had their identity compromised, they will be reported to the commander for a determination of disposition. Commanders will take such action as may be appropriate and, when indicated, will investigate negligence or carelessness and will direct appropriate disposition of the reported items. If destruction is directed, it will be accomplished in the presence of a witnessing officer and such other officials as may be required by regulations. A record of such destruction, signed by the witnessing officer, will be filed in the controlled substances file as authority for dropping the items from the records of the accounts. (AR 40-61 gives procedures for and documentation of this action.)

6. **UCMJ.** In addition to the specific Federal Statutes referred to above, pharmacy technicians are subject to the Uniform Code of Military Justice, Article 134, which includes the wrongful possession or use of habit-forming narcotic drugs.

7. **Prescription ownership.** From the time a patient receives his prescription from the prescriber and surrenders it to the pharmacist for filling, there is no doubt that the patient is the rightful owner of that prescription. Once a prescription has been turned over to the pharmacy for filling and the patient has received his medication, the prescription is a necessary legal document for the pharmacy's records and legally belongs to the pharmacy. The courts also say that if a patient brings a prescription for filling but decides after the medication has been compounded that he does not want it, the written prescription still belongs to him and he may demand that it be returned.

8. **Confidentiality of prescriptions.** Much confidential and privileged information is contained in the prescription file regarding the people of a given community. The nature of prescriptions must not be discussed with unauthorized persons nor may they be permitted to examine the files. If it is important that a person know the contents of a prescription for legal or other reasons, he can obtain a court order to obtain the necessary information. People must not be allowed to examine the files unless they are acting within their official capacity, such as the issuing physician, inventory officer, auditor, or member of an IG team. From the standpoint of pharmaco-medical ethics, it is bad to let one physician examine the prescriptions of another physician; it may also be an invasion of privacy.

9. **Prescription copies.** Frequently, a patient will ask for a copy of his prescription when he is moving to a different area or going on vacation. You may legally provide a patient with a copy of his prescription IF you adhere to the following:

a. All copies must plainly, and in large letters, be marked or stamped "COPY."

b. Prescriptions which cannot be refilled should, in addition to "COPY," bear the words "NOT TO BE REFILLED." Some pharmacists add the notation "FOR INFORMATION ONLY."

c. Those prescriptions which can be legally refilled (that is, those which do not require a prescription initially) or those which are marked to be refilled a specified number of times must bear a marking instructing future pharmacists regarding the number of times the medication may still be refilled.

d. You must be alert for those asking for copies of narcotic, barbiturate, or amphetamine type drugs. It may be wise to ask the prescriber for his consent before doing so. Whenever possible, avoid issuing copies of this type of prescription.

BASIC FUNDAMENTALS OF THE PRESCRIPTION

CONTENTS

BASIC FUNDAMENTALS of the PRESCRIPTION

Section I. PRESCRIPTION LANGUAGE–PHARMACEUTICAL LATIN

1. **Latin in pharmacy and medicine.** Latin in prescription writing is centuries old. Although more and more of the prescription is being written in English today, most prescriptions are in part written in Latin or use the Latin abbreviations. As long as physicians continue to use Latin and Latin abbreviations in prescription writing, the pharmacist will have to be able to read and fully understand the terms that are used. Latin used in medicine and prescription writing may be intended to conceal the nature of the medication from the patient, to reduce the possibility of a patient's tampering with a prescription, or to make the prescription universally legible to pharmacists regardless of their national language. Probably the most outstanding reason for the use of Latin in medicine and pharmacy is through force of habit. It has been done for so long that it is hard to break away from the trend. Medical and pharmacy colleges teach the physician to write prescriptions in Latin and the pharmacist to be able to interpret them.

2. **Commonly used Latin abbreviations, words, and translations.** Since it would be extremely time consuming and of doubtful value to present an entire course in Pharmaceutical Latin here, it is strongly suggested that you read, learn, and *memorize* the words, abbreviations, and meanings on the right. This will familiarize you with the more common terms and phrases used in prescription writing and enable you to understand the physician's or other prescriber's orders. Later, when you have time and a desire to improve your command of Latin, as pertinent to pharmacy, procure a copy of an authoritative pharmacy text. With the aid of such a text, the average individual may become familiar with Latin as it applies to the professions of medicine and pharmacy.

Latin	*Abbreviation*	*English Translation*
ad	ad	to; up to
ad libitum	ad lib.	at pleasure
adde, addendus	add.	add, let them be added
agitata ante usum	agit. ant. us.	shake before using
albus	alb.	white
alternus horis	alt. hor.	alternate hours
amplus	amplus	large
ana	aa.	of each
ante	a.	before
ante cibos; ante cibum	a.c.	before meals; before food
ante meridiem	A.M.	before noon
applicandus	applicand.	to be applied
aqua	aq.	water
aqua bullions	aq. bull.	boiling water
aqua destillata	aq. dest.	distilled water
aqua fervens	aq. ferv.	hot water
aqua frigida	aq. frig.	cold water
aqua forte	aq. fort.	nitric acid
aromaticus	arom.	aromatic
argentum	arg.	silver
aurio	aur.	ear
bene	ben.	well
bibe	bib.	drink
bis in die	b.i.d.	twice a day
bolus	bol.	a large pill
capeat	cap.	let him take
capsula	cap.	a capsule
charta	chart.	paper (powder)
charta cerati	chart. cerat.	waxed paper
cibus	cib.; c.	food
cochleare amplum	coch. amp.	tablespoonful
cochleare infans	coch. inf.	teaspoonful
cochleare magnum	coch. mag.	tablespoonful
cochleare maximum	coch. max.	tablespoonful
cochleare medium	coch. med.	dessertspoonful
cochleare minimum	coch. min.	teaspoonful
cochleare modicum	coch. mod.	dessertspoonful
cochleare parvum	coch. parv.	teaspoonful
cochleare paulus	coch. paul.	teaspoonful
cochleare plenum	coch. plen.	tablespoonful
cola, colatus	col.	strain, strained
collunarium	collun.	nasal douche
collutorium	collut.	mouthwash
collyrium	collyr.	eye lotion
compositus	comp.	compound,

2

Latin	Abbreviation	English Translation
		compounded
congius	cong.	gallon
continuentur remedia	cont. rem.	continue the medication
creta	cret.	chalk
cum	c.; c̄	with
da	d.	give
decem	decem	ten
dentur	dent.; d.	let be given; give
dentur tales doses	d.t.d.	give of such doses
dexter	dext.	right
dies	d.	day
diebus alternis	dieb. alt.	on alternate days
diebus secundis	dieb. secund.	every second day
diebus tertiis	dieb. tert.	every three days
diluo; dilutus	dil.	dilute
dispensa; dispensatur	disp.	dispense; let be dispensed
dividatur	div.	divide
dividatur in partes aequales	div. in par. aeq.	divide into equal parts
dosis	dos.; d.	a dose
drachma	ʒ	a drachm
dura	dur.	hard
e	e	out of; in
et	et	and
e lacte	e lact.	in milk
ex modo praescripto	e.m.p.	in the manner prescribed
fac; fiat; fiant	ft.	make; let be made
ferrum	ferr.	iron
filtra	filtra	filter
flavus	flav.	yellow
folium; folia	fol.	leaf; leaves
fortis; fortior	fort.	strong; stronger
gargarisma	garg.	a gargle
gradatim	grad.	gradually
grossus	gros.	large
gramma	Gm.	gram
granum	gr.	grain
gutta; guttae	gtt.	drop; drops
hora	hor.; h	an hour
hora somni	h.s.	at bedtime
hydrargyrum	hydrarg.	mercury
in aurem sinistram	in aur. sinist.	in the left ear
in die	in d.	in a day
in dies	ind.	daily
in oculo laevo	in ocul. laev; O.L.	in the left eye
inter	inter	between
inter cibos	int. cib.	between meals
inter noctem	int. noct.	during the night
in vitro	in vit.	in glass
lac	lac	milk
levis	lev.	light
libra	lb.	pound
liquor	liq.	liquid; solution
lotio	lot.	lotion
luteus	lut.	yellow
magnus	mag.	large
mane	man.	morning, in the
massa	mass.	a mass
milligramma	mg.; mgm.	a milligram
minimum	♏	a minim
misce	M.	Mix
mistura	mist.	mixture
mitte	mitt.	send
modo praescripto	mod. praes.	in the manner prescribed
mollis	moll.	soft
nasus	n.	nostril
nebula	nebul.	a spray
niger	nig.	black
nocte	noct.	at night
nocte maneque	noct. maneq.; n. et m.	night and morning
non	non	not
non repetatur	non rep.	do not repeat
octarius	O.; oct.	a pint
oculus	ocul.	the eye
oculo dextro	O.D.; ocul. dext.	the right eye, in the
oculo sinistro	O.S.; ocul. sinist.	the left eye, in the
oculo laevo	O.L.; ocul. laev.	the left eye, in the
oculo utro	O.U.; ocul. utro	in each eye
oleum	ol.	oil
omnis	omn.	every
omni altera hora	omn. alt. hor.	every alternate hour
omni hora	omn. hor.	every hour
omni mane	omn. man.	every morning
omni quarta hora	omn. 4 hor.	every four hours
parvus	parv.	small
per	per	by means of
per os	per os	by mouth
phiala	phial.; p.	a bottle
phiala fusca	phial. fusc.	a brown bottle
phiala prius agitata	p.p.a.	the bottle first being shaken
placebo	placebo	I please
plumbum	plumb.	lead
ponderosus	pond.	heavy
post aurum	post aur.	behind the ear
post cibum; post cibos	p.c.	after food; after meals
post meridiem	P.M.	afternoon
praecipitatus	ppt.	precipitated
pro capillis	pro capil.	for the hair
pro recto	pro rect.	rectal
pro re nata	p.r.n.	as occasion arises
pro usa externo	pro us. ext.	for external use
pulvis	pulv.	powder
quantitatim sufficientum	q.s.	a sufficient quantity
quaque	qq.	each, every
quaque die	q.d.	every day
quaque hora	q.h.	every hour
quater in diem	q.i.d.	four times a day
repetatur	rep.	let it be repeated
recipe	Rx; ℞	take thou
ruber	rub.	red
scrupulus	℈	scruple
secundum artem	s.a.	according to the art
secundum legem	s.l.	according to law
semi	sem.	one-half
semissem	ss	one-half
sesqui	sesqui	one and a half

Latin	Abbreviation	English Translation
signa	sig.; S.	write
simul	simul	at one time
sine	s̄	without
sine aqua	sin. q.; s̄ aq.	without water
si opus sit	s.o.s.	if there is need
solve	solv.	dissolve
spiritus frumenti	sp. frum.	whiskey
spiritus vini rectificatus	S.V.R.	alcohol
spiritus vini tenuis	S.V.T.	diluted alcohol
spiritus vini vitis	sp. vin. vit.	brandy
statim	stat.	immediately
succus	suc.	juice
syrupus	syr.	syrup
tabella	tab.	tablet
talis	tal.; t.	of such
ter in die	t.i.d.	three times a day
tres; trium	tres; trium	three
tussis	tuss.	cough
uncia	℥	ounce
unguentum	ung.; ungt.	ointment
ut dictum	ut dict.	as directed
viridis	vir.	green

3. Common names of drugs and the Latin counterpart

Common Name	Latin
Acid	Acidum
Alcohol	Spiritus Vini Rectificatus (SVR)
Belladonna Leaf	Belladonna Folium
Belladonna Root	Belladonna Radix
Bitter	Amari
Cascara	Rhamnus Purshiana
Castor Oil	Oleum Ricini
Charcoal	Carbo
Wood Charcoal	Carbo Ligni
Clove Oil	Oleum Caryophylli
Coal Tar	Pix Carbonis
Coal Tar Solution	Liquor Carbonis Detergens; Liquor Picis Carbonis
Cod Liver Oil	Oleum Morrhuae
Corn Oil	Oleum Maydis
Cottonseed Oil	Oleum Gossypie Seminis
Earth	Terra
Hard Soap	Sapo Duris
Juice	Succus
Lard	Adeps
Lime	Calx
Linseed Oil	Oleum Lini
Medicinal Soft Soap	Sapo Mollis Medicinalis
Oil	Oleum
Ointment	Unguentum
Orange	Aurantium
Peppermint	Mentha Piperita
Peppermint Oil	Oleum Menthal Piperitae
Purified Cotton	Gossypium Purificatum
Rosin	Resina
Seed	Semen
Sherry Wine	Vinum Xericum
Solution	Liquor
Spearmint Oil	Oleum Menthae Viridis
Spermaceti	Cetaceum
Starch	Amylum
Sucrose	Surcrosum; Saccharum
Sweet	Dulcis
Syrup	Syrupus
Turpentine	Terebinthinae
Wax	Cera
Wild Cherry	Prunus Virginiana
Whiskey	Spiritus Frumenti
White Ointment	Ungunentum Alba
White Wax	Cera Alba
Wool Fat	Adeps Lanae
Yellow Ointment	Unguentum Flavum
Yellow Wax	Cera Flava

Section II. THE PRESCRIPTION

The word prescription is a derivation of two Latin words; namely, "prae," meaning "before," and "scribo," meaning "I write." Therefore, the prescription is something written beforehand, hence a rule or direction. It is a written order to the pharmacist by a physician, dentist, veterinarian, or other licensed practitioner, instructing him to compound and/or dispense a specific medication for a specific patient. Through common misuse, the word prescription has also come to mean the completed medication itself. The completed prescription is generally divided into four subdivisions: Superscription, Inscription, Subscription, and Signa. These four parts, in addition to the patient's name, address, and age; the date of writing; and the prescriber's signature, address, and registry number, make up the correct completed prescription.

4. **Superscription.** The superscription is that which is written above. The superscription always consists of, and is in fact represented by the symbol R_x. This symbol is most frequently printed as part of the prescription blank. R_x is taken from the Latin "recipe," meaning "take thou." It is also thought that the slash across the "R" is a sign for Jupiter and is a carry-down of an invocation to the god.

5. **Inscription.** The inscription, or what is written within, contains the actual ingredients and their respective amounts. Each ingredient is placed on a separate line, and all important words are

capitalized. Quantities are written, as will be seen in section III (Pharmaceutical Calculations), in either the metric or the apothecary system. In the apothecary system, the amount is shown by a symbol followed by a roman numeral, e.g., ℥ viii (eight ounces). In the metric system, a symbol is not used, grams or milliliters being written or understood. The inscription may be further subdivided into base, adjuvant, corrective, and vehicle.

a. *Base.* The base is the main or active ingredient or ingredients designed to restore the patient to health.

b. *Adjuvant.* The adjuvant is a substance which increases the efficiency of the base.

c. *Corrective.* The corrective modifies or counteracts any undesirable effects of the base or adjuvant.

d. *Vehicle.* The vehicle may serve several purposes. It may give proper dosage form (producing a liquid, suppository, capsule, etc.). It may dilute so that the patient may take one capsule or one teaspoonful rather than a few grains or a few drops. It may be used to improve taste or appearance. Or it may aid the patient in receiving the proper amount of a potent drug.

6. Subscription. The subscription, or that written below, follows the inscription. It tells the pharmacist the manner of compounding and what the finished product shall be. For example: *M. Fiant solutio* means to mix and let a solution be made. The order of the ingredients on the prescription is not necessarily the order in which they are incorporated into the medication. This is up to the pharmacist and is done according to the art of pharmacy. As you will see later in the course, order of mixing has a pronounced effect on many prescriptions and can be the cause of incompatibilities.

7. Signa (signatura). The signa follows the subscription and means literally to write. It tells the pharmacist the directions to the patient which will be typed on the label. An example of a signa is: ʒ i t. i. d. Since most individuals have no idea of the meaning of a drachm (ʒ), it must be changed to its approximate equivalent, one teaspoonful. The label would then read: "Take one teaspoonful three times a day." Prescriptions should bear exact instructions to the patient as in figure 2-1 rather than the overused "ut dict," which means "as directed." When directions are specified exactly, there is no doubt that the patient understands how much of the medication he is to take, and at what intervals. Also, by using the directions, the pharmacist is able to check more accurately for excessive dosage. Study figure 2-1 to see the relationship of the superscription, the inscription and its parts, the subscription, and the signa.

8. Abbreviations of names of drugs. In writing a prescription, it is always desirable that the official names of agents be used and spelled out completely. Abbreviations or chemical symbols are confusing and can lead to serious error. An abbreviation such as Hyd. Chlor. is not clear. It could be taken for chloral hydrate, for calomel (mercurous chloride), or for mercuric chloride. Chloral hydrate is a hypnotic, used to induce sleep. Calomel is a purgative. Mercuric chloride is a deadly poison even in the smallest doses, and is intended for use as an antiseptic in external preparations to be used on inanimate objects. You can readily see what would happen if one agent were mistaken for another! Imagine the possibilities of confusion with $HgCl$ and $HgCl_2$. $HgCl$ is calomel, the purgative; $HgCl_2$ is mercuric chloride, the poison.

9. Abbreviations in subscription and signa. The more important abbreviations for use in the subscription and the signa are given on the preceding pages.

10. Prescription examples. Read each of the prescriptions shown in figure 2-2 in English and try to pick out the prescription parts previously described in the text and shown in figure 2-1. Note that the prescriptions in figure 2-2 are written in longhand and use abbreviations. This is the form in which you will most likely see them in the pharmacy.

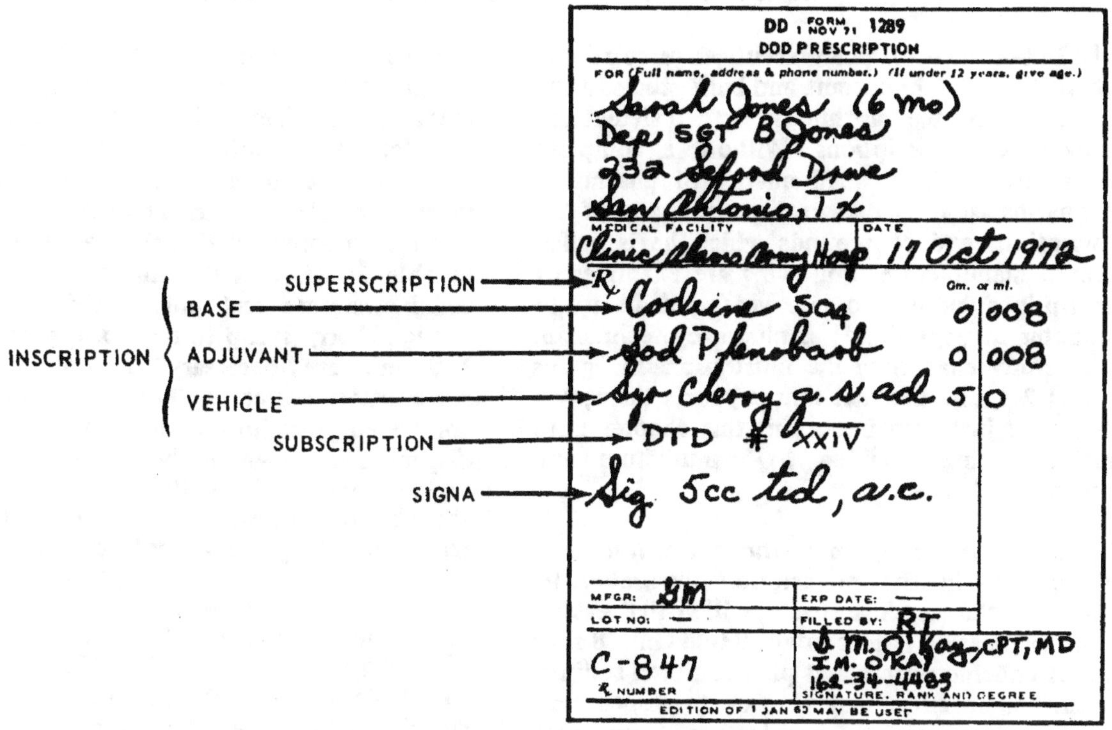

Figure 1. Components of a prescription.

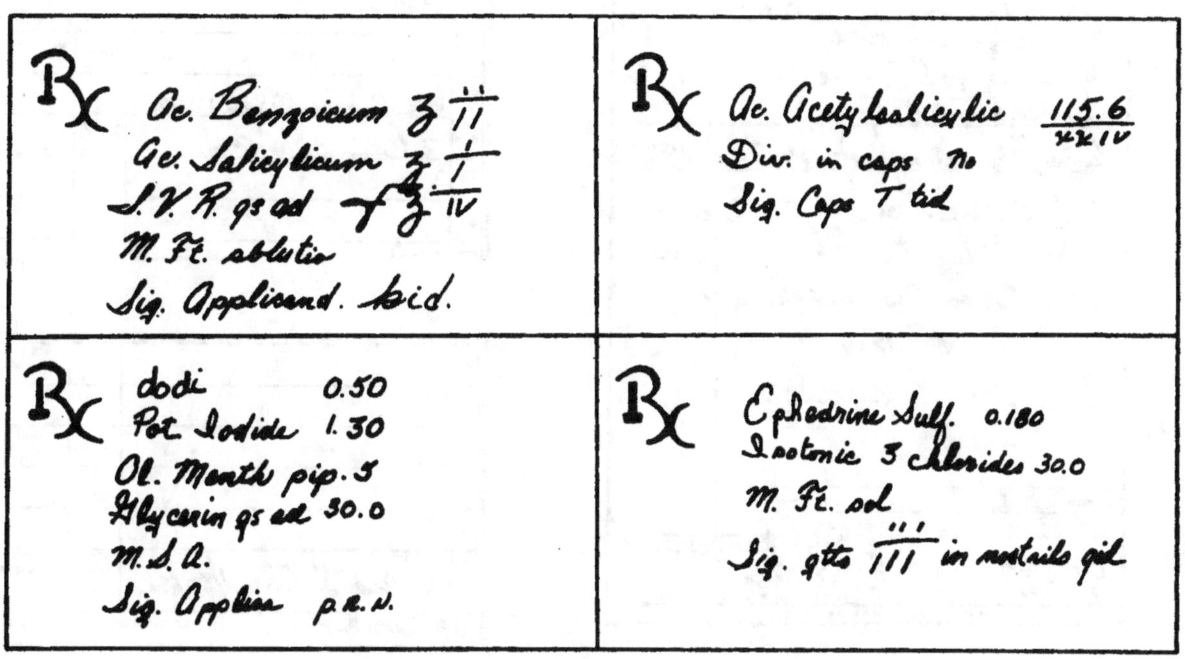

Figure 2. Prescription examples.

Section III. PHARMACEUTICAL CALCULATIONS

11. Importance of pharmaceutical calculations. Perhaps the most important and basic study to the pharmacist is the arithmetic and calculations pertinent to prescriptions. Without a complete understanding of the mathematics of pharmacy, the pharmacist is unable to dispense many of the prescriptions and compounds which he is called upon to manufacture. Following are examples of prescriptions and drug orders which you are apt to encounter in your duties as pharmacy technician. By carefully examining the illustrations in figures 2-3 and 2-4, and the text that supports them, you will realize just how important this chapter is to your becoming qualified to manufacture and dispense medicinals.

a. Example of calculations involved in a prescription. In the prescription illustrated by figure 2-3, the physician has specified that each 5 ml. of medication is to contain 0.008 Gm. (8 mg.) each of codeine sulfate and phenobarbital sodium. He further specifies that you are to dispense 24 doses of this completed medication. How much codeine sulfate, phenobarbital sodium, and cherry syrup will you use in compounding this preparation? What will the total volume of the completed prescription be and what size bottle will be used to contain it? Are the doses of each ingredient safe for this 6-month-old child? When you have completed this chapter, you will readily be able to arrive at the answer: 192 mg. each of codeine sulfate and phenobarbital sodium, and enough cherry syrup to make the product measure 120 ml. are necessary in compounding this prescription correctly. The total volume of the completed prescription will be 120 ml. and will be dispensed in a 4-ounce bottle. The doses are safe for this patient. In addition, you will know that the label for this medication should direct that one teaspoonful be given 3 times a day before meals.

b. Example of calculations involved in a bulk order. Figure 2-4 shows a bulk order for an instrument sterilizer solution. The pharmacist has to calculate how much concentrated benzalkonium chloride solution will be necessary to make 4000

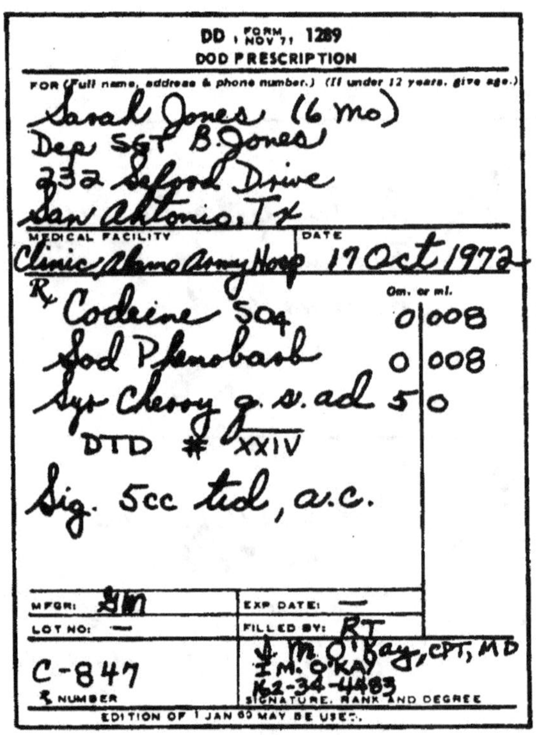
DD FORM NOV 71 1289
DOD PRESCRIPTION
FOR (Full name, address & phone number.) (If under 12 years, give age.)
Sarah Jones (6 mo)
Dep SGT B. Jones
232 Seaford Drive
San Antonio, TX
MEDICAL FACILITY: Clinic, Alamo Army Hosp DATE: 17 Oct 1972
℞ Gm. or ml.
Codeine SO4 0.008
Sod Phenobarb 0.008
Syr Cherry q.s. ad 5.0
DTD # XXIV
Sig. 5cc tid, a.c.
MFGR: GM EXP DATE: —
LOT NO: — FILLED BY: RT
C-847 ℞ NUMBER
J. M. O'Kay, CPT, MD
J. M. O'KAY
162-34-4483
SIGNATURE, RANK AND DEGREE
EDITION OF 1 JAN 60 MAY BE USED.

Figure . 3. Example of calculations involved in a prescription.

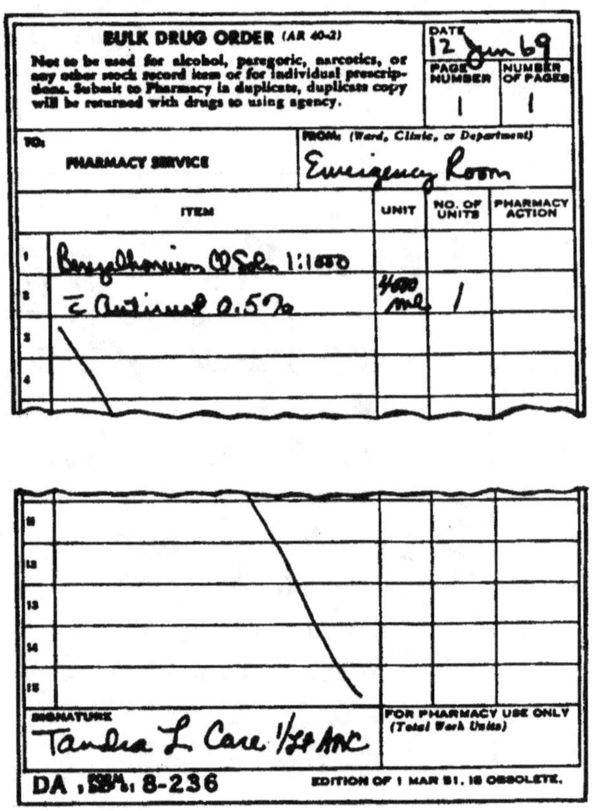
BULK DRUG ORDER (AR 40-2)
Not to be used for alcohol, paregoric, narcotics, or any other stock record item or for individual prescriptions. Submit to Pharmacy in duplicate, duplicate copy will be returned with drugs to using agency.
DATE: 12 Jun 69 PAGE NUMBER: 1 NUMBER OF PAGES: 1
TO: PHARMACY SERVICE FROM: (Ward, Clinic, or Department) Emergency Room

	ITEM	UNIT	NO. OF UNITS	PHARMACY ACTION
1	Benzalkonium Cl Soln 1:1000			
2	c Antirust 0.5%	4000 ml	1	
3				
4				
11				
12				
13				
14				
15				

SIGNATURE: Tandra L. Care 1/Lt ANC
FOR PHARMACY USE ONLY (Total Work Units)
DA FORM 8-236 EDITION OF 1 MAR 51, IS OBSOLETE.

Figure 4. Example of calculations involved in a bulk order.

ml. of a 1:1000 dilution. He will also have to be able to calculate the number of grams of antirust to be used to obtain a 0.5 percent concentration. Upon completing this chapter, it will not be difficult for you to calculate the necessary quantities as being 40 ml. of 10-percent benzalkonium chloride concentrate and 20 Gm. of antirust to make up 4000 ml. of finished solution. These have been but two examples of the absolute necessity of a sound understanding of pharmaceutical arithmetic in pharmacy. As you progress through this chapter, many more will be illustrated and solved.

c. Ground work for pharmaceutical calculations. At first the material that is forthcoming may seem juvenile to you, and you may be inclined to skip over some of the basic aspects. DON'T! Mistakes occur every day in simple addition, subtraction, multiplication, and division. Have you ever caught yourself making such an error? Well, in some places, errors can be allowed for and are not of too much significance, but in pharmacy there is no place for error. First, then, before delving in to the new material, let's begin with a review of fractions and decimals. Here is the place to check yourself on your work. If you work all the problems in fractions and decimals presented in the next few pages, you are well on your way to success in pharmaceutical calculations.

12. Fractions. A fraction represents a simple division problem. It expresses one or more of the equal parts into which a whole number is divided. The fraction $\frac{4}{5}$, then, means five divided into four equal parts of a possible five.

a. Numerator. The number above the separating line is called the numerator. It tells how many parts of the whole are used. In our example' $\frac{4}{5}$, four parts of the whole are used.

b. Denominator. The denominator is the number below the separating line and represents the number of parts into which the whole is divided. Again using $\frac{4}{5}$ as an example, the whole (1) is broken into five equal parts, four of which remain.

c. Mixed numbers. Numbers made up of a whole number plus a fraction are called mixed numbers. For example, $1\frac{4}{5}$ has the whole number, 1, and the fraction, $\frac{4}{5}$, and is consequently a mixed number. It means that we have a whole of 1, plus 4 of the 5 parts of another whole.

d. Proper fractions. A fraction having a numerator which is smaller than its denominator is a proper fraction. It always is less than a whole number. Again, $\frac{4}{5}$ is a proper fraction.

e. Improper fractions. A fraction having a numerator larger than or equal to its denominator is an improper fraction, and it is always equal to or greater than a whole number. For example, $\frac{5}{4}$ is an improper fraction. It is the same as $1\frac{1}{4}$ ($\frac{5}{4} = \frac{4}{4}$ and $\frac{1}{4}$; $\frac{4}{4} = 1$).

f. Relative values of fractions. Let's compare the relative values of several fractions. Of $\frac{1}{5}$, $\frac{1}{6}$, $\frac{1}{3}$, and $\frac{1}{4}$, the smallest is $\frac{1}{6}$. Thus, if fractions have the same numerator, but different denominators, the one with the largest denominator is the smallest in value. Comparing $\frac{2}{5}$, $\frac{3}{5}$, and $\frac{4}{5}$; the largest is $\frac{4}{5}$. Thus, in fractions having the same denominator but different numerators, the one with the largest numerator is the largest. To compare fractions with different numerators and different denominators is more difficult.

13. Rules applying to all fractions. Fractions are division problems and follow three basic rules–

a. Value of fractions maintained. If the numerator and denominator are both multiplied or divided by the same number, the value of the fraction is *not* changed. *Example:* Multiplying both the numerator and denominator of $\frac{1}{3}$ by 3, you get $\frac{3}{9}$ which equals $\frac{1}{3}$; $\frac{3}{9}$ divided by 3 (both numerator and denominator) equals $\frac{1}{3}$ which is equal to $\frac{3}{9}$.

b. Multiplying the value of fractions. If the numerator is multiplied or the denominator divided by a number, the value of the fraction is *multiplied* by that number. *Example:* Multiplying the numerator of $\frac{1}{3}$ by 3 you have $\frac{3}{3}$ which is three times as large; or if you divide the denominator of $\frac{3}{3}$ by 3 you have $\frac{1}{1}$ or 1, which is three times as large.

c. Dividing the value of fractions. If the numerator is divided or the denominator multiplied by a number, the value of the fraction is divided by that number. *Example:* Dividing the numerator of $\frac{3}{9}$ by 3 you have $\frac{1}{9}$, or by multiplying the denominator of $\frac{3}{9}$ by 3 you have $\frac{3}{27}$ which is also $\frac{1}{9}$.

14. Working with fractions. When working with fractions, you often have to reduce a whole number to an improper fraction or reduce an improper fraction to a whole or mixed number.

a. Reducing a whole or mixed number to an improper fraction.

(1) Whole number reduction. To reduce a whole number to an improper fraction, it is necessary to know into how many parts you want to divide the whole (the denominator). If you wish to convert 6, for instance, to an improper fraction having 5 parts, you will have 5 as the denominator. If you reduce 1 to an improper fraction having 5 parts, you would have $\frac{5}{5}$. The whole number, 6, when converted to an improper fraction with 5 as the denominator, would be 6 times as large, or $\frac{5}{5} \times 6 = \frac{30}{5}$.

(2) Mixed number reduction. A mixed number is handled in the same manner. To reduce $8\frac{2}{10}$ to 10ths: $1 = \frac{10}{10}$; then $\frac{10}{10} \times 8 = \frac{80}{10}$ and $\frac{80}{10}$ plus the original $\frac{2}{10} = \frac{82}{10}$, the number of 10ths in $8\frac{2}{10}$.

b. Reducing an improper fraction to a whole or mixed number. As previously stated, a fraction is simply a division problem. For this reason, by dividing the denominator into the numerator, you will get a whole number if the division is even, or a mixed number (whole number plus a remaining fraction) if the division is not even. *Example:* Reduce $\frac{20}{2}$: $\frac{20}{2} = 20 \div 2 = 10$, a whole number; or reduce $\frac{35}{4}$: $\frac{35}{4} = 35 \div 4 = 8\frac{3}{4}$, a mixed number.

15. Lowest terms. A fraction is said to be in its lowest terms when the numerator and denominator cannot be divided by the same number. To illustrate: $\frac{3}{9}$, $\frac{6}{27}$, and $\frac{9}{36}$ are NOT in their lowest terms, for both the numerator and denominator can be divided by a common number. The 3 and 9 in $\frac{3}{9}$ can each be divided by 3 to give $\frac{1}{3}$ which is the lowest terms; the 6 and 27 in $\frac{6}{27}$ by 3 to give $\frac{2}{9}$, the lowest terms; and the 9 and 36 in $\frac{9}{36}$ by 9 to give $\frac{1}{4}$, the lowest terms. These final numbers, then, $\frac{1}{3}$, $\frac{2}{9}$, and $\frac{1}{4}$ are fractions in their lowest terms.

16. Lowest common denominator (LCD). When you add, subtract, or compare fractions, it is necessary to have them in common terms. As apples cannot be added to oranges or automobiles to airplanes, fractions with different denominators cannot be added. By changing apples and oranges to fruit, their common denominator, they can be added. This is also true of fractions. The common denominator can be found by two methods: by multiplying the denominators together, and by a "visual method."

a. Multiplying denominators to find a common denominator. When all the different denominators of the fractions with which you are dealing are multiplied together, the resulting number is common to all. It is not, however, always the lowest number common to all. For example, to find a denominator common to $\frac{1}{4}$, $\frac{1}{3}$, $\frac{1}{2}$, $\frac{1}{8}$, and $\frac{1}{16}$: Multiply the denominators (all of which are different)– $4 \times 3 \times 2 \times 8 \times 16$–you get 3072, the common denominator.

b. Visual method. Visually you can see that 48 is also a denominator common to all the fractions in the preceding example and is much smaller and easier to work with than 3072; 48 is also the *lowest* common denominator. Obtaining the LCD by the visual method is not always easy. The best starting point is to try the denominator which is largest; if it does not work, double it. If doubling the largest denominator does not work, triple it; eventually you will arrive at a common denominator. You must always change the denominators to their LCD before adding, subtracting, or comparing fractions.

c. Expressing fractions in terms of the LCD. After you have established the lowest common denominator for the fractions with which you are working, you must express each fraction in terms of the LCD. This is accomplished by dividing the denominator of the fraction into the LCD and then multiplying both the numerator and denominator by the resulting number. After this has been done for all the fractions involved, you may proceed to add, subtract, or compare.

17. Adding fractions. In the preceding paragraphs we have defined fractions, stated the rules applying to fractions, and given you the necessary information to work with fractions. Now you will work with examples which have been broken down in step procedures to show how this information is used.

a. Proper fractions.

Example: Add $\frac{3}{4}$, $\frac{1}{8}$, and $\frac{5}{6}$.

• *Step 1.* Find the LCD. Visually, you find the LCD to be 24, since 4 will divide into 24, 6 times; 8 will divide into 24, 3 times; and 6 will divide into 24, 4 times.

• *Step 2.* Convert each fraction to similar terms using the LCD. $24 \div 4 = 6$; therefore, $\frac{3}{4} \times \frac{6}{6} = \frac{18}{24}$: $24 \div 8 = 3$; therefore, $\frac{1}{8} \times \frac{3}{3} = \frac{3}{24}$; $24 \div 6 = 4$; therefore, $\frac{5}{6} \times \frac{4}{4} = \frac{20}{24}$.

• *Step 3.* Add the numerators and place the resulting sum over the common denominator. Thus: $18 + 3 + 20 = 41$. Therefore, the sum is $\frac{41}{24}$, which, when reduced to lowest terms, is $1\frac{17}{24}$.

b. Mixed numbers and fractions.

Example: Find the sum of $1\frac{1}{3}$, $2\frac{1}{4}$, and $\frac{1}{2}$.

• *Step 1.* When working with mixed numbers, add all the whole numbers first. $1 + 2 = 3$.

• *Step 2.* Find the LCD for the fractions. By the visual method, you arrive at the LCD as being 12. Change the fractions to common terms. $\frac{1}{3} = \frac{4}{12}$; $\frac{1}{4} = \frac{3}{12}$; $\frac{1}{2} = \frac{6}{12}$.

• *Step 3.* Add the numerator. $4 + 3 + 6 = 13$. Place the resulting number (13) over the LCD: $\frac{13}{12}$, which, reduced to lowest terms, is $1\frac{1}{12}$.

• *Step 4.* Add the $1\frac{1}{12}$ to the whole number from step 1: $1\frac{1}{12} + 3 = 4\frac{1}{12}$.

18. Subtracting fractions

a. Basic method. The procedure for subtracting fractions is basically the same as adding them.

Example: Subtract $\frac{3}{4}$ from $\frac{9}{10}$.

• *Step 1.* Find the LCD. By the multiplication method you find a common denominator to be 40 (4×10). On visual examination, however, you see that 20 is the *lowest* common denominator.

• *Step 2.* Convert each fraction to similar terms using the LCD. Dividing the 4 into 20 you get 5, which when multiplied by the numerator ($5 \times 3 = 15$) gives $\frac{15}{20}$. Doing the same with the $\frac{9}{10}$, 20 divided by $10 = 2$; $2 \times 9 = 18$, therefore, $\frac{18}{20}$.

• *Step 3.* Subtract the two numerators, $18 - 15 = 3$. Place this number (3) over the LCD and arrive at the answer: $\frac{3}{20}$.

b. Subtracting larger from smaller. A problem arises in mixed numbers when the fraction portion of the number being subtracted is larger than the fraction portion of the bigger number.

Example: Subtract $1\frac{2}{3}$ from $3\frac{1}{2}$.

• *Step 1.* Find the LCD. Visually, you see that it is 6.

• *Step 2.* Express both fractions in terms of the LCD. $3\frac{1}{2} = 3\frac{3}{6}$; $1\frac{2}{3} = 1\frac{4}{6}$.

• *Step 3. Subtract:*

$$\begin{array}{r} 3\frac{3}{6} \\ -\ 1\frac{4}{6} \\ \hline \end{array}$$

You can't take $\frac{4}{6}$ from $\frac{3}{6}$. Therefore, you will have to convert the whole number (part of it in this case) to a fraction so that you may subtract. By taking 1 from $3\frac{3}{6}$ and changing it to $\frac{6}{6}$ and adding it to the $\frac{3}{6}$ you already have, you get $2\frac{9}{6}$.

You can now subtract:

$$\begin{array}{r} 2\frac{9}{6} \\ -\ 1\frac{4}{6} \\ \hline 1\frac{5}{6} \end{array}$$

c. Alternate method. An alternate method is to change *all* whole numbers to fractions before subtracting and then reduce the answer to its lowest terms.

Example: Subtract $2\frac{1}{2}$ from $4\frac{1}{4}$.

• *Step 1.* Find the LCD visually, or by the multiplication method, and you arrive at the LCD of 4.

• *Step 2.* Express all numbers (including the whole number portions) in terms of the LCD: $2\frac{1}{2} = \frac{10}{4}$ and $4\frac{1}{4} = \frac{17}{4}$.

• *Step 3. Subtract:*

$$\begin{array}{r} \frac{17}{4} \\ -\ \frac{10}{4} \\ \hline \frac{7}{4} \end{array}$$

• *Step 4.* Reduce to lowest terms: $\frac{7}{4} = 1\frac{3}{4}$, answer.

19. Multiplying fractions. Going back to the three general rules, you know that multiplying the numerator or dividing the denominator by a given number, multiplies the value of the fraction by that number.

a. Multiplying fractions by multiplying the numerator.

Example: Applying the rule, multiply $\frac{3}{4}$ by 8.

• *Step 1.* Multiply the numerator: $3 \times 8 = 24$. Place the resulting number (24) over original denominator: $\frac{24}{4}$

• *Step 2.* Reduce to lowest terms: $\frac{24}{4} = \frac{6}{1} = 6$, answer.

b. Multiplying fractions by dividing the denominator.

Example: Applying the rule, multiply $\frac{3}{4}$ by 2.

• *Step 1.* Divide the denominator: $4 \div 2 = 2$. Placing the original numerator (3) over the new denominator, you have $\frac{3}{2}$.

• *Step 2.* Reduce to lowest terms: $\frac{3}{2} = 1\frac{1}{2}$, answer.

c. Multiplying fractions by fractions. To multiply two or more fractions, multiply the numerators and denominators separately and reduce the obtained fraction to lowest terms.

Example: Multiply $\frac{7}{9}$ by $\frac{6}{14}$.

- *Step 1.* Multiply the numerators: $7 \times 6 = 42$, the new numerator.

- *Step 2.* Multiply the denominators: $9 \times 14 = 126$, the new denominator.

- *Step 3.* Make a fraction of the new numbers: $\frac{42}{126}$.

- *Step 4.* Reduce to lowest terms: $\frac{42}{126} = \frac{1}{3}$, answer.

d. Multiplying fractions by fractions using cancellation. Cancellation is a process of dividing both numerator and denominator of fractions by the same number. It is like reducing to lowest terms. When two or more fractions are to be multiplied (or divided), cancellation between the numerators and denominators not only works, but is time saving in most cases.

Example: Multiply the following: $\frac{7}{9} \times \frac{6}{14} \times \frac{1}{2}$.

- *Step 1.* Here you will divide seven into both numerator and denominator, making the 7 a 1 and the 14 a 2: $\frac{1}{9} \times \frac{6}{2} \times \frac{1}{2} =$

- *Step 2.* Here you will divide both the numerator and denominator by two, making the 6 a 3 and 2 a 1: $\frac{1}{9} \times \frac{3}{2} \times \frac{1}{1} =$

- *Step 3.* Here you will divide both numerator and denominator by three as before. No more such division is possible, so you multiply the numerators together and the denominators together, and if necessary, reduce to lowest terms: $\frac{1}{3} \times \frac{1}{2} \times \frac{1}{1} =$

- *Step 4.* Multiply the numerators and denominators: $\frac{1}{3} \times \frac{1}{2} \times \frac{1}{1} = \frac{1}{6}$, the answer.

In this example, you have made individual steps out of each of the division steps. In a real situation, you would do all of this in one step, as shown in the next two examples.

Example: Multiply $\frac{7}{9} \times \frac{6}{14} \times \frac{1}{2}$; $\frac{\overset{1}{\cancel{7}}}{\underset{3}{\cancel{9}}} \times \frac{\overset{1}{\cancel{\overset{2}{\cancel{6}}}}}{\underset{1}{\cancel{\underset{2}{\cancel{14}}}}} \times \frac{1}{2} = \frac{1}{6}$, answer.

Example: Multiply $\frac{3}{10} \times \frac{9}{26} \times \frac{26}{54}$; $\frac{\overset{1}{\cancel{3}}}{10} \times \frac{\overset{1}{\cancel{9}}}{\underset{1}{\cancel{26}}} \times \frac{\overset{1}{\cancel{26}}}{\underset{2}{\cancel{\underset{18}{\cancel{54}}}}} = \frac{1}{20}$, answer.

e. Multiplying two or more numbers, one or more of which is a mixed number. To multiply mixed numbers, you must change them first to improper fractions, then proceed as with regular fractions.

Example: Multiply $\frac{1}{4} \times 1\frac{5}{8} \times 1\frac{1}{2} \times 5\frac{1}{3}$.

- *Step 1.* Change all mixed numbers to improper fractions: $\frac{1}{4} \times \frac{13}{8} \times \frac{3}{2} \times \frac{16}{3}$

- *Step 2.* Cancel and reduce to lowest terms:

$$\frac{1}{4} \times \frac{13}{\underset{1}{\cancel{8}}} \times \frac{\overset{1}{\cancel{3}}}{\underset{1}{\cancel{2}}} \times \frac{\overset{1}{\cancel{\overset{2}{\cancel{16}}}}}{\underset{1}{\cancel{3}}} = \frac{13}{4} = 3\frac{1}{4}.$$

20. Dividing fractions

a. Again going back to the three general rules, "If the numerator is divided or the denominator multiplied by a given number, the value of the fraction is divided by that number," you have the basis for division among fractions. In order to avoid error, it is best to put a 1 over the whole number, so that you do not inadvertently multiply the numerator instead of the denominator.

Example: Divide $\frac{3}{4}$ by 3. Multiply the denominator of the fraction by 3: $\frac{3}{4} \times \frac{1}{3} = \frac{3}{12} = \frac{1}{4}$.

b. To divide a whole number or a fraction by a fraction, ***invert*** the divisor (the number by which you are dividing). This has the effect of placing a 1 over the fraction. Thus, inverting $\frac{2}{3}$ gives us $\frac{3}{2}$, or: $\frac{1}{\frac{2}{3}} = \frac{\frac{3}{3}}{\frac{2}{3}} = \frac{3}{2}$.

(1) Example: Divide 4 by $\frac{1}{3}$. Invert the fraction by which you are dividing: $4 \times \frac{3}{1} = \frac{12}{1} = 12$.

(2) Example: Divide $\frac{1}{4}$ by $\frac{1}{8}$. Invert the $\frac{1}{8}$; $\frac{1}{\cancel{4}_1} \times \frac{\cancel{8}^2}{1} = 2$.

(3) Example: Divide $2\frac{1}{2}$ by $1\frac{1}{4}$. Here you must first change the mixed numbers to improper fractions, then proceed as before.

$2\frac{1}{2} = \frac{5}{2}$; $1\frac{1}{4} = \frac{5}{4}$.

$$\frac{5}{2} \div \frac{5}{4} = \frac{\cancel{5}^1}{\cancel{2}_1} \times \frac{\cancel{4}^2}{\cancel{5}_1} = \frac{2}{1} = 2.$$

21. Decimals

a. Writing decimals. Fractions that have 10 or any power of 10 for denominators are called decimal fractions. *For example,* $\frac{1}{10}$, $\frac{3}{100}$, $\frac{126}{1000}$, and $\frac{1234}{10000}$ are decimal fractions. In writing decimals, the denominators can be omitted and a decimal point (.) placed in the numerator to show what the denominator is. There are as many digits *after* the decimal point as there were zeros in the denominator. Taking the examples above—

$\frac{1}{10} = 0.1$, $\frac{3}{100} = 0.03$, $\frac{126}{1000} = 0.126$, $\frac{1234}{10000} = 0.1234$.

Where there are less digits in the numerator than there are zeros in the denominator, zeros must be placed between the decimal point and the numerator as in $\frac{25}{10,000} = 0.0025$, and $\frac{21}{100,000} = 0.00021$. Be very careful to place the zeros to the right of the decimal and before (to the left of) the numerator.

b. Movement of decimal point. Any error in the placement of the decimal is serious, for each movement of the decimal point to the right or left produces an error of tenfold. To illustrate what happens, consider the difference between $1.00, $10.00, $100.00, and $1,000.00. In each case, the decimal has been moved one place to the right and in each case, the amount of money represented has been multiplied ten times. Similarly, the dose of nitroglycerin is 0.4 mg.; to give a patient 4.0 mg. is a serious error. For this reason, be extremely cautious and exact when working with decimals.

22. Adding decimals

a. When adding decimals, *always* make sure the decimal points are directly under each other. The actual addition is then the same as with whole numbers.

b. The following three examples demonstrate the necessity of having the decimal points in line under each other. Compare examples (1) and (2) with example (3).

(1) Example: Add $100.25, $50.69, and $18.10.

```
$100.25
  50.69
  18.10
-------
$169.04
```

(2) Example: Add 21.25, 36.17, 18.19, and 7.03.

```
21.25
36.17
18.19
 7.03
-----
82.64
```

(3) Example: Add 1.324, 2347.1, 0.68235, and 11.0001. Remember to line up the decimal points!

```
    1.324
 2347.1
    0.68235
   11.0001
 ----------
 2360.10645
```

23. Subtracting decimals

a. Again the decimal points must be placed directly beneath each other, and again the procedure is the same as with whole numbers.

b. The following two examples also demonstrate the necessity of having the decimal points in line. Study example (2) carefully. Here we must add zeros at the end of the shorter numbers so that we have something to subtract from. Adding zeros at the right of the number after the decimal point has no effect on the value of the number. Zeros cannot, however, be added before the number after a decimal point, or after a number before a decimal point.

(1) Example: Subtract 11.59 from 102.21.

```
 102.21
  11.59
 ------
  90.62
```

(2) Example: Subtract .675061 from 2.31.

```
 2.310000
  .675061
 --------
 1.634939
```

Thus, 2.31 is the same as 2.310000. But 2.31 is NOT equal to 2.0031 or 20.31.

24. Multiplication of decimals. The basic principle in multiplication of decimals is that the number of places to the right of the decimal point in the product (answer) is the *sum* of the decimal points in the factors (numbers being multiplied).

```
Example:  43.789 (3 places to right of decimal)
          x  .02 (2 places to right of decimal)
Product:  .87578 (3 + 2 = 5 places to right of
                 decimal)
```

25. Division of decimals

a. How would you go about determining how much of a powder to pack into each of 12 capsules to evenly divide 64.8 grains of medication? You would divide 64.8 by 12. This division is shown below.

```
     5.4
 12/64.8
    60
     48
     48
```

b. Above you have divided and placed a decimal one place from the right because there was one place in the amount of powder. Division of a decimal by another decimal is basically the same except for one modification. We know that multiplying the numerator and the denominator each by the same number has no effect on the fraction. For this reason, we can eliminate the decimal from the divisor.

(1) Example: Divide 225.6648 by 0.8.

• *Step 1.* Multiply both the numbers by 10 (simply moving the decimal one place to the right in each case): 08/2256.648.

• *Step 2.* Now the decimal will be correctly situated simply by placing it directly above the other decimal.

```
    282.081
 08/2256.648
    16
     65
     64
      16
      16
       064
       064
         08
         08
```

(2) Example: Divide 1.23456 by 0.02.

0.02/1.23456

• *Step 1.* Multiply both numbers by 100 (simply moving the decimal two places to the right in each case).

002/123.456

• *Step 2.* Now the decimal will be correctly situated simply by placing it directly above the other decimal.

```
     61.728
002/123.456
    12
     03
     02
      14
      14
       05
       04
        16
        16
```

26. Roman numerals. Roman numerals are used in writing prescriptions. They are used to specify the amounts of ingredients when the apothecary system is being used, for example, "Codeine Sulfate gr. iii." They are used to specify the number of units (capsules, tablets, powders, or suppositories) to be dispensed, for example, "Disp. xxiv." And, lastly, they are used in the signa or directions to the patient, for example, "tabs. ii stat, then i q iv h." You should therefore be thoroughly familiar with the system of Roman numerals used in pharmacy. The basic symbols or numerals are—

ss or $\overline{ss}$	1/2
i	1
v	5
x	10
L	50
C	100
D	500
M	1000

These basic numerals may be combined to represent *any* number and there are definite rules for the manner in which they are combined. The rules for Roman numerals are as follows:

a. Fractions. Except for "ss" meaning one-half (1/2), all other fractions are represented by the Arabic numeral, for example, 1/4, 3/8, 1/120.

b. Repeating numerals. Numerals may be repeated and when they are, the value of the number is repeated. Thus iii or III is 3, xxx is 30, and ccc is 300. Any numeral that would be the same as another when repeated is NOT repeated. *For example,* vv is NOT used for 10 (5 + 5) because x is 10. LL is NOT used for 100 (C = 100).

c. Smaller numerals before larger. A smaller numeral placed before a larger one is subtracted from that numeral. Only one number can be subtracted in this way. Thus iv (5 – 1) = 4, ix (10 – 1) = 9; XC (100 – 10) = 90; etc. But 3 is *never* written iiv.

d. Smaller numerals after larger. A smaller numeral placed after a larger one is added to it as viii = (5 + 3) = 8; xiii (10 + 3) = 13; CLX = (100 + 50 + 10) = 160.

e. Smaller numeral between two larger. A smaller numeral between two larger ones is ALWAYS subtracted from the larger numeral which follows it as CXL (100 + (50 – 10)) = 140; MCMLXV (1000 + (1000 – 100) + 50 + 10 + 5) = 1965.

f. Dotting the one. A dot over the numeral representing 1(i) is often used to distinguish it from a portion of the numeral v. When poorly written,\ / and v may be very similar. If the ones are dotted however,\ / can never be mistaken for 5. As a further precaution against error, the last i may be replaced by a j; 3 written in this manner would be written iij.

g. Table of Roman numerals. Table 2-1 shows Roman numerals and their equivalents. Memorize this chart. You must know these numerals as well as you do Arabic numerals.

Table 1. The Roman Numerals

ss	=	½	x	=	10	xx	=	20	li	=	51
i	=	1	xi	=	11	xxi	=	21	lix	=	59
ii	=	2	xii	=	12	xxix	=	29	lx	=	60
iii	=	3	xiii	=	13	xxx	=	30	lxx	=	70
iv	=	4	xiv	=	14	xxxi	=	31	lxxx	=	80
v	=	5	xv	=	15	xxxix	=	39	xc	=	90
vi	=	6	xvi	=	16	xl	=	40	c	=	100
vii	=	7	xvii	=	17	xli	=	41	ci	=	101
viii	=	8	xviii	=	18	xlix	=	49	cxxi	=	121
ix	=	9	xix	=	19	l	=	50	d	=	500
									m	=	1000

27. Weights and measures. Metrology is the study of measurement as applied to length, weight, and volume. During your study of pharmacy in your Army career, you will constantly be dealing with it, weighing, measuring, or transposing. To be effective, both while you are learning and while you are practicing pharmacy, you must have certain tables and equivalents *committed to memory.* The time you spend memorizing the tables of weights and measures now will be repaid with interest a hundredfold. Although there are other systems of weight and measure, there are three with which the pharmacist comes into daily contact; the metric system, apothecary system, and avoirdupois system.

28. Metric system. The metric system of weights and measures is the legal standard in the United States. All other systems are referred to it for official comparisons. It is used as the scientific system of measuring, the world over.

a. *Units of length, weight, and volume.*

(1) Meter. The standard unit of length, the meter, may be defined as a multiple (1,650,763.73) of the wave length of the light produced by a gas-discharge lamp filled with Krypton 86. This standard permits measurements to an error of 1 part in 10 million. This extreme accuracy degree is necessary in today's missile programs.

(2) Liter. The unit of volume in the metric system, the liter, is the volume occupied by a kilogram of water at its greatest density (4° C.), and weighed in a vacuum.

(3) Gram. The unit of weight, the gram, is the weight of one cubic centimeter of water at its greatest density (4° C.), and weighed in a vacuum.

NOTE

The internationally recognized symbol for a Gram is "g." This is also the symbol used by *The United States Pharmacopeia*, XVIII, and *The National Formulary*, XIII, which were published in 1970. Previously the official abbreviation for the Gram was "Gm." This was to distinguish the Gram from the grain (gr). Another commonly used abbreviation for the Gram is "gm." The change from the abbreviation "Gm" to "g." for Gram took place while this TM was being revised. The change came too late to convert all the "Gm" abbreviations in this text to "g." As a result, Gram is still abbreviated Gm. throughout even though the accepted abbreviation is "g."

b. *Advantages of the metric system.* There are several definite advantages of the metric system over the other systems–

(1) It has universal use.

(2) Every weight and measure has a simple relation to the meter.

(3) Every unit is multiplied or divided by 10 to reach the next higher or lower unit. As in our system of money, it is a system of decimal progression.

10 mills = 1 cent
10 cents = 1 dime
10 dimes = 1 dollar

(4) It is the only system of weights and measures having a common standard where a unit of weight equals a unit of volume. The common standard is water. Therefore, under the standard conditions of temperature and pressure, 10 ml. of H_2O equals 10 Gm.: 100 ml. of H_2O weighs 100 Gm.

c. *Subdivisions and multiples.* Each table of the metric system has a definite unit around which the subdivision and multiples are based; the meter for length, the liter for volume, and the gram for weight. Subdivisions and multiples of these principal units are indicated respectively by Latin and Greek prefixes.

(1) Subdivisions (from Latin).

$$\frac{1}{1000} = \text{milli}$$

$$\frac{1}{100} = \text{centi}$$

$$\frac{1}{10} = \text{deci}$$

(2) Multiples (from Greek).

10 times = Deka
100 times = Hecto
1000 times = Kilo

d. *Learning the metric system.* When you have learned the subdivisions and multiples above, the metric system will not be difficult for you to understand or to learn. Remember that it works just like our money system. Using tables 2-2, 2-3, and 2-4, those of lengths, weights, and liquid measure, memorize the metric system.

e. *Metric weights set.* Figure 2-5 depicts the standard weight set you will be using in the pharmacy. It consists of weights from 10 milligrams to 100 grams. By combining these weights, it is possible to weight substances between 10 mg. and 201 Gm. *For example,* to weigh 20.750 Gm., you would select a 20 Gm. weight, a 500 mg. weight, a 200 mg. weight, and a 50 mg. weight. The combined total of these weights is 20.750 Gm.

Table 2. Metric Table of Lengths

Lengths			Abbreviations		
10 millimeters	=	1 centimeter	10 mm.	=	1 cm
10 centimeters	=	1 decimeter	10 cm.	=	1 dm.
10 decimeters	=	1 meter	10 dm.	=	1 M.
10 Meters	=	1 Dekameter	10 M.	=	1 Dm.
10 Dekameters	=	1 Hectometer	10 Dm.	=	1 Hm.
10 Hectometers	=	1 Kilometer	10 Hm.	=	1 Km.

The metric table may also be written:

1 meter = 1000 millimeters
= 100 centimeters
= 10 decimeters
= 0.1 Dekameter
= 0.01 Hectometer
= 0.001 Kilometer

Table 3. Metric Table of Weights

Weights			Abbreviations		
10 milligrams	=	1 centigram	10 mg.	=	1 cg.
10 centigrams	=	1 decigram	10 cg.	=	1 dg.
10 decigrams	=	1 gram	10 dg.	=	1 Gm.
10 grams	=	1 Dekagram	10 Gm.	=	1 Dg.
10 Dekagrams	=	1 Hectogram	10 Dg.	=	1 Hg.
10 Hectograms	=	1 Kilogram	10 Hg.	=	1 Kg.

The metric table of weights may also be written:

1 gram = 1000 milligrams
= 100 centigrams
= 10 decigrams
= 0.1 Dekagram
= 0.01 Hectogram
= 0.001 Kilogram

Table 4. Metric Table of Liquid Measures

Liquid measures			Abbreviations		
10 milliliters	=	1 centiliter	10 ml.	=	1 cl.
10 centiliters	=	1 deciliter	10 cl.	=	1 dl.
10 deciliters	=	1 liter	10 dl.	=	1 L.
10 liters	=	1 Dekaliter	10 L.	=	1 Dl.
10 Dekaliters	=	1 Hectoliter	10 Dl.	=	1 Hl.
10 Hectoliters	=	1 Kiloliter	10 Hl.	=	1 Kl.

The metric table of liquid weights may also be written:

1 liter = 1000 milliliters
= 100 centiliters
= 10 deciliters
= 0.1 Dekaliter
= 0.01 Hectoliter
= 0.001 Kiloliter

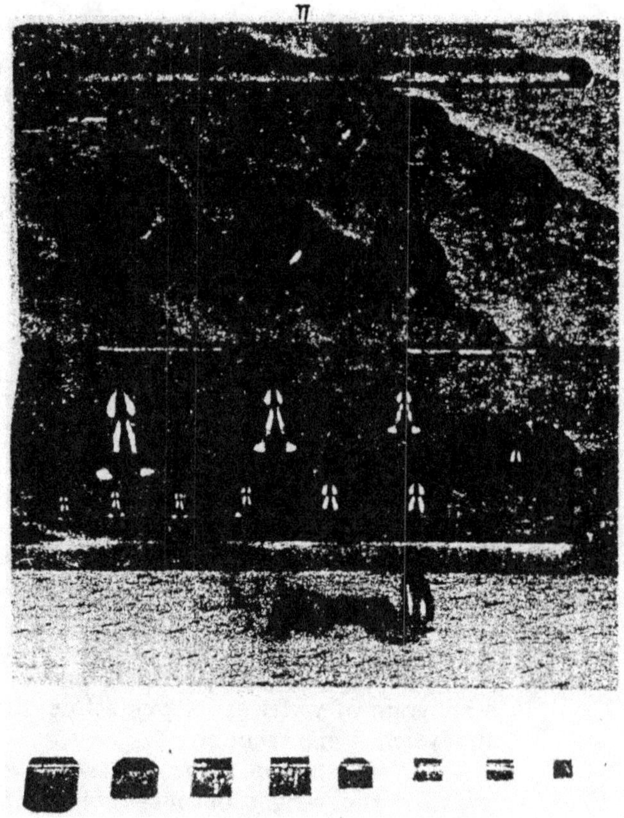

Figure 5. Metric weights.

f. Working with the weights and measures. Now that you have reviewed decimal fractions and have learned the metric system of weights and measures, apply the two as you will be using them in your job.

(1) Example: Addition and subtraction in the metric system. Suppose you dispensed the following amounts of a powder from your stock of 4000 Gm.–28 Gm., 500 mg., 14 cg., and 2 Kg. How much powder would you have remaining?

- *Step 1.* Since you are dealing with four different denominations of weight, you cannot add or subtract until you have a common unit to work with. Since you want the answer in grams (your shelf stock having been specified in grams), it will be simplest to convert all the quantities to grams as follows:

28 Gm. = 28.0 Gm.
500 mg. = .5 Gm.
14 cg. = .14 Gm.
2 Kg. = 2000.0 Gm.
= 2028.64 Gm. amount dispensed

- *Step 2.* You started with 4000 Gm. and dispensed a total of 2028.64 Gm., so by subtracting you will determine the balance on hand. Therefore:

```
  4000.00 Gm.
– 2028.64 Gm.
  1971.36 Gm. remaining
```

NOTE

The same method is applied to liquid measure. How many ml. of alcohol would remain if you dispensed 240 from an original liter?

```
1 liter =  1000 ml.
         –  240 ml.
            760 ml. remaining
```

(2) Example: Multiplication. How many grams of powder would be necessary to manufacture 20 capsules, each containing 300 mg.?

```
  300 mg.
x  20
 6000 mg. = 6.0 Gm.
```

(3) Example: Division. How many 30 ml. bottles of cough syrup can you dispense if you have 3 liters of the syrup on hand?

3 liters = 3000 ml.

3000 ÷ 30 = 100 bottles, answer

29. Apothecary system. Although the Army requires that all Army prescriptions be written in the metric system, the pharmacy technician must also be able to use the apothecary system. In civil practice the apothecary system is widely used and consequently many formulas are specified in terms of apothecary units. Many of the ready-made pharmaceuticals have strength and dosage listed in the apothecary system. Further, you will be filling prescriptions written by civilian prescribers who will use the apothecary system for quantity and dosage. In previous editions of the USP (Revision xiv and before), dosage of the official preparations was listed as an approximation of the apothecary system. The dosage is now completely in the metric system, the apothecary system being completely eliminated.

a. Units of weight and volume.

(1) Apothecary weight. The basic unit in the apothecary system of weight is the grain, which is approximately 64.8 mg. Divisions of the grain are expressed as fractions, for example, $\frac{1}{60}$ gr. Prescriptions will be written with a symbol for the weight denomination and a Roman numeral for the amount of that denomination. Study the table of apothecary weights and abbreviations (table 2-5). Thus, in prescriptions written in the apothecary system, you will see the following written:

℈iii   ʒii   gr iiss   ℥viii

Table 5. Apothecary Weights and Abbreviations

Apothecary weights					Abbreviations		
20 grains	=	1 scruple			gr. xx	=	℈i
3 scruples	=	1 drachm	=	60 grains	℈ iii	=	ʒi
8 drachms	=	1 ounce	=	480 grains	ʒviii	=	℥i
12 ounces	=	1 pound	=	5760 grains	℥xii	=	1 lb.

(2) Apothecary liquid measure. The basic unit of the apothecary system of fluid measure is the minim (♏). Study the table of apothecary liquid measure below in table 2-6. Prescriptions are written with a symbol for the denomination to be used. Thus in prescriptions written in the apothecary system for liquids, you will see quantities such as the following:

f ℥ ss   f ʒ ¼   ♏xii   f ℥ viii

(3) Apothecary weights. Apothecary weights used in pharmacy are of two types—cylindrical weights and coin weights.

(a) Apothecary cylindrical weights. The apothecary cylindrical weights are

Table 6. Apothecary Fluid Measure and Abbreviations

Apothecary fluid measure					Abbreviation		
60 minims	=	1 fluidrachm	=		♏lx	=	fʒi
8 fluidrachm	=	1 fluidounce	=	480 minims	fʒviii	=	f℥i
16 fluidounce	=	1 pint	=	7,680 minims	f℥vxi	=	Oi
2 pints	=	1 quart	=	82 fluidounces	Oii	=	qt i
4 quarts	=	1 gallon	=	128 fluidounces	qt iv	=	Ci

similar to the metric weights depicted in figure 2-5. They usually range from one-half scruple to two drachms. The set contains grain weights in the form of wires; the number of sides indicates the number of grains (fig. 2-6).

(b) Apothecary coin weights. Coin-type weights which have the weight embossed on their surfaces are particularly subject to error and should not be used.

b. Converting between denominations. It is often convenient to express a weight or measure in its equivalent in a lower or higher denomination. This can be easily accomplished by either multiplying or dividing the weight by the number of units that equals either the higher or lower measure.

(1) Example: Express 3/4 quart in its lowest terms in the apothecary system.

- *Step 1.* Since 2 pints = 1 quart; 2 x 3/4 = 1 1/2 pints which can be expressed–pt ii x qt 3/4 = pt iss.

- *Step 2.* Put aside and save the whole number, the one pint, and break the fraction to its next lowest terms.

1 pint = 16 fluidounces
so, 16 fluidounces x 1/2 = 8 fluidounces
or, f℥xvi x pt ss = f℥viii

- *Step 3.* Continue in this manner, changing each remaining fraction to the next lower denomination. In this case, however, you need go no further, 8 ounces is even. Now you have the whole pint saved from step 2, which equals 16 ounces plus the 8 ounces from step 3, or a total of 24 fluidounces for the answer.

(2) Example: Express 2/5 gallon in its lowest apothecary terms.

- *Step 1.* 1 gallon = 8 pints.

8 x 2/5 = 3 1/5 pt
or, pt viii = gal i
pt viii x gal 2/5 = pt iii 1/5

- *Step 2.* Continue in this manner, saving the whole and breaking the fraction to its next lowest terms:

fl℥xvi x pt 1/5 = f℥iii 1/5
flʒxviii x fl℥1/5 = flʒi 3/5
♏lx x flʒ3/5 = ♏xxxvi

- *Step 3.* Putting the numbers previously saved together in sequence, you arrive at the answer: 2/5 gallons = 3 pints, 3 fluidounces, 1 fluidrachm, and 36 minims; or gallon 2/5 = Oiii, fl ℥ iii, fl ʒ i, ♏xxxvi.

(3) Example: In order to proceed from a lower measure to highest terms, the procedure is just opposite. Divide the measure by the number of units of that measure that equals one unit of the next higher measure. Express 57,688 minims in its highest terms.

- *Step 1.* 60 minims = 1 fluidrachm, therefore

```
       961 ——→ 961 flʒ
  60/57688
     540
      368
      360
        88
        60
        28 ——→ 28 minims
```

Save the minims left over and break down the fluidrachms.

- *Step 2.* 8 fluidrachms = 1 fluidounce, therefore

```
    120 ——→ 120 fl℥
  8/961
    8
    16
    16
     01
      0
      1 ——→ 1 fluid ʒ
```

Save the fluidrachms and break down the fluidounces.

- *Step 3.* 16 fluidounces = 1 pint, therefore

```
        7 ——→ 7 pints
  16/120
     112
       8 ——→ 8 fluidounces
```

Save the fluidounces and change the pints to the next higher value (quarts).

- *Step 4.* 2 fluid pints = 1 fluid quart, therefore

```
    3 ——→ 3 quarts
  2/7
    6
    1 ——→ 1 pint
```

- *Step 5.* Now, combine the various quantities you have saved in previous steps. Your answer is:

57,688 minims = 3 qts, 1 pt, 8 f℥ , 1 fʒ , 28 minims.

(4) Checking your answers. You can check your answers in both procedures by just reversing the procedure.

• In example (2), you converted 2/5 gallon to 3 pints, 3 fluidounces, 1 fluidrachm, and 36 minims. Going in reverse to check the accuracy:

60 minims = 1 fluidrachm

$\frac{36}{60}$ minims = 3/5 fluidrachm

3/5 + 1 = 1 3/5 fluidrachms

8 fluidrachms = 1 fluidounce

1 3/5 fluidrachms = 1/5 fluidounce

1/5 + 3 = 3 1/5 fluidounces

16 fluidounces = 1 pint

3 1/5 fluidounces = 1/5 pint

1/5 + 3 = 3 1/5 pints

8 pints = 1 gallon

3 1/5 pints = 2/5 gallon—the answer checks.

• In example (3), you converted 57,688 minims to 7 pints, 8 fluidounces, 1 fluidrachm, and 28 minims. To check this answer, you again proceed in reverse.

7 pt, 8 fl℥ , 1 flʒ + 28 minims ⟶ 28 minims

7 pt, 8 fl℥ , 1 flʒ

1 flʒ = 60 minims ⟶ 60 minims

7 pt, 8 fl℥

8 fl℥ = 64 flʒ (8 × 8)

64 flʒ = ⟶ 3,840 minims

(64 × 60)

7 pt = 112 fl℥ = 896 flʒ = ⟶ 53,760 minims

(112 × 8) (896 × 60)

adding the columns of minims ⟶ 57,688 minims

our answer checks.

c. Addition and subtraction. The arithmetic involved in the apothecary system is slightly more involved than that of the metric system. In the metric system, the units increase by multiples of ten. However, the apothecary system has no uniform scale of variation. You are again confronted with the problem that quantities of like denomination must be added or subtracted first, then converted to lowest terms. To illustrate this, look at the following addition problem.

(1) Example:

4 lb, 3℥ , 4ʒ , 1℈ , 18 gr.
+ 8 lb, 2℥ , 3ʒ , 2℈ , 19 gr.

• *Step 1.* By simple addition, adding pounds to pounds, ounces to ounces, you get—

4 lb, 3℥ , 4ʒ , 1℈ , 18 gr.
+ 8 lb, 2℥ , 3ʒ , 2℈ , 19 gr.
12 lb, 5℥ , 7ʒ , 3℈ , 37 gr.

• *Step 2.* This answer is not in its reduced terms, because 37 grains equals one scruple plus 17 grains, 3 scruples equal a drachm, and so on. To reduce this answer, begin at the right and work to the left, changing each quantity possible to the next higher denomination. Twenty grains equals one scruple, leaving 17 grains and adding 1 scruple to the 3 previously in the column. Likewise, since there are 3 scruples to the drachm, you must convert 3 of the 4 scruples you now have in this column to 1 drachm, leaving 1 ℈ and increasing the drachms to 8. There being 8 drachms to the ounce, you have no drachms remaining, but increase the ounces to 6. The final reduced answer then beomes 12 lb, 6℥ , 1℈ , 17 gr.

(2) Example: Subtract 4 lb, 6℈ , 4ʒ , 1℈ , 19 gr. from 6 lb, 8℥ , 5ʒ , 2℈ , 15 gr.

• *Step 1.* Set up for subtraction.

6 lb, 8℥ , 5ʒ , 2℈ , 15 gr.
− 4 lb, 6℥ , 4ʒ , 1℈ , 19 gr.

Since you could not take 19 grains from 15 grains, it is necessary to convert one scruple to grains, reducing the number of scruples in the upper figure to 1 and increasing the grains to 35. You may never have a negative number in subtracting weights and measures.

• *Step 2.* Having converted the scruple to grains, your problem becomes:

6 lb, 8℥ , 5ʒ , 1℈ , 35 gr.
− 4 lb, 6℥ , 4ʒ , 1℈ , 19 gr.
2 lb, 2℥ , 1ʒ , 0℈ , 16 gr.

d. Multiplication and division.

(1) Example: Multiplication. Multiplication of compound numbers such as arise in the apothecary system may be accomplished in several ways, the easiest of which is to multiply each denomination individually, then reduce the answer. Multiply 2 gal, 3 qt, 1 pt, 9 f℥ , 7 fʒ , 18 min. by 6.

• *Step 1.*

2 gal, 3 qt, 1 pt, 9 f℥ , 7 fʒ , 81 min.
× 6
12 gal, 18 qt, 6 pt, 54 f℥ , 42 fʒ , 108 min.

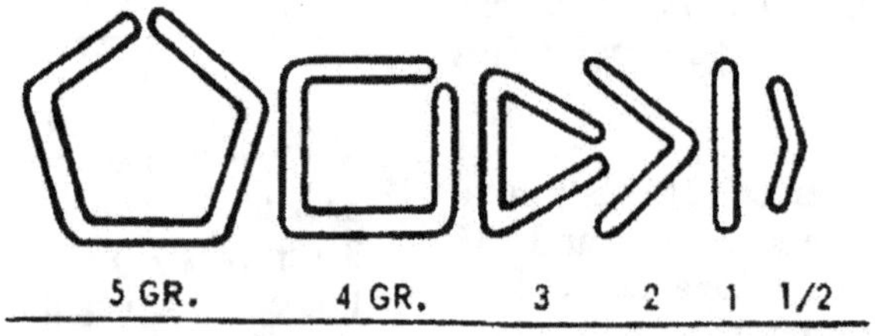

Figure 6. Apothecary grain weights.

Table 7. Approximate Equivalents

Weight

Metric	Approx apothecary	Metric	Approx apothecary	Metric	Approx apothecary
0.1 mg.	1/600 gr.	6 mg.	1/10 gr.	0.1 Gm.	1-1/2 gr.
0.2 mg.	1/300 gr.	8 mg.	1/8 gr.	0.12 Gm.	2 gr.
0.3 mg.	1/200 gr.	10 mg.	1/6 gr.	0.15 Gm.	2-1/2 gr.
0.4 mg.	1/150 gr.	12 mg.	1/5 gr.	0.2 Gm.	3 gr.
0.5 mg.	1/120 gr.	15 mg.	1/4 gr.	0.3 Gm.	5 gr.
0.6 mg.	1/100 gr.	20 mg.	1/3 gr.	0.5 Gm.	7-1/2 gr.
1 mg.	1/60 gr.	25 mg.	3/8 gr.	0.6 Gm.	10 gr.
1.2 mg.	1/50 gr.	30 mg.	1/2 gr.	1 Gm.	15 gr.
2 mg.	1/30 gr.	50 mg.	3/4 gr.	1.5 Gm.	22 gr.
3 mg.	1/20 gr.	60 mg.	1 gr.	2 Gm.	30 gr.
4 mg.	1/15 gr.	75 mg.	1-1/4 gr.	3 Gm.	45 gr.
5 mg.	1/12 gr.	90 mg.	1-1/2 gr.	4 Gm.	60 gr. (1 drachm)
				5 Gm.	75 gr.
				7.5 Gm.	2 drachms
				15 Gm.	4 drachms
				30 Gm.	1 ounce

Liquid Measure

Metric	Approx apothecary	Metric	Approx apothecary	Metric	Approx apothecary
0.03 ml.	1/2 minim	0.6 ml.	10 minims	15 ml.	4 f. drachms (1/2 oz)
0.05 ml.	3/4 minim	0.75 ml.	12 minims	30 ml.	1 f. ounce
0.06 ml.	1 minim	1 ml.	15 minims	60 ml.	2 f. ounces
0.1 ml.	1-1/2 minims	2 ml.	30 minims	120 ml.	4 f. ounces
0.2 ml.	3 minims	3 ml.	45 minims	250 ml.	8 f. ounces
0.25 ml.	4 minims	4 ml.	60 minims	500 ml.	16 f. ounces (1 pint)
0.3 ml.	5 minims	5 ml.	1 f. drachm	1000 ml.	1 quart
0.5 ml.	8 minims	10 ml.	2 f. drachms		

N.B. These are *approximate* equivalents. They may be used to compare prepared dosage forms such as tablets, capsules, and solutions. For converting *specific* quantities as are called for in formulas, use the exact equivalents provided in the U.S.P. For prescription compounding, use the exact equivalents rounded to 3 significant figures.

• *Step 2.* Simply reduce the above answer to the lowest terms as previously explained.

17 gal, 2 qt, 1 pt, 11f℥ , 3fʒ , 48 min.

(2) Example: Division (usual method). Division of compound numbers is best done by dividing the highest measure first, keeping the whole number obtained and converting any remainder to the next smaller denomination and adding it to the given quantity. Then continue the division. Divide 8 gal, 2 qt, 1 pt by 3.

• *Step 1.*

8 gal ÷ 3 = 2 gal (+ 2 gal remainder)
2 gal = 8 qt + original 2 qt = 10 qt.

• *Step 2.*

10 qt ÷ 3 = 3 qt (+ 1 qt remainder)
1 qt = 2 pt + original 1 pt + 3 pt.

• *Step 3.*

3 pt ÷ 3 = 1 pt.

• *Step 4.* Add the products from all steps (not the remainders!).

2 gal, 3 qt, 1 pt, answer.

(3) Example: Division (alternate method). An alternate method is to convert the amounts to their lowest form; in this case, pints, then convert back to highest terms after dividing. Divide 8 gal, 2 qt, 1 pt by 3.

• *Step 1.*

8 gal = 64 pt
2 qt = 4 pt
1 pt = 1 pt
total = 69 pt

• *Step 2.* Divide.

69 ÷ 3 = 23 pt

• *Step 3.* Convert back to highest terms.

23 pt = 11 qt, 1 pt
11 qt = 2 gal, 3 qt
2 gal, 3 qt, 1 pt, answer.

30. Avoirdupois system. In the United States all items sold by weight are commercially bought and sold by avoirdupois weight. Exceptions to this rule include gems and precious metals. The weight which appears on a scale when you weigh yourself is avoirdupois weight. Unless expressly stated, all drugs and chemicals are bought and sold by avoirdupois weight. Therefore, it is *extremely* important to note that in receiving narcotics from the warehouse, an ounce bottle contains 437.5 grains (avoirdupois ounce), not 480 grains (apothecary ounce). As you can readily see, serious error could result in your narcotic records if you did not understand this principle. The grain is common to BOTH the avoirdupois and the apothecary system, *but* the ounces and pounds are different. Study the comparison below.

Apothecary ounce = 480.0 grains
Avoirdupois ounce 437.5 grains
= 42.5 grains *difference*

Apothecary pound = 12 oz x 480 grains = 5760 grains
Avoirdupois pound = 16 oz x 437.5 grains = 7000 grains
1240 grains *difference*

31. Relationship and approximate equivalents. The metric system, apothecary system, and avoirdupois system are all used extensively by the pharmacy technician. Because you have and use three separate systems of weight and measure, it is necessary to understand their relationship and know how to convert from one to the other quickly and accurately.

a. Some relationships to remember.

• *Remember:* The pharmacist receives drugs and chemicals by avoirdupois weight at 437.5 grains per ounce, 16 ounces per pound.

• *Remember:* The pharmacist dispenses prescriptions in the metric or apothecary system. The apothecary system has 480 grains per ounce and only 12 ounces per pound.

• *Remember:* One apothecary fluidounce (H_2O) weighs 454.6 grains at 25° C. There are 480 minims in an apothecary fluidounce. It follows, then, that 1 minim of water at 25° C. weighs $\frac{454.6}{480} = 0.95$ grains.

b. Approximate equivalents. Table 2-7 should be thoroughly memorized. These equivalents will allow conversion between systems with a *relative degree of accuracy.* A facsimile of this table should be conspicuously placed near the work area in your pharmacy as a reference and check.

c. Exact conversion. Exact accuracy in conversion from one system to another as is needed for compounding prescriptions cannot be accomplished using approximate equivalents. Nearly exact conversion equivalents are given in a table in the USP.

32. **Ratio and proportion**

a. Ratio. Ratio is an expression of the relationship of one thing to another. For the purpose of arithmetic, ratio is the relation showing the amount by which one thing is different from another. Thus, if you have a solution of 9 grams of sodium chloride in 1000 grams of water, the ratio of NaCl to water is 9:1000 or $\frac{9}{1000}$, and is read "9 to 1000." The value of a ratio is the number obtained by dividing the first term (antecedent) by the second term (consequent); therefore, the value of 12:4 is 3.

(1) Ratios remain constant. Multiplying or dividing BOTH terms of a ratio does not change its value. Therefore, multiplying both terms of 10:5 by 5 gives us 50:25. In either case, the ratio is the same, 2:1. The terms of a ratio taken together are called a couplet.

(2) Equal units. Ratio can exist only between numbers of the same unit value—as ratio of percent to percent or weight to weight—but never weight to percent. (*Exception:* In pharmacy, we often make solutions which are expressed as weight to volume.) The comparing of numbers of the same unit volume follows as certainly as apples can be compared to apples and oranges to oranges, but never oranges to apples.

(3) Examples of ratio problems:

- What is the value of the ratio 10:100? Divide the first term by the second to get 1/10.
- Simplify 6:36. Divide both terms by 6 to get 1:6.
- What is the ratio between 18 percent and 9 grams? No ratio! Percent cannot be compared to grams.
- What do the following three ratios have in common? 1:5, 3:15, 5:25. When simplified, each is 1:5 or 1/5.

b. Proportion. 15:3 :: 10:2 is a proportion. It is read "15 is to 3 as 10 is to 2." Proportion is a means of showing equality between ratios. 15 ÷ 3 = 5 and 10 ÷ 2 = 5; they have the same value. The first and fourth terms of a proportion are called the *extremes* and the second and third terms are called the *means.* In the example cited above, 15 and 2 are the extremes; 3 and 10 are the means. The product of the extremes (15 x 2) equals the product of the means (3 x 10).

(1) Example: 50:10 :: 25:5
50 x 5 = 250;
10 x 25 = 250.

Thus, it is apparent that if one of the numbers were an unknown, it could easily be determined as follows:

(2) Example: If it takes 50 grains of powder to make 5 capsules, how many grains are necessary to make 3 capsules? This problem is nothing more than a proportion in which one of the terms is an unknown.

50:x :: 5:3
5x = 150 (arrived at by multiplying the means and extremes)
x = 30 grains, answer (to make 3 capsules)

It is customary to let x or y represent the unknown number in proportions. Thus you find that 30 grains would be necessary to make 3 capsules.

(3) Example: Rule of Words. Putting this example into a rule of words—"To find either extreme, multiply the means (2nd and 3rd numbers) and divide by the known extreme." Likewise, "To find either mean, multiply the extremes (1st and 4th numbers) and divide by the known mean." Notice how you progress from a statement of problem to a written proportion. If 500 Gm. of a salt solution contains 10 percent salt, to what weight must you evaporate the solution to make it 20 percent salt?

- *Step 1.* Write down the facts.

500 Gm. is 10%
? Gm. is 20%

• *Step 2.* Let x represent the unknown (?) quantity. Arbitrarily, let x take the fourth position.

• *Step 3.* Since we can compare only like articles, put the number with the same denomination as x in the third position.

• *Step 4.* Determine if the unknown is to be larger or smaller than the third number. In the preceding example, you are evaporating a solution and thus it will be smaller. Since the smaller follows the larger in the 3rd and 4th positions, the *same* must hold true of the 1st and 2d. Therefore, the larger number will be in first position, and the smaller in second position.

• *Step 5.* From the preceding 4 steps, you may conclude that–

$$20:10 :: 500:x$$

• *Step 6.* Cross multiply (multiply the means and extremes).

$$20\,x = 5000$$

• *Step 7.* Solve for x.

$$x = 5000 \div 20$$

x = 250 Gm., the weight of the 20% solution, answer.

33. Percentage preparations. Many of the calculations you will be required to make in the pharmacy will be for the compounding and dispensing of percentage preparations (solutions or powders). The most important factor to keep in mind here is that *slight* errors in dilute preparations may be considered negligible, whereas even a slight error in a concentrated preparation may be serious. To firmly impress this in your mind, consider the difference between losing one quarter from your pocket containing ten quarters and losing ten quarters from another pocket containing 100 quarters. The loss in each case is 10 percent. In the first instance, 10 percent loss amounted to only 25 cents, while in the second instance the 10 percent loss amounted to $2.50. Thus, as the percentage of a solution or other preparation becomes greater, the error becomes more severe. The strength of a solution is the ratio of active ingredient to solvent and can be expressed as a percent or as a ratio.

a. Percent solutions. The Latin "per centum" literally means "by hundreds." Ten percent, then, refers to 10 hundreds or 10 parts out of 100 parts. A 10-percent solution could be broken down as follows:

Total volume of solution – 100% or 100 parts
Solute (active ingredient) – 10% or 10 parts
Solvent – 90% or 90 parts

In solutions of solids or gases in a liquid, the solid or gas being dissolved is called the solute, and the liquid is the solvent. In solution of liquids in liquids, we arbitrarily say that the liquid present in greater quantity is the solvent and the liquid of lesser quantity is the solute. Thus we say that in mixing 25 percent water and 75 percent alcohol, we obtain a solution of water in alcohol. Reversing the situation, 25 percent alcohol and 75 percent water, we would term a solution of alcohol in water.

(1) Variable meaning of percentage. Percentage in solutions can have different meanings under different circumstances. In solution, you are dealing with solids which are weighed, and liquids which can be weighed or measured; thus, it is necessary to define the expression of percentage concentration of solutions. There are three different percentage solutions:

(a) Percent weight in weight (w/w)–expresses the number of grams of a constituent in 100 grams of solution.

(b) Percent weight in volume (w/v)–expresses the number of grams of a constituent in 100 ml. of solution, and is used in prescription practice regardless of whether water or another liquid is used.

(c) Percent volume in volume (v/v)–expresses the number of milliliters of a constituent in 100 ml. of solution.

(2) Rules for percentage solutions. Unless specifically stipulated otherwise, the following rules hold true for prescriptions of percentage solutions:

- Mixtures of solids are weight in weight.
- Solids in liquids are weight in volume.
- Liquids in liquids are volume in volume.
- Gases in liquids are weight in volume.

For example, to make a 10-percent solution, dissolve 10 Gm. of a solid or 10 ml. of a liquid in the amount of solvent necessary (qs) to make 100 ml. of finished solution. In the apothecary system, 45.6 grains of a solid or 48 minims of a liquid dissolved in enough solvent to make 1 fluidounce would yield a 10-percent solution. Slight changes in volume attributable to changes in room temperature are negligible and may be disregarded.

b. Percent weight in volume solutions. Weight in volume (w/v) percentage may be called the "key" to percentage and ratio solutions. You are dissolving a weight of solid in a volume of liquid (water, unless otherwise specified).

(1) Metric system rule. Multiply the specified percentage, expressed as a decimal fraction, times the required number of ml. The resulting number will represent the number of grams of solid in the solution, or percent (decimal) x ml. = grams solute.

(2) Apothecary system rule. Multiply the percent, expressed as a whole number times 4.5457 times fluidounces of solution required. The answer you obtain will be the number of grains of solute to be used. The weight of 1 fluidounce of water at 25° C. is 454.57 grains. Therefore, 4.5457 grains is the amount of solute necessary to prepare a 1-percent solution of 1 ounce. Expressed as a formula, this rule becomes percent (whole number) x 4.5457 x fl oz. required = grains of solute.

(3) Example: Prepare 300 ml. of 20-percent (w/v) solution of sodium thiosulfate. How many grams of solute are necessary? How much solvent is used?

- *Step 1.* Formula.
  % (decimal) x ml. = grams solute

- *Step 2.* Substitute.
  .20 x 300 = 60 grams of solute

- *Step 3.* Since the total solution is to be 300 ml., you add enough water to the 60 grams of solute to make the finished product measure 300 ml. If you assumed that 60 grams took up 60 ml. of volume, you could deduce that 240 ml. of liquid added to the 60 grams of solute would make 300 ml. This does not hold true. Many solids when dissolved do not take up a volume equal to their weight, so you must always add enough water to make the volume up to the required amount. This bringing up to the required volume is expressed in prescriptions as "qs ad" from the Latin, and means "add a sufficient quantity."

(4) Example: Work this similar problem in the apothecary system. Make ℥ iv (4 fluidounces) of a 20-percent solution of sodium thiosulfate.

- *Step 1.* Formula.
  % x 4.5457 x fl. oz. = grains of solute.

- *Step 2.* Substitute.
  20 x 4.5457 x 4 = 363.6 grains = (ʒ vi gr iiiss)

The prescription could have been written:

Rx Sod. Thiosulfate grs 363.6
Pur. Water qs ad ℥ iv.

c. Percent volume in volume solutions. To calculate percentage of solutions of one liquid in another, multiply the desired percent, as a decimal fraction, of the active ingredient times the amount of total solution desired.

Example: How many ml. of an active ingredient must be used to produce 480 ml. of a 3-percent solution?

480 x .03 = 34.4 ml., answer

d. Percent weight in weight solution. In some cases, a definite finished weight of solution is required. To find the percent of solid in the solution, multiply the total weight of the finished solution desired by the percent desired, expressed as a decimal. Written as a formula this would be–Gm. total solution x % (decimal) = Gm. of active solute. By subtracting this weight (the weight of the solute) from the weight of the total solution, the weight of the liquid required as solvent is found. This weight may be converted to volume by dividing the weight of liquid required by the specific gravity of the liquid. Specific gravity will be discussed below.

(1) Example: How many grams of acriflavine are required to manufacture 200 Gm. of a 10-percent (w/w) solution? How much glycerin will you use as the solvent? Express the amount of glycerin in both weight and volume (Sp. Gr. glycerin = 1.25).

200 x 0.10 = 20 Gm. acriflavine
200 – 20 = 180 Gm. glycerin
180 ÷ 1.25 = 144 ml. glycerin

(2) Example: Prepare 4 fluidounces of a 10-percent (w/w) solution of acriflavine in glycerin. This problem takes on more difficulty in the apothecary system. First reduce the total weight of solution to grains.

- *Step 1.* Reduce solution to grains.
  4 fl oz x 454.6 = 1818.4 grains (total solution)

- *Step 2.* 10 % of 1818.4 = 181.84 grains of acriflavine.

- *Step 3.* 1818.4 – 181.84 = 1636.56 grains of glycerin.

- *Step 4.* 1 fl oz of water weighs 454.6 grains; therefore, 1 fluidounce of glycerin weighs 454.6 x 1.25 = 568.25 gr.

- *Step 5.* Since you need 1636.56 grains of glycerin, by dividing this by the number of grains of glycerin in a fluidounce, you will obtain the volume of glycerin required in terms of fluidounces.

1636.56 ÷ 568.25 = 2.88 fluidounces or
f℥ ii fʒ vii ♏ ii

34. Ratio preparations. Ratio is similar to percent, the entire solution is the total, the active ingredient is a certain part of the total, and the solvent or diluent is the remainder. Ratio solutions are expressed as so much in so much; for example, 1 in 10; 1 in 100; 1 in 1000. It means exactly what it says, 1 part in a total of 10 parts, or 1 part in a total of 100 parts; it does not mean 1 part plus 10 parts to give 11 parts. It is obvious that a 1 in 10 solution, therefore, is identical to a 10 percent solution. A ratio solution is expressed by parts—so many parts in a total of so many parts; 1 part in 10 parts = 1 in 10. The number of parts of active ingredient is taken as 1, and the total parts possible is variable as in 1 in 10, 1 in 20, 1 in 100. You remember in percentage, the total mixture was always 100 and the active part was variable, as 10 percent (10/100), 20 percent (20/100), or 50 percent (50/100).

a. Weight in volume solution by ratio. The following proportion is used in making ratio solutions of the weight in volume type.

$$\frac{\text{weight of solute}}{\text{wt of given volume of solution if it were water}} :: \frac{\text{one part of solute}}{\text{No. of parts of completed solution containing 1 part of solute}}$$

(1) Example: What is the ratio strength (w/v) of a solution containing 25 Gm. of solute in 250 ml. of solution?
Substitute in the preceding formula.

$$\frac{25}{250} :: \frac{1}{x}$$

$$25x = 250$$

x = 10; ratio strength, then, is 1 in 10 (1/10)

Using this formula, any one of the four parts can be found, if the other three are known.

(2) Example: If the ratio strength (w/v) of a solution is 1:25, and it contains 50 Gm. of solute, what is the total volume of the solution? Substitute:

$$\frac{50}{x} :: \frac{1}{25}$$

x = 1250 ml., the total volume of solution.

b. Volume in volume solution by ratio. Again, a simple proportion can be used to solve this type of problem.

$$\frac{\text{vol. of ingredient}}{\text{vol. of total solution}} :: \frac{\text{parts of ingredient}}{\text{parts of whole}}$$

CAUTION

The two volumes concerned *must* be expressed in the same denomination; that is, if one is expressed in ml., the other must also be ml.

(1) Example: What amount of active ingredient must be used to produce 500 ml. of a solution (v/v) with a ratio strength of 1:20? Substitute:

$$\frac{x}{500} :: \frac{1}{20}$$

$$20x = 500$$

x = 25 ml., answer

(2) Example: What is the ratio strength of a solution which contains 5 ml. of active ingredient in a total of 250 ml.? Substitute:

$$\frac{5}{250} :: \frac{1}{x}$$

$$5x = 250$$

$$x = 50$$

strength is 1 in 50 (1:50)

c. Weight to weight solution by ratio. For w/w solutions, two proportions may be expressed;

one shows the relationship between active ingredient and the total solution, the other between ingredient and diluent.

$$\frac{\text{wt ingredient}}{\text{wt mixture}} :: \frac{\text{parts of ingredient}}{\text{parts total mixture}}$$

or

$$\frac{\text{wt ingredient}}{\text{wt diluent}} :: \frac{\text{parts of ingredient}}{\text{parts of diluent}}$$

(1) Example: What is the weight in grams of a 1:10,000 (w/w) solution containing 150 mg. of active ingredient? Substituting in first formula:

$$\frac{150}{x} = \frac{1}{10{,}000}$$

$$x = 1{,}500{,}000 \text{ mg.}$$

$$x = 1500 \text{ Gm. (wt of solution)}$$

(2) Example: If 8 Gm. of a substance is dissolved in 128 ml. of water, what is the w/w ratio strength of the solution? Substituting in second formula:

$$\frac{8}{128} :: \frac{1}{x}$$

$$8x = 128$$

$$x = 16$$

1 in 16 (1:16)

35. Specific gravity. Specific gravity, abbreviated Sp. Gr., is the relation between the weights of two substances, one of which is a standard. Determination of Sp. Gr. is accomplished under specific conditions, namely, 25° C. and normal barometric pressure. Distilled water is the standard for liquids and solids, and air for gases. Specific gravity is always expressed as a decimal; the standard substance has a Sp. Gr. of 1.000. Comparing equal volumes of glycerin and water, for example, we find that glycerin is 1-1/4 times as heavy. Since the Sp. Gr. of water is 1.000, the Sp. Gr. of glycerin is 1.250.

36. Specific gravity of liquids. There are several instruments used for determination of the specific gravity of liquids. We will discuss only two here, the pycnometer and the hydrometer.

a. Pycnometer. The pycnometer (fig. 2-7) is a specific gravity bottle. Pycnometer is derived from the Greek word pykno, meaning dense, and meter, meaning measure. It is, therefore, a device for measuring density. Any small, long-necked flask made of thin glass will serve as a pycnometer. It is preferable for simplicity of calculation that the pycnometer hold some simple unit volume of

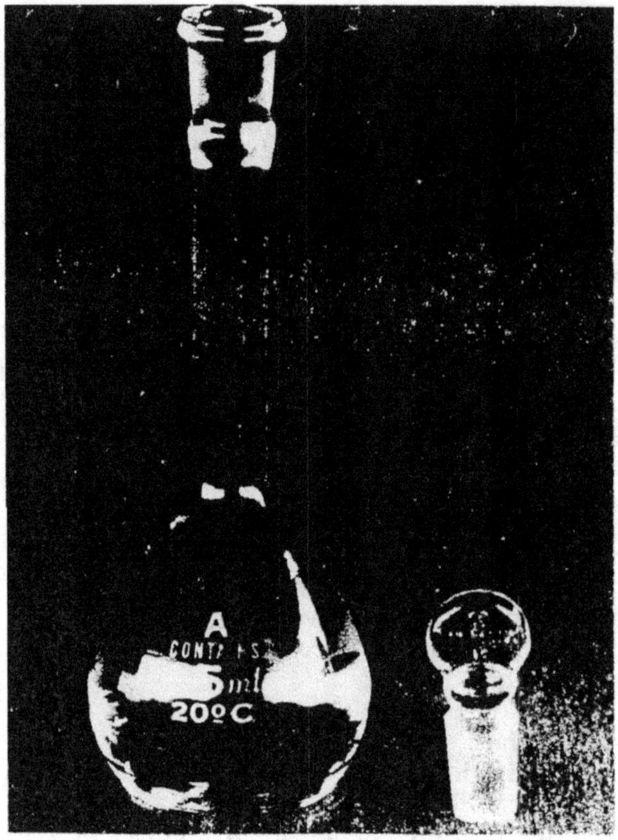

Figure 7. The pycnometer.

water, 25 Gm., 50 Gm., or 100 Gm. You will see the benefit of this in the following paragraphs. To find specific gravity using a pycnometer, proceed as follows:

(1) First, we must know the exact weight of the empty pycnometer. This is called the "tare" or "tare weight." Since dirt and moisture will affect this tare weight, it is important that the vessel be clean and dry. Make a note of the tare weight.

(2) Distilled water is then poured into the pycnometer until it reaches a convenient level in the neck. A line is marked on the pycnometer at the level of the lower edge of the meniscus (concave or convex surface of the liquid).

(3) Note the temperature of the water and record it. Now carefully weigh the pycnometer and its contents and record the combined weight.

(4) The weight of the water alone can be calculated by subtracting the tare weight of the pycnometer from the combined weight recorded in step *(3)* above. This is the weight of the water at the recorded temperature. The tare weight, temperature, and weight of the water may be permanently etched on the side of the flask for

future calculations. These figures will remain constant for all future specific gravity determinations.

(5) When the flask is again clean and dry, the specific gravity of any liquid may be taken by filling it to the same point with the liquid to be tested.

(6) Weigh the pycnometer, now containing a liquid to be tested, and subtract the tare weight of the vessel. The number resulting will be the weight of the liquid you are testing.

(7) Determine the specific gravity by substituting in this formula:

$$\text{Sp. Gr.} = \frac{\text{weight of known volume of substance}}{\text{weight of equal volume of distilled water}}$$

(8) Example: A pycnometer weighs 20.123 Gm. when clean and dry. When filled to a convenient level with water at 25° C., it weighs 44.678 Gm. The same bottle filled to the same level with glycerin at 25° C. weighs 50.816 Gm. What is the specific gravity of the glycerin?

• *Step 1.*

weight of glycerin + bottle	=	50.816 Gm.
minus tare weight of bottle		– 20.123 Gm.
the weight of glycerin		30.693 Gm.

• *Step 2.*

weight of water + bottle	=	44.678 Gm.
minus tare weight of bottle		– 20.123 Gm.
the weight of water		24.555 Gm.

• *Step 3.* Formula:

$$\text{Sp. Gr.} = \frac{\text{weight substance}}{\text{weight equal volume of water}}$$

• *Step 4.*

$$\text{Sp. Gr.} = \frac{30.693}{24.555} = 1.25 \text{ the Sp. Gr. of glycerin}$$

b. Hydrometer. The hydrometer is an instrument which gives us a quick but not as accurate a determination of specific gravity as the pycnometer. It can also be used to measure density of liquids and percent of solutions, such as the alcoholic content of liquids or the radiator of an automobile. The hydrometer consists of a closed glass tube, blown at one end and having a long stem at the other. The blown end is filled with a heavy weight (usually mercury or shot) to keep it erect when floated in a liquid. The long stem is internally calibrated with a graduated scale. For increased accuracy, there are hydrometers calibrated for use in light liquids and others for heavy liquids.

(1) Theory of the hydrometer. All floating bodies displace their own weight of a liquid in which they are immersed and sink to a depth proportionate to the volume of liquid displaced. Since this volume equals the weight of the immersed object, specific gravity can be determined by comparison of the volumes displaced. Thus a hydrometer is marked 1.000 at the level it sinks in distilled water at normal temperature. The scale is then carried above and below the 1.000 mark. When the instrument is placed in a different liquid, the specific gravity of that liquid can be read directly from the scale.

(2) Testing the hydrometer. Do not accept hydrometers as you receive them. Always test them first. By immersing your hydrometer in a number of liquids of known specific gravity, including water, you can observe its degree of accuracy. In the event a particular hydrometer shows consistent deviation of one or two points, you need not discard it as useless. Make a notation of the deviation on its box and merely add or subtract the error from the reading as you use it.

(3) Hydrometer jar. The hydrometer is generally floated in a hydrometer jar to take the reading (fig. 2-8). This device lessens the amount of liquid necessary for a reading because it is tall and narrow. It also facilitates cooling of the liquid to specified temperature, the jar being easily immersed in ice water.

(4) Other applications of the hydrometer:

(a) Urinometer–this hydrometer has a special scale for the determination of specific gravity of urine.

(b) Saccharometer–generally measures the percent of syrups rather than the specific gravity.

(c) Alcoholometer–determines alcoholic strength of hydroalcoholic solutions.

(d) Lovi's beads–also called specific gravity beads, are balloon-like, hollow globes of glass. They are of different sizes and weights and have a specific gravity number etched on their sides. When dropped into a liquid, those heavier than the liquid sink to the bottom; the ones lighter than the liquid float to the top; and the one which hovers in the liquid, neither floating nor sinking, represents the specific gravity. They must be used at a definite temperature for which they have been calibrated.

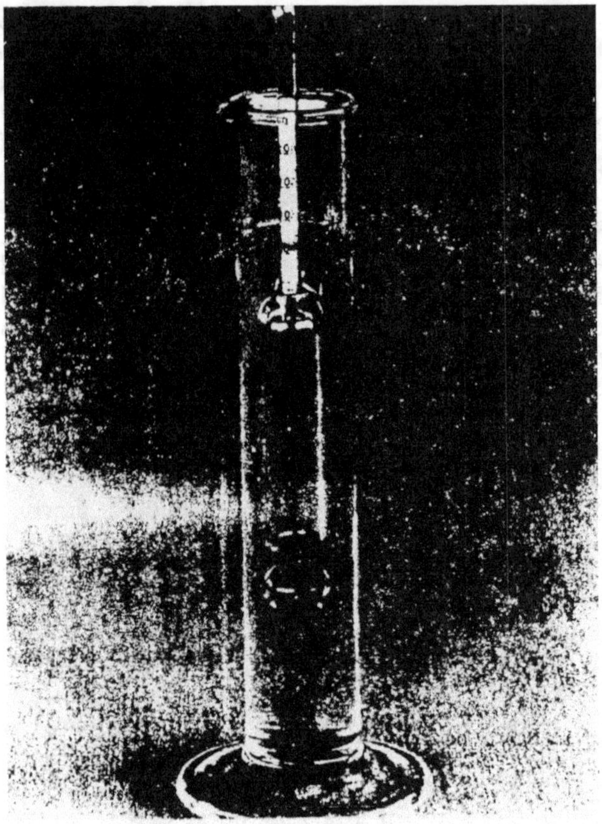

Figure 8. Hydrometer and jar.

37. Specific gravity of solids. Although various procedures must be used for determining the specific gravity of different solids, the formula used is always the same:

$$\text{Sp. Gr.} = \frac{\text{weight of solid in air}}{\text{weight of equal volume of water}}$$

Because of slight variations of technique necessary to establish the specific gravity of solids with different physical properties, we will break solids into groups according to their solubility and weight relative to water. Thus we have—

- Solids insoluble in and heavier than water.
- Solids soluble in and heavier than water.
- Solids insoluble in and lighter than water.
- Solids soluble in and lighter than water.

a. Solids insoluble in and heavier than water.

(1) When solid is a single piece. First, consider a solid in one piece, such as a block of metal or a strip of wire. The easiest method for determining specific gravity of a single piece of solid insoluble in and heavier than water is by using a balance.

- *Step 1.* Accurately weigh the sample to be tested on a good Rx or analytical balance and record this weight as the weight of the substance in air.

- *Step 2.* Attach a horsehair or fine, water-proofed, silk thread to the sample and to the beam of the scale. Immerse the sample in a beaker of water so that it is covered by the water, but not touching the bottom or sides of the beaker. The weight of the sample must be entirely supported by the beam of the balance. Make sure no air bubbles are attached to the sample which would provide buoyancy and make the weighing in water inaccurate. Record the weight of the sample in the water.

- *Step 3.* Apply the formula. *For example,* if a sample of copper weighs 10.52 Gm. in air and 9.34 Gm. when suspended in water, to find the specific gravity of the copper:

Weight in air	=	10.52 Gm.
Weight in water		9.34 Gm.
		1.18 = loss of weight in water

$$\text{Sp. Gr.} = \frac{\text{weight in air}}{\text{weight of equal volume of water}}$$

Since the loss of weight in water equals the weight of an equal volume of water, substitute in the formula:

$$\text{Sp. Gr.} = \frac{10.52}{1.18}$$

$$\text{Sp. Gr.} = 8.92 \text{ (copper)}$$

(2) When solid is fragmentary. Another method of determining the specific gravity of solids insoluble in and heavier than water is by the use of a pycnometer. This method is convenient when the solid is in fragments or smaller particles.

- *Step 1.* Weigh the sample in air and record the weight.

- *Step 2.* Drop the material into a tared pycnometer and fill with distilled water at 25° C. Weigh again, making sure that no water remains on the exterior of the vessel. This weight represents the weight of the pycnometer, the water, and the sample. Subtracting the tare weight, you have the weight of the sample plus the water in the bottle.

- *Step 3.* Apply the formula. *For example,* a sample weighing 10.5 Gm. is placed in a pyconometer which has been determined to hold

100 Gm. of water. You determine the weight of the sample plus the water plus the bottle to be 206.2 Gm. The tare weight of the bottle is 100 Gm.

206.2 Gm. weight of bottle, water, sample
− 100.0 Gm. weight of bottle
106.2 Gm. weight of water and sample
10.5 Gm. weight of sample in air
100.0 Gm. weight of water held by bottle
110.5 Gm. weight of water plus sample
− 106.2 Gm. weight of water and immersed sample
4.3 Gm. loss of weight in water

$$\text{Sp. Gr.} = \frac{10.5}{4.3} = 2.442, \text{ the specific gravity}$$

NOTE

The specific gravity of insoluble powders can also be determined by this method. Care should be taken to shake the powder with a quantity of water before filling the pycnometer to eliminate air bubbles and the error they can cause.

b. Solids insoluble in and lighter than water. The problem here is to make the solid sink into the water so that you can find out how much water it displaces. A weight or sinker, insoluble in water and heavy enough to cause the lighter sample to sink beneath the surface, can be attached. Since the loss of weight in water of the sample and sinker combined equals their total individual losses, it will be easy then to determine the loss of weight of the sample.

Example: A block of wax weighs 21.5 Gm. in the air. To this you attach a lead sinker which you have predetermined to lose 1.1 Gm. when immersed in water. Together they lose 25.8 grams when immersed in water. What is the specific gravity of the wax?

- *Step 1.*

Loss of weight of wax + sinker	=	25.8 Gm.
Loss of weight of sinker	−	1.1 Gm.
Loss of weight of wax	=	24.7 Gm.
Weight of wax in air	=	21.5 Gm.

- *Step 2.* Apply the formula.

$$\text{Sp. Gr.} \frac{21.5}{24.7}$$

$$\text{Sp. Gr.} = 0.87$$

c. Solids soluble in and heavier than water. The problem here is solubility. By substituting a liquid in which the sample is not soluble for the water, you can then determine by proportion what the loss of weight in water would be. The following proportion will apply:

$$\frac{\text{Sp. Gr. of oil}}{\text{Sp. Gr. of water}} :: \frac{\text{loss of weight in oil}}{\text{loss of weight in water}}$$

Example: 20.311 Gm. of Copper Sulfate immersed in an oil having a specific gravity of 0.865 filling a 100 Gm. pycnometer weighs 98.859 Gm. Find the specific gravity of copper sulfate.

- *Step 1.*

Weight of $CuSO_4$ in air	=	20.311 Gm.
Weight of oil in pycnom.	=	86.5 (100 x 0.865)
Weight of $CuSO_4$ + oil		106.811 Gm.
Weight of oil + immersed $CuSO_4$	=	98.859 Gm.
Weight of oil displaced		7.952 Gm.

- *Step 2.* Substitute in proportion.

$$\frac{\text{Sp. Gr. of oil}}{\text{Sp. Gr. of water}} :: \frac{\text{loss of weight in oil}}{\text{loss of weight in water}}$$

$$\frac{0.865}{1} :: \frac{7.952}{x}$$

$$865x = 7952$$

$x = 9.193$, the loss of weight in water

- *Step 3.* Substitute in Sp. Gr. formula.

$$\text{Sp. Gr.} = \frac{20.311}{9.193}$$

$$\text{Sp. Gr.} = 2.209$$

NOTE

If the copper sulfate were in one solid lump, you could measure the loss of weight in oil directly by suspending it from a balance into the oil.

d. Solids soluble in and lighter than water. Here, the problem, and not a slight one, is to find a liquid lighter than the solid and one in which it is not soluble. When this is accomplished, the procedure is the same for solids soluble in and heavier than water (*c* above).

38. Application of specific gravity to pharmaceutical problems. Specific gravity, when known, is of great assistance to us as pharmacists in reducing metric and apothecary volumes to weight and, conversely, in reducing weights to volumes.

a. Metric.

- 1 ml. of water weighs 1 Gm.
- Sp. Gr. of water is 1.000.
- 1 ml. of any liquid with Sp. Gr. of 1.000 weighs 1 Gm.
- 1 ml. of a liquid with Sp. Gr. of 2.000 weighs (1 x 2.000) 2 Gm.
- 1 ml. of a liquid with Sp. Gr. of 1.5 weighs 1 x 1.5 or 1.5 Gm.

Therefore, the volume in ml. times specific gravity = weight in Gm.

(1) Example: What is the weight in grams of 1 liter of glycerin (Sp. Gr. 1.25)?

- *Step 1.* 1 liter = 1000 ml.

- *Step 2.* 1000 ml. x 1.25 = 1250 Gm., the weight of 1 liter of glycerin.

(2) Example: How many ml. of chloroform are there in 1480 Gm.? (Sp. Gr. of chloroform = 1.48).

$$x \text{ ml.} \times 1.48 = 1480 \text{ Gm.}$$

$$x = \frac{1480}{1.48} = 1000 \text{ ml. or 1 liter of chloroform}$$

b. Apothecary. There is no convenient weight-to-volume comparison in the apothecary system. However, you may derive a working formula from the steps below.

- *Step 1.* In the metric system, 1 gram of water or any liquid with a specific gravity of 1.000, has a corresponding volume of 1 ml. In the apothecary system, a fluidounce of water or any fluid with a specific gravity of 1.000 does not weigh 1 ounce, nor does a fluidrachm weigh a drachm, nor a minim weigh a grain.

- *Step 2.* BUT, 1 fluidounce of water at 25° C. weighs 454.6 grains. Since there are 480 minims in 1 fluidounce, a minim of water weighs 454.6 ÷ 480 = 0.95 grain.

- *Step 3.* 1 fluidounce of any liquid having a specific gravity of 1.000 weighs 454.6 grain. 1 fluidounce of any liquid having a specific gravity of 2.000 weighs 454.6 x 2.

- *Step 4.* Conclusion. 1 fluidounce of any liquid weighs (in grains) 454.6 x specific gravity. Thus the following formula:
454.6 x Sp. Gr. x number of fluidounces = weight in grains.

(1) Example: How much does f℥ii, ʒiv of glycerin weigh? Sp. Gr. of glycerin is 1.25.

- *Step 1.* f℥ii, ʒiv = 2.5 fluidounces.

- *Step 2.* Substitute in formula:
454.6 x 1.25 x 2.5 = weight in grains

```
  454.6          568.25
x 1.25           x 2.5
 22730          284125
  9092          113650
 4546           1420.625, weight of glycerin
568.250
```

- *Step 3.* Convert to highest terms.
1420.625 rounded off (.625 → .63 grains)
20 gr./℈, so 1420 ÷ 20 = 71℈
3 ℈/ʒ, so 71 ÷ 3 = 23ʒ + 2℈ remainder
8 ʒ/℥, so 23 ÷ 8 = 2℥ + 7ʒ remainder

- *Step 4.* Collect the amounts.
℥ii ʒvii ℈ii gr ss(.63)

(2) Example: What is the volume of 250 grains of a liquid with a specific gravity of 0.942?

- *Step 1.* Formula.
454.6 x 0.942 x y (No. fluidounces) = weight in grains
454.6 x 0.942 x y = 250

```
   0.942
 x 454.6
    5652
   3768
  4710
 3768
428.2332
```

$$y(428.233) = 250$$

$$y = \frac{250}{428.233}$$

$$y = .583 \text{ fluidounce}$$

- *Step 2.* Reduce to correct terms.
8 fʒ = 1f℥
therefore, .583 x 8 = 4.664 fluidrachms
60 minims = 1 fʒ
therefore, .664 x 60 = 40 minims

- *Step 3.* Combine the quantities:
fʒ iv ♏ x l

39. Specific volume

a. Identification. Specific volume is much like specific gravity, except the comparison is between volumes rather than weights. Specific volume can be described as the ratio of the volume of one substance to the volume of an equal weight of a standard substance. As in specific gravity, the standard is water and the standard temperature is 25° C.

$$\text{Since Sp. Gr.} = \frac{\text{weight of substance in air}}{\text{weight of equal volume of water}}$$

$$\text{Sp. Vol.} = \frac{\text{volume of substance}}{\text{volume of equal weight of water}}$$

$$\text{Then, Specific Gravity} = \frac{1}{\text{Sp. Vol.}} \text{ and}$$

$$\text{Sp. Vol.} = \frac{1}{\text{Sp. Gr.}}\text{; they are reciprocals}$$

b. Sample problems.

(1) Problem: What is the specific volume of 750 Gm. of chloroform measuring 510.2 ml.?

- *Step 1.* Volume of chloroform = 510.2 ml.
  Volume of equal weight water = 750.0 ml.

- *Step 2.* Substitute in formula

$$\text{Sp. Vol.} = \frac{\text{volume of substance}}{\text{volume of equal weight water}}$$

$$\text{Sp. Vol.} = \frac{510.2}{750}$$

$$\text{Sp. Vol} = 0.68$$

(2) Problem: Using the information in the previous problem, what is the specific gravity of chloroform?

Using the reciprocal formula:

$$\text{Sp. Gr.} = \frac{1}{\text{Sp. Vol.}}$$

$$\text{Sp. Gr.} = \frac{1}{0.68}$$

Sp. Gr. = 1.47, answer

```
      1.47
68/100.00
    68
    32 0
    27 2
     4 80
     4 76
```

40. Density

a. Identification. Density is the ratio between weight and volume of a substance; or, density = weight divided by volume, and is expressed not as a relative number, as specific gravity was, but with specific units as Gm./ml., lb/cu.ft., or gr./fl.oz.

From the formula:

$D = \frac{w}{v}$, we see that if we know density and volume we can determine weight; knowing density and weight, we can find volume; and knowing weight and volume, we can find density.

b. Sample problems.

(1) Problem: What is the density of alcohol if 250 ml. weigh 200 Gm.?

$$\text{Density} = \frac{\text{weight}}{\text{volume}}$$

$$D = \frac{200}{250}$$

$$D = 0.80 \text{ Gm./ml.}$$

(2) Problem: How many ml. of mercury (density 13.6) would there be in a sample weighing 2000 Gm.?

$$D = \frac{w}{v}$$

$$13.6 = \frac{2000}{v}$$

$$13.6\,v = 2000$$

$$v = \frac{2000}{13.6}$$

$$v = 147.06 \text{ ml.}$$

41. Temperature

a. Definition. What exactly is temperature? Temperature can be stated as being the degree of hotness or lack of hotness, or the *intensity of heat.* Relative temperatures can be sensed by touch in some cases, but the sense of touch can be very misleading. A piece of cloth and a piece of metal, although exactly the same temperature will feel differently to the touch. The cloth will not seem as warm or as cold as the metal. This is due to the rate at which the substance dissipates heat.

b. Measurement of temperature. Temperature, therefore, must be measured by a device which gives accurate degrees of heat. Such instruments are called thermometers. The thermometer is based on the principle of expansion and contraction of substances with change in temperature. The most common thermometers utilize alcohol or mercury. In order for readings obtained from expansion and contraction to be valid, the expansion and contraction must be uniform.

c. *Liquid thermometer.* The liquid thermometer consists of a fine capillary tube, hermetically sealed, with a bulb at one end. The tube is filled to a point on the capillary, the bulb serving as a reservoir. Upon elevating the temperature, the liquid expands and rises in the tube to a new level. Thus, calibrating the tube with known constant temperatures and dividing the space between with equal degrees, we have an instrument that will measure temperature. Figure 2-9 shows two liquid thermometers discussed below.

42. Temperature calculation. There are two different scales by which liquid thermometers can be calibrated–the Centigrade scale and the Fahrenheit scale.

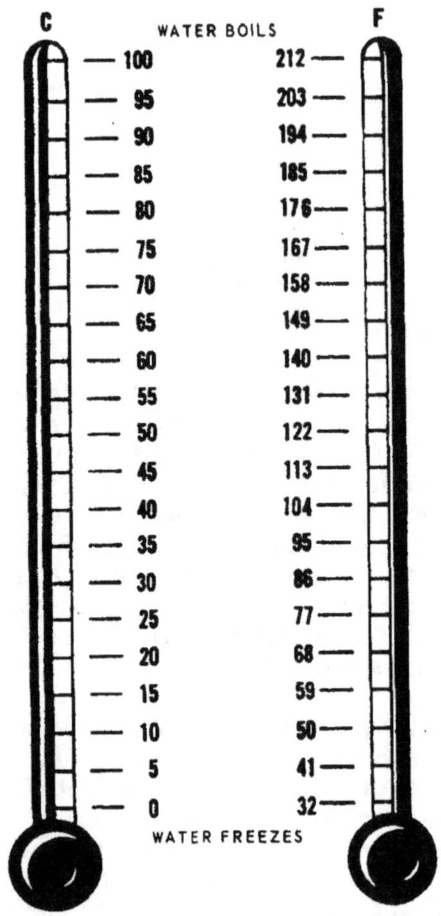

Figure 9. Thermometer comparison.

a. *Centigrade.* The Centigrade thermometer is so calibrated that the melting point of ice is 0° C. and the boiling point of water is 100° C. By this scale, there is a difference of 100 degrees between the freezing and boiling points of water. The Centigrade scale has been adopted by the USP and NF as the official temperature standard. In fact, it is the standard temperature measuring device the world over.

b. *Fahrenheit.* The Fahrenheit thermometer is calibrated so that 32° F. is the melting point of ice and 212° F. is the boiling point of water. The difference between freezing and boiling on this scale is 180°. The Fahrenheit scale is used mainly for household purposes.

c. *Importance of stating the scale.* Because of the great difference between these two scales, you can see the importance of always stating which scale you are using when referring to a temperature. By itself, 40° means nothing; 40° Fahrenheit is approximately 4.4° Centigrade; 40° Centigrade is 104° Fahrenheit, a considerable difference.

d. *Absolute temperature.* We, as pharmacists, will not deal with the absolute temperature scale; however, you should be familiar with what it is. Remember only that *absolute* degree equals Centigrade degrees plus 273°. Expressed as a formula this becomes–

$$A^\circ = C^\circ + 273^\circ.$$

43. Temperature conversion. Knowing that the range in degrees between the freezing and boiling points of water is 100° in the Centigrade scale and 180° in the Fahrenheit scale, it is obvious that one Centigrade degree is equal to 1.8 (9/5), the size of a Fahrenheit degree. Therefore, a 5-degree change in Centigrade temperature is a 9-degree change in the Fahrenheit scale. Since 0° C. equals 32° F., 1° C. must equal 32° plus 9/5° or 1.8°, or 33.8° F. Thus, we can derive several formulas. However, the basic formula is: $9C = 5F - 160$, or $5F = 9C + 160$.

a. *Example:* Convert −5° Centigrade to Fahrenheit.

- *Step 1.* Formula: $5F = 9C + 160$
- *Step 2.* Substitute: $5F = 9(-5) + 160$

$$5F = -45 + 160$$
$$5F = 115$$
$$F = 115 \div 5$$
$$F = 23^\circ F$$

b. Example: Convert --40° Fahrenheit to Centigrade.

- *Step 1.* Formula: 9C = 5F – 160
- *Step 2.* Substitute: 9C = 5 (–40) – 160

$$9C = -200 - 160$$
$$9C = -360$$
$$C = -360 \div 9$$
$$C = -40^{\circ}\ C$$

c. Example: Convert 80° Fahrenheit to Centigrade.

- *Step 1.* Formula: 9C = 5F – 160
- *Step 2.* Substitute: 9C = 5(80) – 160

$$9C = 400 - 160$$
$$9C = 240$$
$$C = 240 \div 9$$
$$C = 26.6^{\circ}\ C$$

44. Dosage

a. Importance of dosage calculation to the pharmacist. When a prescription reaches the pharmacist from the desk of a prescriber, the ingredients are specified, the quantities listed (perhaps in specific amounts, perhaps as ratio, perhaps as percentages), and the instructions to the patient are written in Latin, in pharmaceutical or medical terminology. The pharmacist must (1) fill the prescription, (2) check the prescriber for possible error of amounts and dosage, and (3) write the directions upon the label in terms which can be easily understood by the patient. For these reasons, an accurate knowledge of dosage is mandatory for the pharmacist. Imagine the consequences of the following:

(1) Error in converting a percent ingredient to the specific amount.

(2) Prescriber's inadvertent error in amount of ingredient to be used in preparation of a medicinal (with the accompanying error of the pharmacist not observing the error).

(3) Prescriber's error in calculation of dosage (again combined with the pharmacist's missing the error). Although errors are the exception rather than the rule, the pharmacist must be forever on his guard against them. It is not his privilege to look for errors, but his *duty*. The pharmacist is held responsible equally with the erring physician. Overdose, even though it may originate at the prescriber, if not corrected by the pharmacy technician may constitute negligence.

b. Approximate household equivalents. The approximate household equivalents shown in table 2-8 are useful in making calculations for number of doses in a medication and for translating directions into terms understandable to the patient. These approximate equivalents are in obvious discrepancy due to approximating equivalency between three different measures. In table 2-8, one teasp, 1 fʒ (approx 4 ml.) and 5 ml. are not equal at all. However, the directions to the patient cannot read "Take 1 drachm" or "4 ml." or "5 ml." They must be written in some language that all literate persons can understand–thus, "one teaspoonful."

c. Medicine glass. Because of inaccuracy in household equivalents and because household spoons, cups, and glasses vary considerably in size, the patient should be strongly advised to purchase a medicine glass (fig. 2-10) for accurate dosage.

d. Calculation of dosage. Some of the dosage calculations you will be making most frequently are listed below. The following proportion can be established which will aid in solving dosage problems:

$$\text{Total doses} = \frac{\text{total amount}}{\text{size of each dose}}$$

(1) Calculating the size of an individual dose. When given the total amount of medication and the number of doses to be made, the size of each can be calculated by dividing. *Example:* A

Table 8. Approximate Household Equivalents

Metric measure	Apothecary equivalent (approximate)	Household measure
2 ml	fʒss	½ teaspoonful
5 ml	fʒi	1 teaspoonful
8 ml	fʒii	1 dessertspoonful
15 ml	fʒiv	1 tablespoonful
30 ml	fʒviii (f℥i)	2 tablespoonfuls
60 m	f℥ii	1 wineglassful
120 ml	f℥iv	1 teacupful
240 ml	f℥viii	1 tumblerful

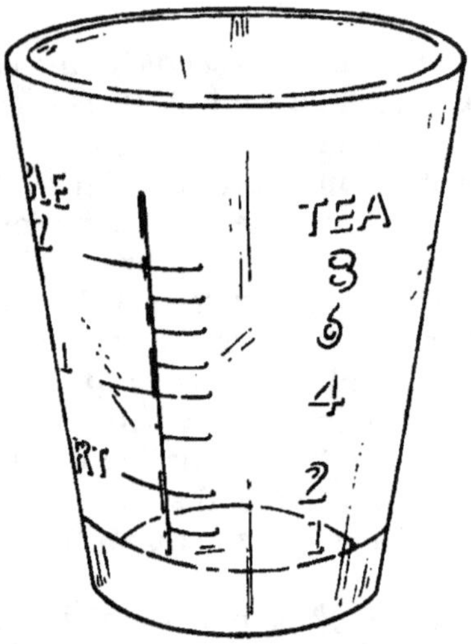

Figure 10. A medicine glass.

particular medication is to be taken 4 times daily for 1 week, and a total of 280 grains is being dispensed. What is the amount of this medication in a single dose?

- *Step 1.* What is the total number of doses?
  4 doses daily x 7 days = 28 doses, total

- *Step 2.* Formula.

$$\text{Total doses} = \frac{\text{total amount}}{\text{size of each dose}}$$

- *Step 3.* Substitute—

$$28 = \frac{280 \text{ gr.}}{x}$$

$$28x = 280$$

$$x = 10 \text{ grains in each dose.}$$

NOTE

The answer will always be in the same denomination as the total amount, or if the total amount is the unknown, in the same denomination as the individual dose.

(2) Calculating number of doses. The number of doses in a specific amount can be calculated if you are given the total amount and the size of the dose.

(a) Example: How many doses of 5 grains each will result from a total of 75 grains of total medication?

- *Step 1.* Formula.

$$\text{Total doses} = \frac{\text{total amount}}{\text{size of each dose}}$$

- *Step 2.* Substitute.

$$x = \frac{75 \text{ gr.}}{5}$$

$$x = 15 \text{ doses}$$

(b) Example: If the dose of a medication is to be one-half fluidrachm, how many doses will a patient receive, given an 8-ounce bottle of medication?

- *Step 1.* Since there are 8 fluidrachms to the fluidounce, 8 fluidounces would contain 8 x 8 = 64 fluidrachms.

- *Step 2.* Formula.

$$\text{Total doses} = \frac{\text{total amount}}{\text{size of each dose}}$$

- *Step 3.* Substitute.

$$x = \frac{64 \text{ fluidrachms}}{.5}$$

$$x = 128 \text{ doses, answer}$$

(3) Calculating total amount of medication. If you know the size of the dose and the number of doses prescribed, you can determine the total medication to be dispensed.

Example: A patient is to receive 1 fluidounce of whisky morning, noon, and night for an indefinite period of time. What quantity would be dispensed for 1 week's medication?

- *Step 1.* 1 ounce dose x 3 doses per day x 7 days per week equals 21 ounces. The formula may also be used as shown in step 2 below.

- *Step 2.* Formula.

$$\text{Total doses} = \frac{\text{total amount}}{\text{size of each dose}}$$

$$21 = \frac{x}{1}$$

$$x = 21 \text{ ounces, answer}$$

(4) Calculating amount of a single ingredient. The amount of a single ingredient present in a dose of a mixture of several medicinal agents can be determined by dividing the amount of that ingredient by the total doses.

(a) Example: Calculate the amount of *each* ingredient in a single dose of the following prescription.

Rx Acetylsalicylic acid ʒii ℈i gr vii
Acetophenetidin ʒi ℈ii gr v
Caffeine gr xss
M. Ft. M.
Div in caps, no. xxi
Sig: Cap i q 4 h, prn.

- *Step 1.* Reduce all ingredients to *grains.*

Acetylsalicylic acid equals

2 x 60 grains (per drachm)	= 120	gr.
1 x 20 grains (per scruple)	= 20	gr.
7 grains	= 7	gr.
	147	gr.

Acetophenetidin equals

1 x 60 grains (per drachm)	= 60	gr.
2 x 20 grains (per scruple)	= 40	gr.
5 grains	= 5	gr.
	105	gr.

Caffeine equals

10 1/2 grains	= 10.5	gr.

- *Step 2.* You know that the total amount is for 21 capsules; therefore, the amount in a single capsule would be–

$$\text{Total doses} = \frac{\text{total amount}}{\text{size of each dose}}$$

$$21 = \frac{147}{x} = 7 \text{ grains acetylsalicylic acid per capsule}$$

$$21 = \frac{105}{x} = 5 \text{ grains acetophenetidin per capsule}$$

$$21 = \frac{10.5}{x} = 1/2 \text{ grain caffeine per capsule}$$

NOTE

To check this prescription for possible errors, consult the USP or Remington for the dose of each of the ingredients and compare the dose with the amounts you have calculated to be in each capsule.

(b) Example: A solution contains 4/5 grain of a potent drug in 4 ounces. What dose must be given to provide 1/120 grain of the drug?

- *Step 1.* Formula.

$$\text{Total doses} = \frac{\text{total amount}}{\text{size of each dose}}$$

- *Step 2* Substitute.

$$x \text{ doses} = \frac{\frac{4}{15}}{\frac{1}{120}}$$

- *Step 3.* Remember that you can divide fractions by inverting the divisor and multiplying. Thus,

$$x \text{ doses} = \frac{4}{15} \times \frac{120}{1}$$

$$x = \frac{480}{15} = 32 \text{ doses}$$

- *Step 4.* Since you are to get 32 doses from 4 ounces, each dose must be one fluidrachm (8 fluidrachms = 1 ounce).

e. Children's doses. Enough emphasis cannot be placed upon the calculation of dosage for children. Because of their size, weight, and incomplete development, they are not able to tolerate as much medication as adults. Although many factors besides weight and age play an important part in dosage, only these two will be discussed here. (Chapter 9 explains dosage factors in more detail.)

(1) Formulas for calculating children's doses. Several formulas can be employed for calculating doses for children and infants; however, because of different degrees of response by children to different medications (e.g., children are extremely susceptible to morphine), it is best to become familiar with the correct doses through experience and to memorize doses as they present themselves. If at all in doubt about the size of a dose, ALWAYS check with the pharmacy officer or the prescriber. The most generally used formulas for calculation of doses for children are–

(a) Young's rule (most widely used).

$$\frac{\text{child's age}}{\text{child's age} + 12} \times \text{adult dose} = \text{child's dose}$$

(b) Clark's rule.

$$\frac{\text{weight of child (lb)}}{150} \times \text{adult dose} = \text{child's dose}$$

(2) Example problems. Study the following examples carefully to see the application of the above rules.

(a) Example: What would be the dose of elixir of phenobarbital for a child 3 years old? (Elixir phenobarbital contains 400 mg. of phenobarbital per 100 ml. Adult dose of

phenobarbital is 30 mg., up to 4 times a day.) Use Young's rule.

- *Step 1.* Rule.

$$\frac{\text{child's age}}{\text{child's age} + 12} \times \text{adult dose} = \text{child's dose}$$

- *Step 2.* Substitute.

$$\frac{3}{3 + 12} \times 30 \text{ mg.} = \text{child's dose}$$

$$\frac{90}{15} = 6 \text{ mg., the child's dose}$$

- *Step 3.* Since 100 ml. of phenobarbital elixir contains 400 mg., 1 ml. would contain 4 mg. Therefore; 1:x :: 4:6.

$$4x = 6$$

$$x = 1.5 \text{ ml., the dose for 3-year-old child.}$$

(b) Example: What would be the dose of tetracycline hydrochloride for a 3-year-old girl weighing 30 pounds? Usual adult dose is 500 mg. Use Clark's rule.

- *Step 1.* Formula.

$$\frac{\text{weight of child (lb)}}{150} \times \text{adult dose} = \text{child's dose}$$

- *Step 2.* Substitute.

$$\frac{30}{150} \times 500 \text{ mg.} = \text{child's dose}$$

$$\frac{15{,}000}{150} = 100 \text{ mg., the child's dose}$$

45. Concentration and dilution. Many times in pharmacy it is necessary to dilute or concentrate a substance in order to dispense the right dosage; the dilution of nose drops is one of the most frequently seen examples. Phenylephrine hydrochloride solution is a standard nose drop preparation. Its strength as it comes to us is 1 percent. Most of the prescriptions for phenylephrine solution will call for 1/4 percent. You can see, then, that it will have to be diluted before dispensing.

a. Mechanics of dilution. If 1 ounce of a 1 percent-solution of phenylephrine hydrochloride solution was diluted to a new volume of 2 ounces, the percent of the new solution would be 1/2 of the original 1 percent, that is, 1/2 percent. Perhaps it will be more apparent if you consider that 1 ounce of a 1-percent solution contains approximately 4.5 grains of active ingredient. By diluting the solution to a volume of 2 ounces, you still have only 4.5 grains of active ingredient in a volume of 2 ounces. Thus, you have halved the percentage. If the active ingredient remains constant and the volume of the solution increases, the percentage decreases. And if the active ingredient remains constant and the volume of the solution decreases, the percentage increases. The percentage strength and the volume of a solution are inversely proportional to each other.

b. Concentration–dilution proportion. Since volume and percentage strength of solutions are inversely proportional, the following formula or proportion applies.

$$\frac{\text{\% concentration of original solution}}{\text{\% concentration of new solution}} :: \frac{\text{new volume}}{\text{original volume}}$$

This proportion can be used to solve any concentration or dilution problem arising in the pharmacy.

(1) Example: You have 30 ml. of a 10-percent solution and want to make a 1-percent solution. To what volume must you dilute the original solution? Substituting in the proportion you have—

$$\frac{10 \text{ (original \%)}}{1 \text{ (new \%)}} :: \frac{x \text{ (unknown new volume)}}{30 \text{ (original new volume)}}$$

$$x = 300 \text{ ml., the new volume}$$

In a practical situation, then, you would dilute the original 30 ml. of 10-percent solution to a total volume of 300 ml. to prepare the desired 1-percent solution.

(2) Example: Make a 4-percent solution from 60 ml. of a 2-percent solution by concentrating the volume. Again, substituting in the proportion, you have—

$$\frac{2\%}{4\%} :: \frac{x}{60}$$

$$4x = 120$$

$$x = 30 \text{ ml.}$$

You must concentrate the 60 ml. of 2-percent solution to a new volume of 30 ml. in order to obtain the 4-percent solution.

46. Alligation. Alligation is a process for finding the value of a combination containing known quantities of known strengths; *for example,* to determine the strength of a solution resulting from the mixture of 100 ml. of 20-percent alcohol and

20 ml. of 10-percent alcohol. Actually, alligation is two different processes, alligation medial and alligation alternate. Alligation medial is used for determining percentage strength and alligation alternate for proportional number of parts.

a. Alligation medial. Alligation medial is used in determining the percentage strength of a mixture of two or more ingredients of different strengths. Alligation medial can also be used to determine the resulting specific gravity of a mixture of two or more substances with different specific gravities.

(1) Example: What percentage of codeine sulfate is contained in a mixture of 60 grams of a 15-percent codeine powder and 15 grams of a 40-percent codeine powder?

• *Step 1.* Find the amount of codeine sulfate in the total mixture.

60 x .15 = 9.0 Gm. of codeine sulfate
15 x .40 = 6.0 Gm. of codeine sulfate
15.0 Gm. total codeine in mixture

• *Step 2.* Find the weight of the total mixture.

60 Gm. + 15 Gm. = 75 Gm. total weight of mixture

• *Step 3.* Divide the amount of codeine by the total weight to find the percent of codeine in the mixture.

$$\frac{15.0}{75.0} = .20 \text{ or } 20\% \text{ codeine sulfate}$$

(2) Example: You prepare a mixture of 3 ounces of liquid A and 13 ounces of liquid B. What is the cost per ounce of the resulting mixture if liquid A costs $4.00 per pint and liquid B costs $1.44 per pint?

• *Step 1.* Find the cost per ounce of each ingredient.

A = $4.00/pint ÷ 16 = $ .25/ounce
B = $1.44/pint ÷ 16 = $ .09/ounce

• *Step 2.* Find the number of ounces in the total mixture.

3 ounces of A + 13 ounces of B = 16 ounces

• *Step 3.* Find the total cost of these two ingredients.

3 ounces at $0.25 = $ .75
13 ounces at $0.09 = $1.17
$1.92 total cost of mixture

• *Step 4.* Find the cost per ounce of the mixture.

$1.92 ÷ 16 = $0.12, cost per ounce

(3) Example: What is the specific gravity of a mixture of 250 ml. of Glycerin (Sp. Gr. 1.25) and 500 ml. of chloroform (Sp. Gr. 1.48)?

• *Step 1.* Find the number of grams in each of the volumes.

250 ml. x 1.25 = 312.5 Gm. of glycerin
500 ml. x 1.48 = 740.00 Gm. of chloroform

• *Step 2.* Find the total volume and total weight of the mixture.

250 ml. + 500 ml. = 750 ml., total volume
312.5 Gm. + 740 Gm. = 1052.5 Gm., total weight

• *Step 3.* Divide weight by volume to find Sp. Gr.

$$\frac{1052.5}{750} = 1.403, \text{ the Sp. Gr. of mixture}$$

b. Alligation alternate. Alligation alternate is a method of determining the proportionate number of parts of two or more ingredients of known strength when they are to be mixed to form a desired strength. The parts can then be changed to represent volume or weight. A substance of greater strength is mixed with one of lesser strength to form a mixture of a strength somewhere between that of the two ingredients. For example, 50-percent alcohol can be mixed with 25-percent alcohol to produce 30-percent alcohol. It is not possible to mix 50-percent alcohol with 25-percent alcohol to get less than 25-percent or more than 50-percent alcohol. The increase in percentage from the smaller ingredient to the percentage desired, equals the parts of the higher percent ingredient, and the decrease in percentage of the higher to the desired equals the parts of the lower percent ingredient.

(1) Example: What must be the proportion of 50-percent alcohol and 25-percent alcohol, mixed to obtain 30-percent alcohol?

• *Step 1.* Examine the situation. We desire a 30-percent alcohol solution from a 50-percent and a 25-percent solution. The 50-percent solution is 20 percent too strong and the 25-percent solution is 5 percent too weak. In other words, the 50-percent solution must decrease 20 percent and the 25-percent increase 5 percent.

• *Step 2.* Prepare a diagram and place the percentage you desire at completion in the center block. Place the highest percent ingredient (50 percent) on the left and the lowest percent ingredient (25 percent) on the right.

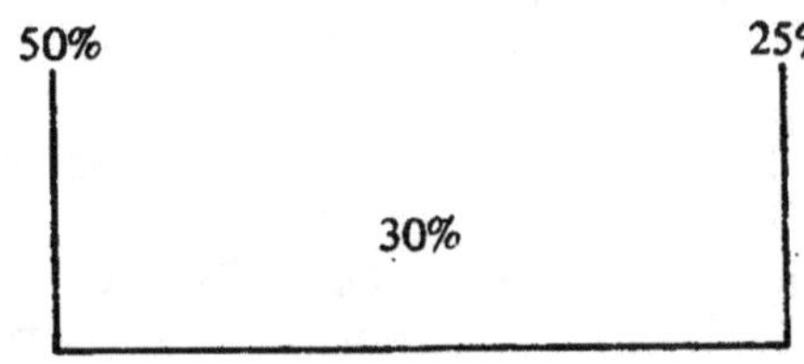

• *Step 3.* Subtract the percent you desire (center block) from the high percent and place your answer below the low percent. This answer represents the parts of the LOW percent you will need to make the desired strength solution.

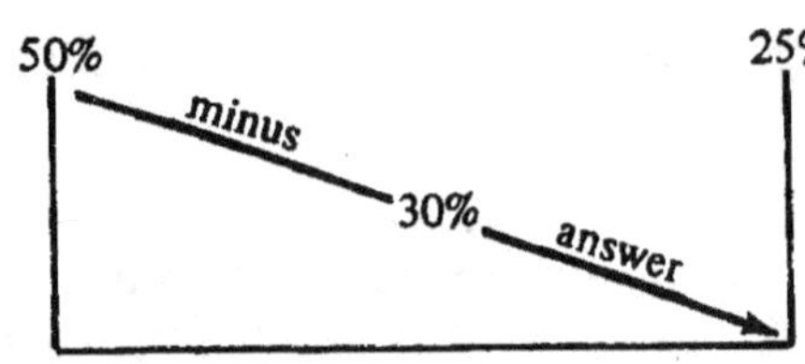

• *Step 4.* Subtract the low percent from the desired percent (center block) and place your answer below the high percent. This answer represents the parts of the HIGH percent you will need to make the desired strength solution.

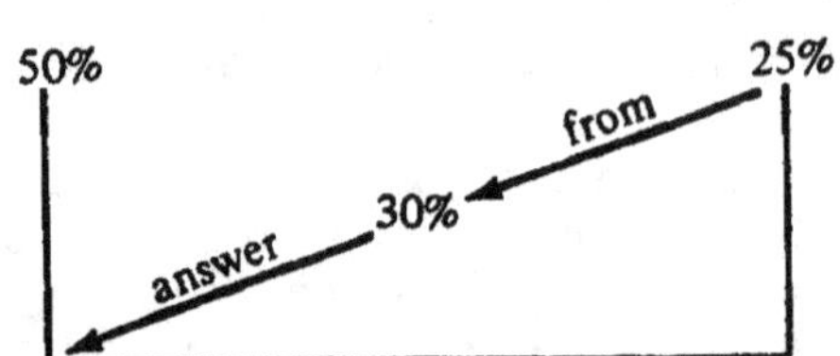

5 = Parts of high percent

The paperwork from your completed problem, then, should look like this. It indicates that to make a 30-percent solution from 50-percent and 25-percent alcohol, you will need 5 parts of the 50 percent and 20 parts of the 25 percent.

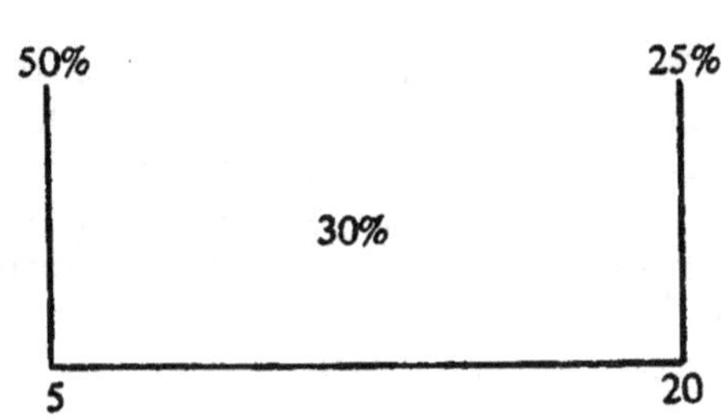

• *Step 5.* Express the number of parts in the denomination most suitable, such as ml., grains, grams, or ounces. Thus, 20 ml. of the 25 percent + 5 ml. of the 50 percent will make a 30-percent mixture; 20 ounces of the 25 percent + 5 ounces of the 50 percent will also make a 30-percent mixture.

(2) Example: In what proportion must you mix 95-percent, 10-percent, 50-percent, and 30-percent alcohol to make 40-percent alcohol?

• *Step 1.* Examine the situation. You desire a 40-percent solution by combining so many parts each of 95 percent, 50 percent, 30 percent, and 10 percent.

• *Step 2.* Although the setup looks a little different because there are 4 ingredients in this problem, use the same procedure, that is, to subtract the lesser percents from the desired to get the number of parts, and to subtract the desired percent from the higher percents to get the number of parts. This problem has been broken down into four diagrams to show each segment of subtraction. However, the problem should be worked from one diagram.

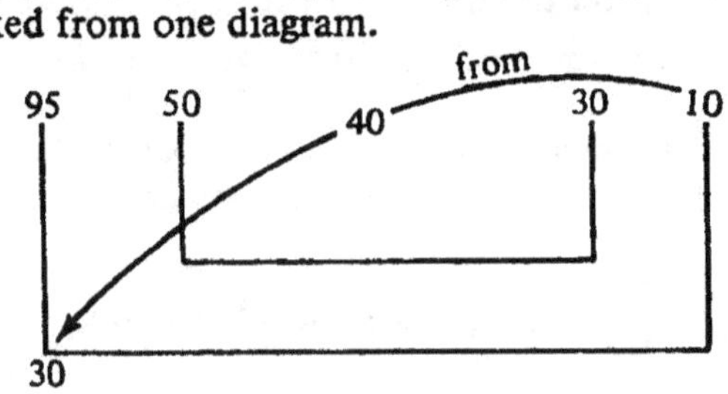

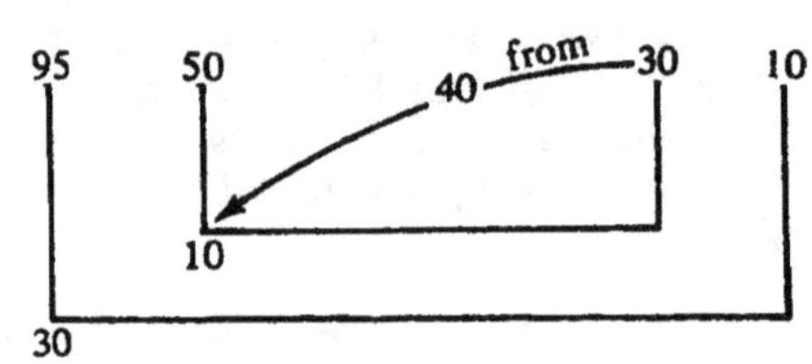

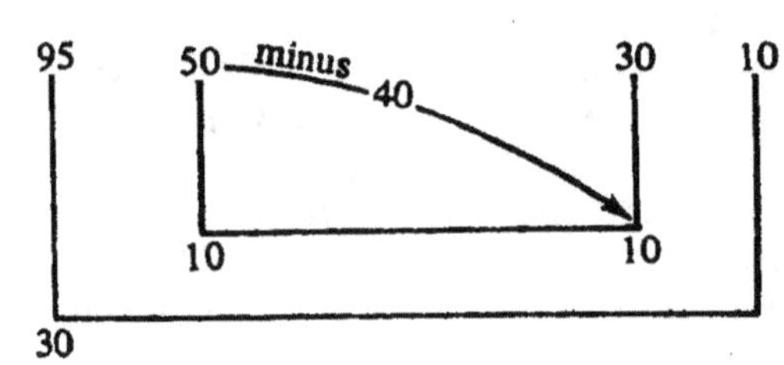

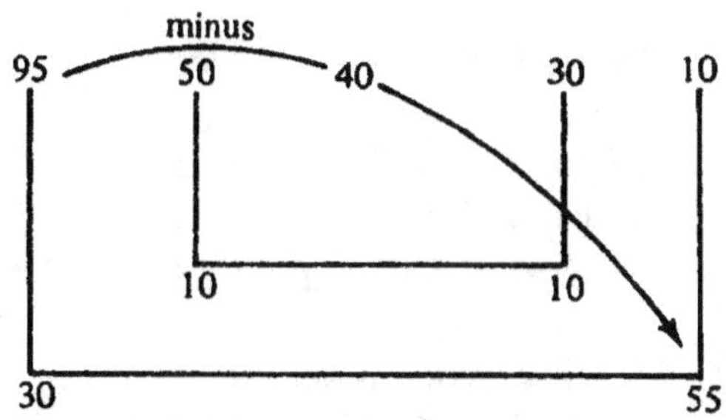

You therefore need–

30 parts of 95% alcohol
55 parts of 10% alcohol
10 parts of 50% alcohol
10 parts of 30% alcohol
105 parts of 40% alcohol

• *Step 3.* By expressing the parts as ounces, you mix 30 ounces of 95 percent, 55 ounces of 10 percent, 10 ounces of 50 percent, and 10 ounces of 30 percent to produce 105 ounces of 40-percent alcohol.

(3) Example: How many ml. of 10-percent, 20-percent, and 30-percent sodium hydroxide solution must be mixed to make a quart of 25-percent solution?

• *Step 1.* Examine the situation. You desire a 25-percent solution from the combination of 10-percent, 20-percent, and 30-percent solutions of sodium hydroxide.

• *Step 2.* Set up.

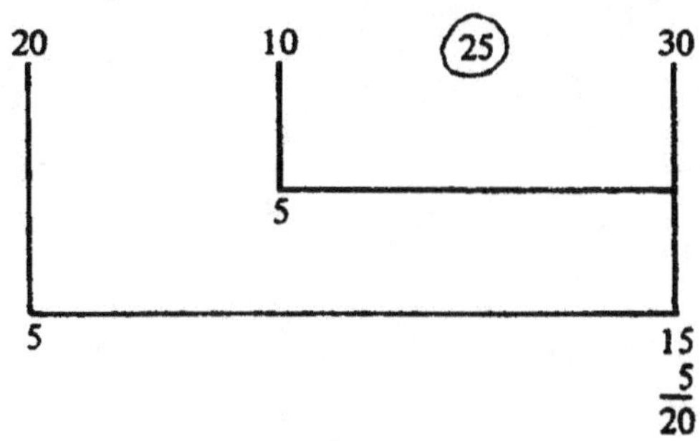

• *Step 3.* Thus you need–

5 parts of 20%
5 parts of 10%
20 parts of 30%
30 parts of 25% will result

• *Step 4.* Find what one part would equal. You know that there are 473 ml. in 1 pint, and therefore 946 ml. in 1 quart. The total number of ml. to be made is 946. You have a total of 30 parts of the solutions which are to equal 946 ml.; 1 part, then, would equal 946 ÷ 30 = 31.53 ml. per part.

• *Step 5.* Multiply the numbers of parts by the 31.53 ml. to find the number of ml. of each to be used.

31.53 x 5 = 157.65 ml. of 20%
31.53 x 5 = 157.65 ml. of 10%
31.53 x 20 = 630.60 ml. of 30%

(4) Example: How much water must be added to a pint of 95-percent ethyl alcohol to make 70-percent alcohol?

• *Step 1.* Examine the situation. You desire to make a 70-percent solution of alcohol from a 95-percent solution and a 0-percent solution (water).

• *Step 2.* Set up.

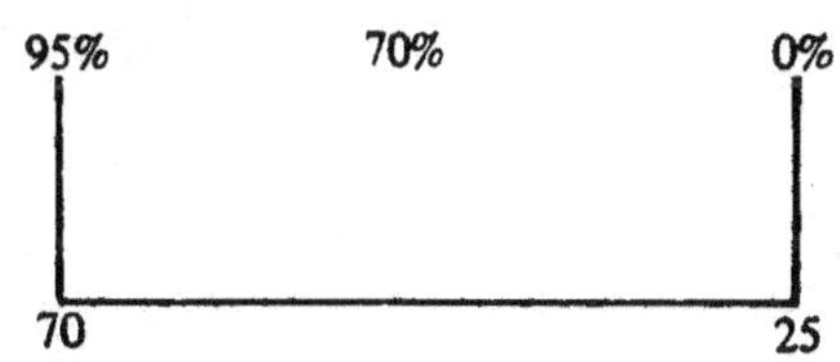

• *Step 3.* Thus you need–

70 parts of 95% alcohol
25 parts of 0% alcohol (water)
95 parts of 70% alcohol

• *Step 4.* Solve. One pint contains 473 ml.

70 : 473 :: 25 : x
70x = 473 x 25
70x = 11,825
x = 168.93 ml. of water required.

(5) Example: How many ml. of a 60-percent sulfuric acid by volume solution must be added to 344 ml. of 30-percent sulfuric acid and 172 ml. of 15-percent sulfuric acid to make 50-percent sulfuric acid?

• *Step 1.* Examine the situation. You desire to make a 50-percent solution of sulfuric acid by combining 344 ml. of 30-percent sulfuric acid, 172 ml. of 15-percent sulfuric acid, and x number of ml. of 60-percent sulfuric acid.

• *Step 2.* Find the percent strength of the mixture formed by combining the acids of known strength and volume.

$$\begin{array}{rl} 344 \times 0.30 = & 103.2 \text{ Gm.} \\ 172 \times 0.15 = & 25.8 \text{ Gm.} \\ \hline 516 \text{ ml.} & 129.0 \text{ Gm.} \end{array}$$

$129.0 \div 516 = .25$, or 25%, the strength of the mixture of the two acids.

• *Step 3.* Set up for a mixture of the 25 percent and the 60 percent to be added.

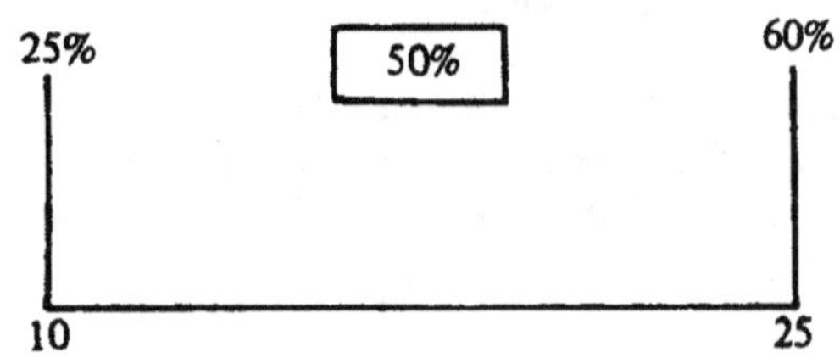

• *Step 4.* Thus you need–

25 parts of 60% sulfuric acid
10 parts of 25% sulfuric acid
35 parts of 50% sulfuric acid

• *Step 5.* Since you have 516 ml. of the 25-percent strength solution, which represents 10 parts, find how many ml. will represent 25 parts.

$$10 : 25 :: 516 : x$$
$$10x = 516 \times 25$$
$$10x = 12{,}900$$

x = 1,290 ml. of the 60% sulfuric acid required.

NOTES AND RESOURCES

CONTENTS

NOTES AND RESOURCES

I - Glossary of Drugs With National Nomenclatures

ANESTHETICS

United States	Germany	Netherlands	France
Chloroprocaine N.F	....	Chloroprocaine	
Cocaine hydrochloride U.S. P.	Cocainhydrochlorid DAB 7....................	Cocaine hydrochloride	Cocaine chlorhydrate.
Cyclopropane U.S.P	....	Cyclopentaan	Cyclopropane.
Droperidol	Dehydrobenzperidol	Droperidol	Haldol.
Ether U.S.P	Aether pro narcosi DAB 7 . .	Ether U.S.P.............	Ether pur pour . anesthesie.
Halothane U.S.P	Halothan	Halothaan	Halothane.
Lid.ocaine hydrochloride .... U.S.P.	Lidocainii hydrochloridum .... Ph. Int.	Lidocaine hydrochloride	Xylocaine.
Mepivacaine hydrochloride .... N.F.	Scandicain...............	Mepivacaine hydrochloride.	
Nitrous oxide U.S.P.	Distickstoffoxide, Lachgas	Lachgas, distikstofoxide....................	Protoxyde d"azote.
Prilocaine hydrochloride .... N.F.	....	Prilocaine hydrochloride................	
Procaine hydrochloride .... U.S.P.	Procainhydrochlorid DAB 7.	Procaine hydrochloride.	Lignocaine.
Proparacaine hydrochloride .... U.S.P.	....	Proparacaine hydrochloride, ... proxymetacaine.	
Tetracaine hydrochloride .... U.S.P:	Tetracainhydrochlorid DAB 7.	Tetracaine hydrochloride	Tetracaine.
Thiopental sodium U.S.P.	Trapanal	Thiopental-natrium..	Penthiobarbital injectable.

MUSCLE RELAXANTS

United States	Germany	Netherlands	France
Curare	....	Curare.	
Pancuronium bromide	....	Pancuronium bromide.	
Succinylcholine U.S.P	Suxamethonium chloridum .... Ph.Int.	Succinylcholine	Succinylcholine.
Tubocurarine chloride U.S.P.	D-Tubocurarini chloridum Ph.Int.	Tubocurarine chloride	Tubocurarine.

NARCOTICS

Codeine phosphate U.S.P	Codeinphosphate DAB 7...	Codeine fosfaat	Codeine.
Meperidine hydrochloride U.S.P.	Pethidini hydrochloridum Ph.Int.	Pethidine hydrochloride.	Pethidine chlorhydrate.
Methadone hydrochloride U.S.P.	Methadoni hydrochloridum Ph.Int.	Methadon hydrochloride.	
Morphine sulfate U.S.P	Morphini sulfas Ph.Int.....	Morfine sulfaat..	Morphine.
Papaverine hydrochloride .... N.F.	Papaverinhydrochlorid DAB 7.	Papaverine hydrochloride	Papaverine.

HYPNOTICS

Amobarbital U.S.P...	Amobarbitalum Ph.Int.....	Amobarbital........	Amobarbital.
Paraldehyde U.S.P..	Paraldehyd DAB 7	Paraldehyde	Paraldehyde.
Pentobarbital U.S.P.	Neodorm........................	Pentobarbital......	Nembutal.
Phenobarbital U.S.P	Phenylaethylbarbitursaure DAB 7.	Fenobarbital.......	Phenobarbital.
Secobarbital U.S.P..	....	Secobarbital	Secobarbital.

ANTIBIOTICS

United States	Germany	Netherlands	France
Ampicillin U.S.P.......	Amblosin, Binotal.....	Ampicilline	Ampicilline. ....
Bacitracin U.S.P.......	Bacitracin	Bacitracine	Bacitracine.
Carbenicillin.............	Anabactyl	Carbenicilline.	
Cephaloridine	....	Cefaloridine............	Cephaloridine.
Cephalothin U.S.P...	Cefalotin	Cefalotine	CepHalotine........
Chloramphenicol U.S.P	Chloramphenicol DAB 7............................	Chlooramfenicol	Chloramphenicol.
Colistin N.F.............	Colistin	Colistine	Colistine.
Erythromycin U.S.P .	Erythromycinum Ph. Int.	Erythromycine	Erythromycine.
Gentamicin sulfate U.S.P....................	Refobacin	Gentamicine sulfaat	Gentamycine.
Kanamycin U.S.P	Kanmytrex, Kanamycin, ... Resistomycin.	Kanamycine	Kanamycine.
Lincomycin U.S.P	Cillimycin	Lincomycine.	
Methicillin U.S.P	Cinopenil	Methicilline...............	Methicilline.
Neomycin sulfate U.S.P	Neomycin, Bykomycin	Neomycine sulfaat .	Neomycine.
Oxacillin U.S.P.........	Cryptocillin, Stapenor	Oxacilline	Oxacilline.
Polymyxin B sulfate U.S.P...	Polymyxini B-sulfas Ph.Int..	Polymyxine B sulfaat	Polymyxine B.

Potassium penicillin G, ... U.S.P.	Penicillin G-Kalium DAB 7.	Kalium penicilline B . . .	Penicilline.
Potassium phenoxymethyl .... penicillin U.S.P.	Beromycin, Immunocillin, ... Isocillin, Aracil.	Kalium fenoxymethyl penicilline.	
Streptomycin sulfate U.S.P.., ...	Streptomycinsulfat DAB 7..	Streptomycine sulfaat .	Streptomycine sulfate.
Tetracycline U.S.P ...	Tetracyclinum Ph.Int .	Tetracycline	Oxytetracycline.

DRUGS AFFECTING SYMPATHETIC NERVOUS SYSTEM AND NERVE ENDINGS

Atropine sulfate U.S.P	Atropinsulfat DAB 7	Atropine sulfaat	Atropine sulfate.
Cyclopentolate hydrochloride U.S.P.	....	Cyclopentolaat hydrochloride.	
Epinephrine U.S.P	Adrenalin DAB 7	Adrenaline	Adrenaline. .....
Homatropine hydrobromide U.S.P.	Homatropinhydrobromid .... DAB 7.	Homatropine hydrobromide.	Homatropine bromhydrate.
Isoproterenol U.S.P	Isoprenalini hydrochloridum Ph.Int.	Isoprenaline	Isuprel, isoprenaline.
Levarterenol bitartrate U.S.P.	Noradrenalinhydrogentartrat .... DAB 7.	Levarterenol bitartraat.	Noradrenaline.
Physostigmine salicylate U.S.P.	Physostigminsalicylat DAB 7	Fysostigmine salicyclaat................	
Pralidoxime chloride U.S.P..	Pralidoximi methiodidum .... Ph.Int.	Pralidoxime chloride	Pralidoxime.
Scopolamine U.S.P	Scopolaminhydrobromid DAB 7.	Scopolamine U.S.P	Scopolamine.

ELECTROLYTES

Calcium gluconate injection .... U.S.P.	Calcium gluconicum 10%	Calcium gluconaat injectie.	Calcium levulinate.
Dextrose injection U.S.P	Traubenzuckerlösung 10%	Glucose injectie	Solution injectable de glucose, isotonique.
Lactated Ringer's injection .... U.S.P.	Ringer-Lactat-Lösung	Ringer lactaat injectie	Lactate de calcium.

Ringer's injection U.S.P.	Ringer-Lösung	Ringer injectie .	Solution de Ringer.
Sodium chloride injection .... U.S.P.	Natriumchloridlösung, isotonisch, pyrogenfrei, steril (DAB 7).	Natrium chloride injectie.	Solution injectable de chlorure de sodium, isotonique.

PLASMA EXPANDERS

United States	Germany	Netherlands	France
Normal human serum albumin U.S.P.	Humanalbumin 20%	Normal humaan albumine uit serum.	Albumine humaine.
Plasma protein fraction U.S.P.	PPL, Humanalbumin 5%.................	Protein fractie uit plasma..........	Gamma globuline.

MISCELLANEOUS DRUGS

Acetylsalicyclic acid U.S.P	Acetylsalicylsaure DAB 7	Acetylsalicyl zuur ..	Acetylsalicylique acide.
Amyl nitrite N.F	....	Amyl nitriet	Nitrite d'amyle.
Chlorpromazine U.S.P	Chlorpromazini hydrochloridum Ph.Int.	Chloor promazine	Chlorpromazine.
Digitalis U.S.P	Digitalisblatter DAB 7	Digitalis	Digitaline.
Digoxin U.S.P..........	Digoxinum Ph.Int	Digoxine.	
Ethacrynic acid U.S.P	....	Ethacryne zuur.	
Furosemide U.S.P...	Lasix	Furosemide	Furosemide-Lasilix.
Hydrocortisone sodium succinate injection U.S.P.	Hydrocortisonhemisuccinat	Hydrocortison natrium .... succinaat injectie.	Hydrocortisone hemisuccinate.
Mafenide	Marfanil	Mafenide.	
Mannitol U.S.P	D-Mannit	Mannitol.	
Oxygen U.S.P	Sauerstoff	Zuurstof	Oxygene.
Petrolatum U.S.P.	Paraffinum solidum DAB 6, Paraffinum durum DAB 7.	Vaseline	Vaseline.
Probenecid U.S.P ...	Benemid	Probenecide.	
Silver nitrate U.S.P .	Silbernitrat DAB 7 ..	Zilvernitraat	Nitrate d'argent.
Sodium nitrite U.S.P	Natriumnitrit DAB 7.	Natrium nitriet	Nitrite de sodium.
Sodium polysterene sulfonate U.S.P.	Kationen-Austauscherharz	Natrium polystyreen sulfonaat.	
Sodium thiosulfate U.S.P.	Natriumthiosulfat DAB 7	Natrium thiosulfaat	Hyposulfite de sodium.

VACCINES AND ANTITOXINS

Gas gangrene antitoxin, pentavalent.	Gasoedem- Antitoxin, polyvalent.	Gas gangreen-antitoxine pentavalent.	Serum antigangreneux polyvalent. ....
Tetanus immune globulin (human) U.S.P.	Tetanus-Immunglobulin	Tetanus-immuno globuoline (menselijk).	
Tetanus toxoid U.S.P.	Tetatoxoid	Tetanus vaccin .	Vaccin antitetanique.

ANTISEPTICS

Alcohol U S P	Aethanol DAB 7	Alcohol	Alcool ethylique.
Hexachlorophene U.S.P	Hexachlorophen WHO	Hexachlorophene .	Exophene.

II - Useful Tables

TABLE 1.— *Atomic weights, valences, and equivalent weights of certain elements*

Element	Atomic weight	Valence	Equivalent weight
Sodium	23.0	1	23.0
Potassium	39.0	1	39.0
Magnesium	24.0	2	12.0
Calcium	40.0	2	20.0
Chlorine	35.5	1	35.5
Phosphorus	31.0	3	10.3
Sulfur	32.0	2	16.0

TABLE 2. *Milliequivalent per gram of certain elements and compounds*

Element or compound	Mini-equivalent	Element or compound	Mini-equivalent
Sodium	43.5	Potassium chloride:	
Potassium	26.0	Potassium	13.5
Magnesium	85.0	Chloride	13.5
Calcium	50.0	Sodium lactate:	
Chloride	29.0	Sodium	9.0
Sodium chloride:		Lactate	9.0
Sodium	17.0		
Chloride	17.0		

364

TABLE 3. *Normal range of concentration of serum constituents*

Constituent		Concentration per 100 -milliliters	Milliequivalent per liter
Sodium	...milligram	310-340	135-148
Potassium	.........do.........	13.6-20.7	3.5-5.3
Magnesium	.........do.........	1.8-3.0	1.5-2.5
Calcium	.........do.........	9.6-11.0	4.8-5.4
Chloride	.........do.........	348-383	98-108
Urea nitrogen....................	.........do.........	8-26	
Carbon dioxide		101-132	23-30 mM
Total protein	.........gram..	6.0-8.2	
Albumin	.......do.........	3.8-5.0	
Globulin	.......do.........	2.3-3.5	

TABLE 4. *Normal range of concentration of whole blood gases and pH values*

Constituent	Concentration
pO_2 Arterial	90-100 torr[1]
Venous	30 torr
pCO_2 Arterial	35-16 torr
Venous	38-49 torr
pH	7.35-7.45

[1] One torr = 1 mm Hg at sea level.

TABLE 5. *Equivalent United States and imperial weights and measures*

Unit of measurement	Abbre-viation	United States measure	Imperial measure
1 milligram	mg	0.015432 grain	0.015432 grain.
1 gram	g	15.432 grains	15.432 grains.
1 kilogram	kg	{35.274ounces(avoirdupois) { 32.150ounces(apothecary)	35.274 ounces (avoir-dupois) 35.274 ounces (apothecary).
1 grain	gr	{0.0648gram {64.8milligrams	0.0648 gram. 64.8 milligrams.
480 grains	gr	31.1035 grams	31.1035 grams.
1 ounce	oz	{437.5 grains {28.350 grams	437.5 grains. 28.350 grams.
1 milliliter	ml	16.23 minims	16.894 minims.
1 liter	1	33.814 fluid ounces............	35.196 fluid ounces.
1 minim	min	0.0616 milliliter	0.0592 milliliter.
1 fluid ounce	fl oz	29.573 milliliters	28.412 milliliters.
1 pint[1]	Pt	473.17 milliliters	568.25 milliliters.

[1] Sixteen fluid ounces, U.S. measure; 20 fluid ounces, imperial measure.

USEFUL TABLES

TABLE 6. *Approximate equivalent metric and imperial doses*

Milliliters	Minims	Grams	Grains	Milligrams	Grains
0.1	1%	0.1	1%	0.1	1/600
0.12	2	0.12	2	0.125	1/480
0.15	2y2	0.15	2%	0.25	1/240
0.2	3	0.2	3	0.3	1/200
0.25	4	0.25	4	0.5	1/120
0.3	5	0.3	5	0.6	1/100
0.4	6	0.4	6	1	1/60
0.5	8	0.5	8	1.5	1/40
0.6	10	0.6	10	2	1/30
1	15	1	15	2.5	1/24
1.3	20	1.3	20	3	1/20
2	30	2	30	5	1/12
3	45	3	45	8	1/8
4	60	4	60	9	3/20
5	75	5	75	10	1/6
6	90	6	90	12	1/5
8	120	8	120	16	1/4
10	150	10	150	20	1/3
15	225	15	225	25	2/5
20	300	20	300	30	1/2
25	375	25	375	50	3/4
				60	1
				75	1 1/4

TABLE 7. *Equivalent avoirdupois and metric weights*

Pounds	Kilograms	Pounds	Kilograms
100	45.359	155	70.306
105	47.627	160	72.574
110	49.895	165	74.842
115	52.163	170	77.110
120	54.431	175	79.378
125	56.698	1 80	81.646
1 30	58.966	185	83.914
1 35	61.234	190	86.182
140	63.502	195	88.450
145	65.770	200	90.718
150	68.038	....	

TABLE 8. *Equivalents of centigrade and Fahrenheit thermometric scales*

Degrees C	Degrees F	Degrees C	Degrees F	Degrees C	Degrees F
-10	14.0	31	87.8	72	161.6
-9	15.8	32	89.6	73	163.4
-8	17.6	33	91.4	74	165.2
-7	19.4	34	93.2	75	167.0
-6	21.2	35	95.0	76	168.8
-5	23.0	36	96.8	77	170.6
-4	24.8	37	98.6	78	172.4
-2	26.6	38	100.4	79	174.2
-2	28.4	39	102.2	80	176.0
-1	30.2	40	104.0	81	177.8
0	32.0	41	105.8	82	179.6
1	33.8	42	107.6	83	181.4
2	35.6	43	109.4	84	183.2
3	37.4	44	111.2	85	185.0
4	39.2	45	113.0	86	186.8
5	41.0	46	114.8	87	188.6
6	42.8	47	116.6	88	190.4
7	44.6	48	118.4	89	192.2
8	46.4	49	120.2	90	194.0
9	48.2	50	122.0	91	195.8
10	50.0	51	123.8	92	197.6
11	51.8	52	125.6	93	199.4
12	53.6	53	127.4	94	201.2
13	55.4	54	129.2	95	203.0
14	57.2	55	131.0	96	204.8
15	59.0	56	132.8	97	206.6
16	60.8	57	134.6	98	208.4
17	62.6	58	136.4	99	210.2
18	64.4	59	138.2	100	212.0
19	66.2	60	140.0	101	213.8
20	68.0	61	141.8	102	215.6
21	69.8	62	143.6	103	217.4
22	71.6	63	145.4	104	219.2
23	73.4	64	147.2	105	221.0
24	75.2	65	149.0	106	222.8
25	77.0	66	150.8	107	224.6
26	78.8	67	152.6	108	226.4
27	80.6	68	154.4	109	228.2
28	82.4	69	156.2	110	230.0
29	84.2	70	158.0		
30	86.0	71	159.8		

BASIC FUNDAMENTALS OF ORGANIC CHEMISTRY

CONCISE TEXT

CONTENTS

BASIC FUNDAMENTALS of ORGANIC CHEMISTRY

CONCISE TEXT

For years, chemistry was divided into two main categories: inorganic chemistry, dealing with substances of mineral origin, and organic chemistry, dealing with those derived from living organisms. It was widely accepted that some "vital force" was necessary in the making of organic compounds and although man could manufacture inorganic compounds, he would have to be satisfied with a role of merely analyzing substances of organic nature, leaving their manufacture up to the plants and animals with the "vital force." Since the synthesis of urea, a recognized organic substance, chemists have had to modify their thinking and organic chemistry has become the study of the compounds of carbon, regardless of whether or not they are derived from plants or animals. Since then, scientists have been able to produce hundreds of thousands of organic compounds.

1. The importance of organic chemistry

a. Organic substances important to life. From the simplest, one-celled organisms to the grossly complex human being, all living organisms are made up of organic materials. Protoplasm, the basis for life itself, is a highly complex mixture of organic compounds. Organic chemistry is of primary importance, then, in the composition and function of living things. Most of the things essential in our everyday life are also of organic nature.

(1) Food. Fundamental to our existence is the food which we ingest to produce energy and growth. Our food is organic in nature. Further, the foods required by the plants and animals which supply us our food are organic. Proteins ... carbohydrates ... fats ... vitamins ... these are all organic compounds.

(2) Housing. Many of the materials used in the construction of our houses and the furnishings within are organic. Wood ... plastic ... rubber ... all are organic.

(3) Clothing. It is hard to find a single garment or article of clothing that is not of organic material. Cotton ... wool ... silk ... rubber ... nylon ... leather ... plastic ... dacron, and many, many other synthetic materials make up almost 100 percent of our garments.

b. Organic substances important to health. A great majority of the items used by man to promote and sustain health are organic in nature.

(1) Medicinals. List every medicinal you and your family have ever taken, touched, heard of, or seen. When you have finished, you will have a lengthy list; more than 90 percent of the items will be organic or have organic ingredients. Less than 10 percent of our medicinal agents are of inorganic origin.

(2) Agents related to medicine and pharmacy. In addition to the medications given to treat and prevent disease, there are many adjunct items. Sterile dressings, sutures, and prostheses may also be of organic origin. More than a million organic compounds have been made and studied. Infinitely more are possible, whereas inorganic compounds synthesized and studied number only about 50,000. In years to come, there will be a far greater spread between the number of organic and inorganic compounds. This is so because carbon has the ability to form infinitely long and high molecular weight chains.

c. Advances in medicine and pharmacy. In the past 35 years, more advances have been made in medicine than since the beginning of civilization, and the vast majority of these have been through the efforts conducted in organic synthesis. Certainly, then, the field of organic chemistry is important to man, and even more important to the pharmacist and physician.

2. Sources of organic compounds. Before the synthesis of urea by Wohler in 1828, all the organic compounds in use were naturally occurring and produced by the plant or animal kingdom. Today, we have three possible sources for organic substances: natural, synthetic, and semisynthetic.

a. Natural. Mother nature has been kind to us in supplying many useful organic substances "readymade." Proteins, carbohydrates, and fats, our important food substances, along with vitamins, essential food supplements, are all naturally occurring in plant and animal life. Fibrous material for clothing manufacture is available, as are alkaloidal drugs, fuels, and building materials. We need only harvest and process these naturally occurring products.

b. Synthetic. The synthetic organic products used widely today may be compounded by chemical action of naturally occurring organic substances to produce new substances, or they may be entirely synthesized from raw elements. Organic chemists have been able to make in the laboratory not only exact duplicates of organic compounds occurring in nature, but also myriads of new compounds which do not occur naturally.

c. Semisynthetic. Some of the medicinal agents used today are neither natural nor synthetic, but combinations of the two. These may be thought of as semisynthetic compounds. The most impressive of these semisynthetics are the antibiotics. In 1928, Sir Alexander Fleming noticed that a foreign mold in a culture plate caused the inhibition of a staphylococcus culture. Through subculturing, he isolated penicillin, a widely used antibiotic. A number of the antibiotics used today are synthetic; others must still be derived semisynthetically with the help of the microorganisms.

3. Important basic principles of organic chemistry. Before we can learn about the organic compounds important to pharmacy, it is necessary that we know some basic principles and properties pertaining to all organic substances.

a. General properties of organic compounds. With a field so large, it is difficult to classify the hundreds of thousands of compounds that have been isolated and studied to date. They differ widely in structure, action, and use. The following general statements, however, apply to all organic compounds:

(1) The number of organic compounds possible is almost limitless, whereas inorganic compounds are held within a restricted field.

(2) Molecular structure of organic substances is far more complex than the structure of inorganic materials.

(3) Organic compounds favor covalent bonding, while most inorganic bonding is of the electrovalent type.

(4) Organic compounds are generally insoluble in water, but soluble in the organic solvents such as alcohol, carbon tetrachloride, carbon disulfide, chloroform, or ether.

(5) Most organic compounds are thermolabile; that is, they are sensitive to destruction by heat.

(6) Organic reactions are difficult to predict. You remember that in inorganic chemistry, reactions took place rapidly, yielding definite products. Organic reactions may take hours or even days and the yield of intended products is rarely more than 50 percent. There may be many compounds formed in a single reaction.

b. Unique properties of carbon. The unique properties of carbon compared to the other elements is the basis and reason for organic chemistry. Carbon, the first member of the fourth group in the periodic table, has six protons, six neutrons, and six orbital electrons. The electron configuration, as you should imagine, is two electrons in the K shell and four in the L shell. If you look carefully at the periodic table, you will see that carbon is the lowest atomic weight element exactly midway between two inert elements. In reacting, carbon can attain stability either by accepting four electrons or losing four electrons, and because of this it is equally liable to be oxidized or reduced. Actually, since carbon forms compounds by covalent bonding, the electrons are neither gained nor lost, but shared.

c. Purification of organic compounds. The purity of organic compounds may be determined by a number of tests, including specific gravity determination, refraction index, crystal form, and other physical constants. The customary way of determining the purity of organic compounds, however, is by determination of their boiling and melting points. Impurities lower melting points and make the range in temperature between starting and completion of melting rather wide. Moreover, the boiling point of pure organic compounds is constant. Variations from this constant indicate impurities.

(1) Purification by crystallization. Crystallization is the method generally employed for the purification of solid organic substances. A solvent is chosen in which the solid is much more soluble when the solvent is hot than cold. The substance to be purified is dissolved in the hot solvent and any insoluble material is filtered off. The solution is then cooled, depositing crystals of the pure substance. The liquid is filtered off; the crystals are washed with more pure solvent and dried.

(2) Purification of extraction with an immiscible solvent. Liquids containing small amounts of impurities can be effectively purified by extracting the impurities with another solvent. The solvent chosen for the extraction should be immiscible with the liquid to be purified. It must also be one in which the impurity is much more soluble than in the liquid to be purified. The two liquids are shaken together and the impurity transfers to the liquid in which it is more soluble. Upon standing, the two liquids separate into layers which can then be separated by physical means.

(3) Fractional distillation. Mixtures of liquids or solutions of solids in liquids may be purified by fractional distillation. The impure substance is placed in a flask and by slowly increasing the temperature, the different substances are distilled off. The collecting vessels are changed with each rise in the temperature fraction to receive the various substances.

(4) Other methods. Other methods for eliminating impurities from organic substances are steam distillation and sublimation.

d. Tests for organic compounds. To determine if a compound is organic, it generally suffices to heat the compound. If it decomposes at a relatively low temperature, leaving a black, charred residue, it is very probably an organic compound. Compounds which sublime cannot be tested in this manner. Specific procedures for the qualitative and quantitative analysis of organic compounds are of no practical value to you as a pharmacy technician and will not be covered here. Most texts on organic chemistry and all laboratory manuals in the field will answer any questions you may have on the analysis of organic materials.

e. Skeleton structure. As previously stated, carbon possesses the ability to link together to form complex molecules. These molecules may form continuous chains, branching chains, closed chains (rings), or rings with separating elements other than carbon. The following are examples of these structures:

(1) Continuous or straight chain.

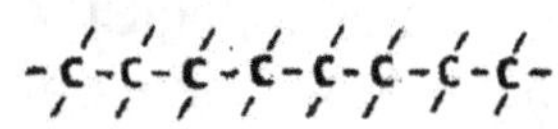

(2) Branching chain.

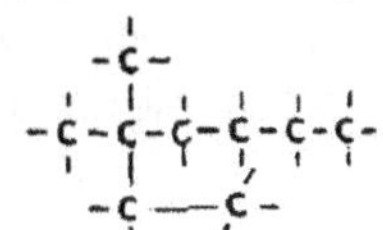

(3) Closed chains or rings.

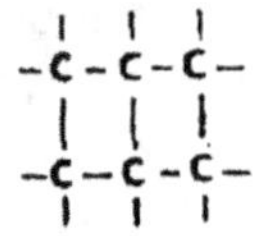

(4) Rings including other elements.

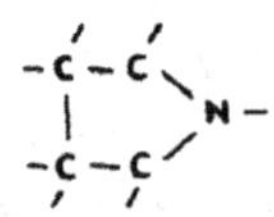

f. Bonds.

(1) Valence bonds. The study of organic compounds is immeasurably simplified by the graphic representation of their formulas. In writing these formulas, lines or dots (called bonds) are commonly used to show how the atoms are joined together in the molecule. These bonds represent the valence, and the number of bonds attached to each element symbol represents the valence of that atom in the molecule. Thus, in the formula-

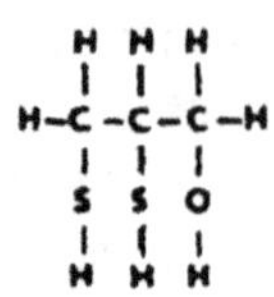

the valence of each C atom is 4, that of the S atom is 2, each O atom has a valence of 2, and each H atom has a valence of 1. It is also written-

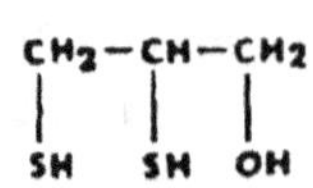

to represent the same formula. These written formulas show not only that the elements are bonded together, but how they are bonded. Therefore, it is advisable to include here a brief description of the more important kinds of valence bonds in terms of their electron meanings.

(2) Electrovalent bond. This type of bond is most frequently seen in electrolytes such as sodium chloride, NaCl. An actual electron transfer from one atom to another occurs in the electrovalent bond. In sodium chloride, the Na atom loses, transfers, or gives its single valence electron to the Cl atom.

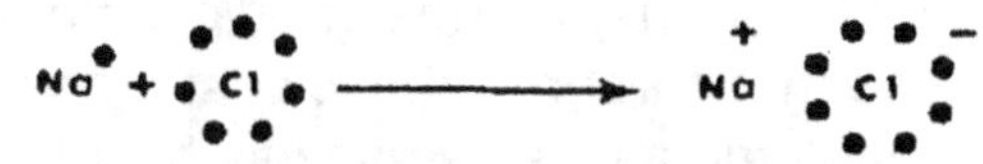

Since the Na atom loses a negative charge, it takes on a positive charge of one. The chlorine atom, gaining the electron, takes on a negative charge of one. The two elements, Na and Cl, are held together by the attraction of the opposite charges. These charged particles in solution will transmit an electric current and therefore are termed electrolytes. The electrovalent bond is not very common in organic molecules. An example of a bond which is at least partly electrovalent is the bond between the O and the H in carboxylic acids and phenols.

(3) Covalent bond. This is the type of bond found in organic compounds between carbon atoms and in such inorganic molecules as H_2 O, H_2, or Cl_2.

(a) Sharing electron pairs. In the covalent bond, the atoms involved "share," rather than transfer, one or more pairs of electrons. In the case of the chlorine molecule, each element has seven outer electrons. Two atoms are combined to form a stable molecule, with each atom sharing two electrons (one from each atom).

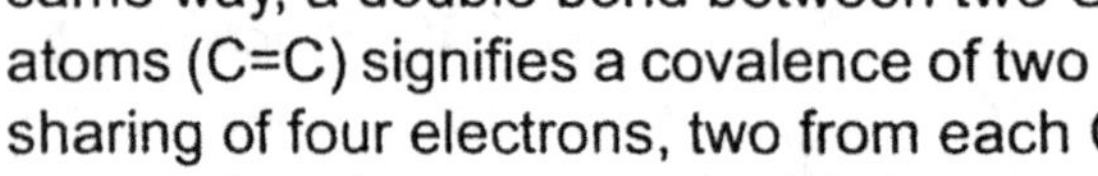

(b) Single, double, and triple bonds. A single bond between two C atoms signifies a covalence of one or a sharing of two electrons, one from each atom. In the same way, a double bond between two C atoms (C=C) signifies a covalence of two or a sharing of four electrons, two from each C atom. A triple bond (C≡C) would then show a covalence of three or a sharing of six electrons, three from each atom.

(c) Illustration of covalent bonding. To illustrate this bonding, the following electron formulas are shown. The electrons belonging originally to C are designated by circles, those originally part of H

by dots, and those belonging originally to O by

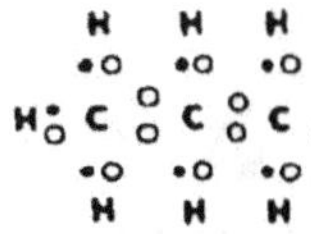

Propane

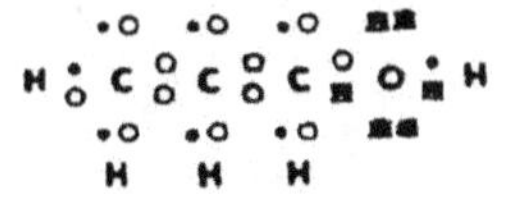

Propanol

Note that in both molecules, each element has attained a stable configuration. Hydrogen has attained two electrons in the outer orbit and both carbon and oxygen have eight electrons in their outer orbits.

g. Isomerism. Compounds that have the same composition; that is, the same number and kind of atoms but in different arrangement, are called isomers. Below are diagrams for three isomers of the same formula (octane). Eighteen are possible. For the sake of simplicity, the hydrogen atoms normally saturating the carbon atoms have not been shown.

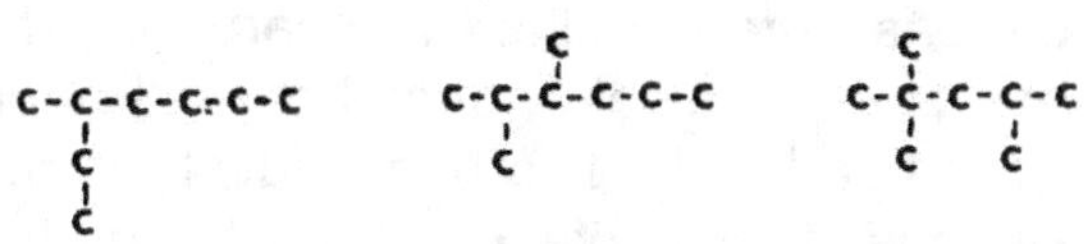

The atoms of octane can be arranged in 18 different ways, although there are always the same number and kind of atoms. Each different arrangement is an isomer. Each has the formula C_8H_{18}. As the complexity of the organic material involved increases, so does the number of possible isomers. These isomers are not identical in their properties or actions and consequently there are billions of possible arrangements for the hundreds of thousands of organic structures known.

h. Graphic formula. The best way to show the complete atomic relationships of the molecule is by graphic formulas. The formulas shown in the explanation of isomerism are examples of graphic formulas, except that the hydrogen atoms have been omitted. The following is an example of a full graphic formula:

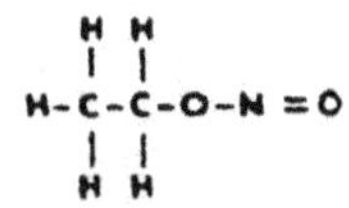

i. Linear formula. A linear formula is a simplification of a graphic formula. Although the linear formula is easier to write, unlike the graphic formula it does not show the complete molecular structure. In most cases, the graphic formula is preferred. The following examples compare three types of linear formulas with a graphic formula:

(1) Graphic formula.

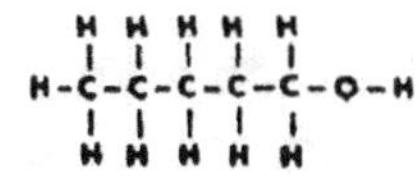

(2) Linear formula (dashes represent bonds).

CH_3 -CH_2 -CH_2 -CH_2 -CH_2 -OH

(3) Linear formula (dots represent bonds).

CH_3•CH_2•CH_2•CH_2•CH_2•OH

(4) Linear formula (bonds not shown). CH_3 CH_2 CH_2 CH_2 CH_2 OH

j. Classification of organic compounds. Practically all organic compounds are grouped into the following classes:

(1)	Hydrocarbons	(6)	Esters
(2)	Alcohols and phenols	(7)	Ethers
		(8)	Carbohydrates
(3)	Aldehydes	(9)	Alkaloids
(4)	Ketones	(10)	Nitrogenous
(5)	Acids products		

These ten classes may be broadly considered as derivatives of either methane or benzene. The methane derivatives, which are straight or branched chain compounds, are termed aliphatic compounds. The benzene derivatives are cyclic compounds and are classified as aromatic compounds.

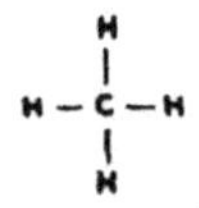

Methane

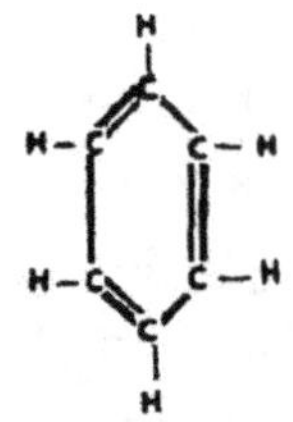

Benzene

4. Hydrocarbons. Compounds composed solely of carbon and hydrogen are called hydrocarbons. They may be either aliphatic, that is, straight or branched formations, or cyclic, i.e., arranged into a ring or closed cycle.

a. Terminal carbon atoms. The straight chain hydrocarbons have two terminal carbon atoms; the branched chain hydrocarbons have three terminal carbon atoms or more; and the closed ring or cyclic hydrocarbons have no terminal carbon atoms, since each carbon is joined to another in the ring. The following structures illustrate the terminal carbon atoms in the various formations.

(1) Straight chain hydrocarbon showing two terminal carbons.

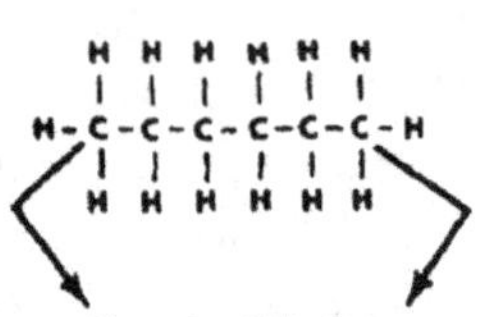

(2) Branched chain with three terminal carbons.

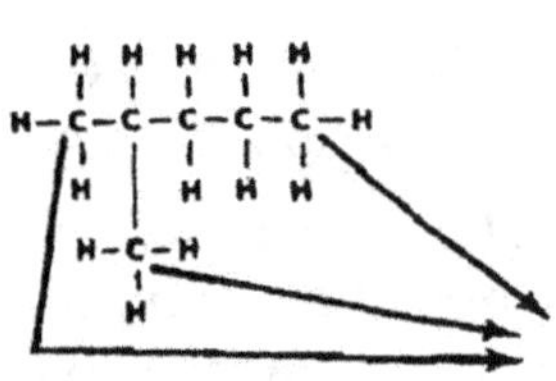

(3) Branched chain with four terminal carbons.

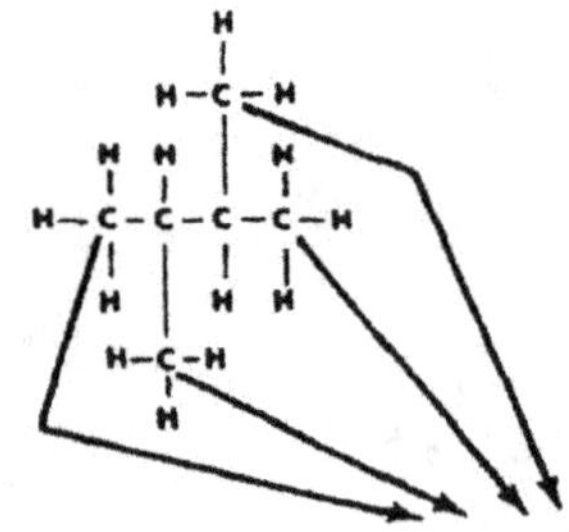

(4) Cyclic hydrocarbon showing no terminal carbons.

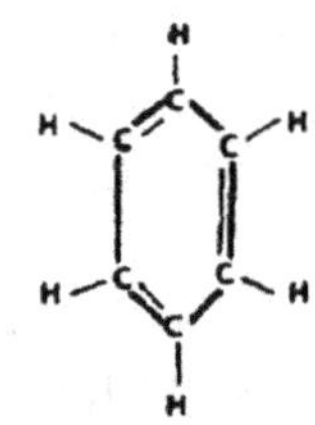

b. Aliphatic hydrocarbons. We will discuss in this portion of the chapter only the aliphatic hydrocarbons. The cyclic hydrocarbons will be discussed later with other cyclic compounds.

(1) Alkanes (paraffins, methane series, saturated hydrocarbons). This is the basic group of the hydrocarbons. They are composed solely of carbon-hydrogen bonds and carbon-carbon single bonds. Because they contain only single bonds, they are referred to as ìsaturated hydrocarbons.î This is a very stable bond and not reactive. The term paraffin comes from this property. The Latin word ìparumî means ìlittleî and ìaffinisî means affinity. Paraffins do not easily react with other chemicals.

(a) Homologous series. The alkanes form a homologous series. Each member differs from the preceding one by the addition of CH_2. Members next to each other are called homologs. Ethane and methane differ by CH_2 and are homologs of each other. The smallest alkane is methane, thus the term "methane series." The following list of the first ten alkanes form the basis for all other organic compounds and should be learned.

- methane, CH_4
- ethane, C_2H_6
- propane, C_3H_8
- hexane, C_6H_{14}
- heptane, C_7H_{16}
- octane, C_8H_{18}

- butane, C_4H_{10}
- pentane, C_5H_{12}
- nonane, C_9H_{20}
- decane, $C_{10}H_{22}$

(b) Naming simple alkanes. Looking at the first ten members, you can see a pattern developing. All alkanes end in -ane. This indicates a saturated hydrocarbon. The first four members have common names but starting with the fifth member, pentane, the name indicates how many carbon atoms are present. For example, the Greek word for the number of carbon atoms is followed by ìaneî: hexane has six carbons (hexa) each connected to another by a single bond (ane).

(c) General formula of alkanes. All alkanes conform to the general formula C_nH_{2n+2} (where n = the number of carbon atoms). If we know the number of carbon atoms, we can determine the number of hydrogen atoms in the alkane. Example: What would be the formula for eicosane (eico stands for 20) according to the general formula?

$$n = 20$$
$$C_nH_{2n+2}$$
$$C_{20}H_{2\times 20+2} = C_{20}H_{42}$$

(d) Empirical formula. The formula above tells us only how many carbon and hydrogen atoms are present; it does not tell us how they are arranged. It is called an empirical formula. In order to identify the exact compound, we must use either a graphic formula or a linear formula. This is necessary as several isomers may exist.

(e) Isomers. Isomerism is possible from the fourth member of this series on. These are structural isomers; that is, they differ in arrangement of the atoms. Thus, butane may exist in the two following isomeric forms:

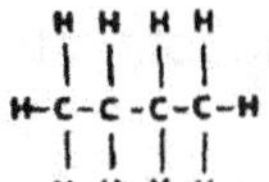

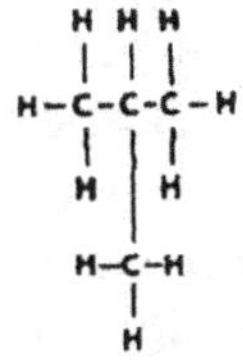

Both compounds have the empirical formula C_4H_{10}, but differ in arrangement. As the length of the carbon chain increases, the number of isomeric possibilities increases.

(f) Nomenclature of the alkanes. Because of the vast number of possible isomeric structures, it is necessary to have a system for naming these compounds. It would be hopeless to try to remember common names for all the members. The International Union of Chemists has devised the following system for naming any alkane.

1. All the straight chain alkanes have the ending *ane,* and except for the first four members, are named for the number of carbon atoms they possess.

2. Groups branching off a straight chain are named by using the stem of the alkane with the same number of carbon atoms, and changing its *ane* ending to *yl.* Thus we have the following groups or radicals: CH_3 = Meth*yl*, same number of C atoms as meth*ane*; C_2H_5 = eth*yl*, same number of C atoms as eth*ane*, and so on.

3. Branching alkanes are named on the basis of the longest straight chain they contain. The groups or radicals attached are listed alphabetically, preceding the base name. If the same radical appears more than once, it is given a prefix to show the number of times; for example, "di" for twice, "tri" for thrice, and "penta" for five times.

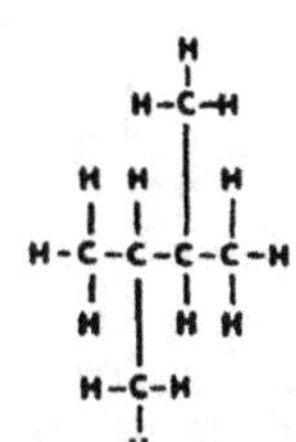

In the preceding graphic formula we have a branching chain isomer of hexane. The longest straight chain consists of four carbon atoms and therefore will be named on the basis of butane. There are two methyl groups attached and consequently this structure will be dimethyl butane.

4. It is important to know just where these methyl groups are attached, so the chain must be numbered. Only the longest chain is numbered, and always from the most branched end. In the case above, both ends are equally branched, so it makes no difference from which end you number.

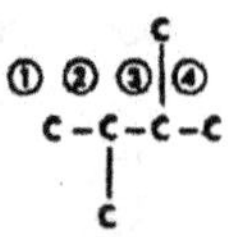

We can now further identify the compound as 2,3-dimethyl butane. How would you name the following compound?

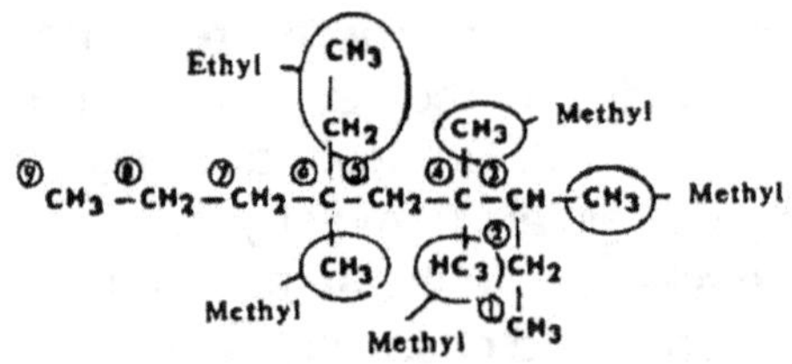

This compound is numbered for you, and the longest chain is 9 carbon atoms long. It will, then, be named as a nonane. Its name-6-ethyl-3, 4, 4, 6-tetramethylnonane.

5. In the event it is not obvious which end of the chain is most branching, number from both ends, name the compound both ways, and the compound whose numbers total the smaller figure when added will be the correct name. To illustrate this, let's number the above compound from the other end and see which is correct.

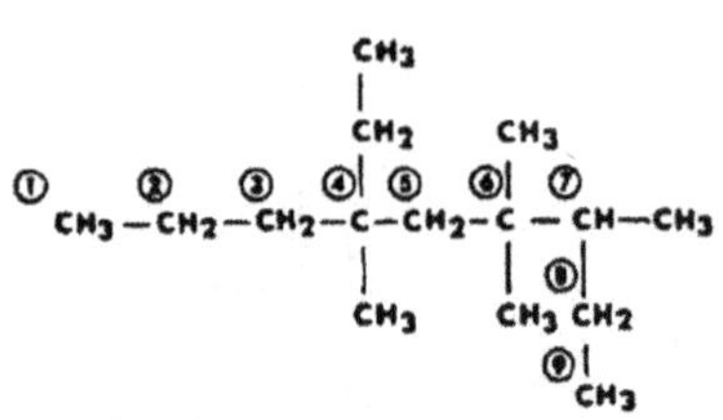

Numbered in this fashion, the name would be 4-ethyl-4, 6, 6, 7-tetramethylnonane. Adding the numbers 4, 4, 6, 6, and 7, we get a total of 27. The previous name's numbers (6, 3, 4, 4, and 6) when totaled give a sum of 23. Since 23 is the lower number, that name is correct.

6. Just as we can name a structure from its formula, we can construct the graphic formula, given its name. To illustrate, let's draw the formula for 2, 4-dimethyl hexane. This name tells us that the longest chain is six carbons long, and that there are two methyl groups attached, one at the number two carbon and one at the number four carbon. Thus we draw the structure

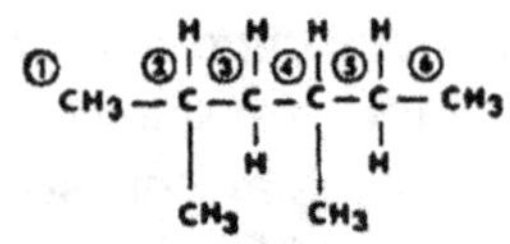

(2) Alkenes (ethylene series, olefins, unsaturated hydrocarbons). The first member of the alkene series is ethylene ($C_2 H_4$), which is also called ethene. You should guess from the number of carbons and hydrogens in this compound that the general formula for the alkenes is C_nH_{2n}. The number of hydrogen atoms is exactly twice the number of carbons.

(a) Reason for the general formula. The general formula for the alkenes (C_nH_{2n}) has two less hydrogens than that for the alkanes ($C_n H_{2n+2}$). This is because the alkenes are unsaturated; somewhere in the molecule a double bond exists. For each double bond, two pairs of electrons are required. Thus, bonds which were attached to a hydrogen in the alkanes are paired between two carbons in the alkenes, causing two less hydrogen atoms in the alkene molecule.

(b) Reactivity. Because the alkenes are unsaturated, having at least one double bond which is strained and unstable when compared to a single bond, they are quite reactive. Unsaturated compounds seek to gain saturation and thus enter into chemical reaction easily.

(c) Alkene nomenclature. Alkenes are named from the corresponding alkane; that is, from the alkane having the same carbon content. In adapting the proper alkane name to fit its corresponding alkene, the *ane* ending is dropped and *ene* or *ylene* is added. There is no alkene corresponding to methane, so the alkene series progresses in the following manner:

- Ethylene or ethene (C_2H_4)
- Propylene or propene (C_3H_6)
- Butylene or butene (C_4H_8)
- Pentylene or pentene (C_5H_{10})
- Hexylene or hexene (C_6H_{12})

(d) Naming complex alkenes. Naming alkenes is basically the same as naming the alkanes. The longest chain containing the double bond is selected as the base. The chain is numbered from the end that gives the double bonded carbon atoms the lowest numbers. The number of the carbon closest to the end of the chain is prefixed to the base name to indicate where the double bond is located. Radicals attached to the chain are named in the same manner as the alkanes. The formula below would be named 3-methyl-2-pentene:

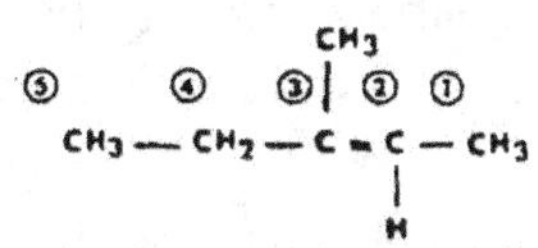

(3) Alkynes (alkines). This homologous series contains a triple bond and has the general formula C_nH_{2n-2}. The alkynes are even more unstable than the alkenes because of the triple bond. They react explosively. The first and simplest member of this group is ethyne, generally called by its common name, acetylene.

$$HC{\equiv}CH$$

Nomenclature for the alkynes is basically the same as for the alkenes.

(4) Occurrence of the hydrocarbons in nature. Petroleum, or crude oil as it is sometimes called, is a mixture of hydrocarbons varying greatly in composition. It is obtained from beneath the surface of the ground, and is the result of decomposition of various forms of marine life over thousands of years.

(a) Gaseous hydrocarbons. The first four alkanes (methane, ethane, propane, and butane) are gases. Natural gas is a mixture of about 80 percent methane with small amounts of ethane and propane. As the number of carbons increase, the compounds become denser, and pentane is the first liquid member of the series.

(b) Pentane and hexane. The first fraction to be distilled from crude oil is a mixture of pentane and hexane, two very volatile liquids. This combination of hydrocarbons is commercially known as petroleum benzin or petroleum ether, and is generally the substance used in cleaning fluids and lighter fluids.

(c) Heptane, octane, and nonane. The next fraction to distill off from the petroleum is a combination of heptane, octane, and nonane. This is the mixture known as gasoline. Normal heptane, the worst possible gasoline, has an octane rating of 0. The best gasoline is isooctane (2, 2, 4-trimethylpentane) and has an octane rating of 100.

(d) Kerosene. The next fraction to come off is not so volatile as the previous ones. This mixture has 10 or 11 carbon atoms and is commercially sold as kerosene. It is used as a fuel for heaters, kerosene stoves, and lanterns.

(e) Fuel oil and dieselene diesel oil). These are the next mixtures to be distilled from the petroleum and they range from 12 to 16 carbon atoms in composition.

(f) Other fractions. Progressing in molecular composition and at the same time becoming thicker and more nearly solid are-

1. Light lubrication oils *(Example:* 3-in-1 oil).
2. Light motor oil.
3. Heavy motor oil.
4. Transmission grease.
5. Axle grease.
6. Petroleum tar.
7. Waxes or paraffins.

Those fractions containing 30 or more carbon atoms are solids.

(5) Pharmaceutical products of the hydrocarbons.

(a) Ethylene (ethene) $CH_2 = CH_2$, C_2H_4. Ethylene, a very volatile gas, is highly flammable when mixed with oxygen. In concentrations of 85-90 percent, it is used as a surgical anesthetic that is power-

ful enough to permit any level of surgery. Because it is highly combustible, it must not be used near an open flame and extreme precautions must be taken against ignition by static electricity. Ethylene is used in the synthesis of ethyl alcohol and ethylene glycol and, because it destroys chlorophyll, it is used in the artificial ripening of oranges, lemons, and other fruits.

(b) Cyclopropane (trimethylene), C_3H_6.

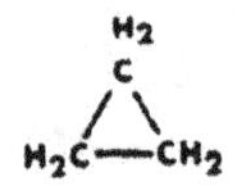

Although this is not an aliphatic hydrocarbon, it is usually considered with the aliphatics because it resembles them in properties and uses. This gas is also used as a general inhalation anesthetic, and since it is effective in concentrations of only 15-20 percent, it is safer for the patient than ethylene. It, too, is explosive and every precaution must be taken to prevent open flames or sparks from occurring in the operating room where it is being used.

(c) Ichthammol (ammonium ichthosulfonate). Ichthammol is a black, tarlike substance of natural occurrence. It can be manufactured by destructive distillation of bituminous substance, sulfonation, and neutralization of the product with ammonia. It is water miscible and is often incorporated into ointments for its anti-infective and irritant properties.

(d) Paraffin. Paraffin is a purified mixture of solid hydrocarbons obtained from petroleum. It is a waxy substance, insoluble in water and mainly used in pharmacy to stiffen ointments and suppositories. It is classified as a pharmaceutical necessity.

(e) Petrolatum (petroleum jelly; yellow petrolatum). Petrolatum is a purified mixture of semisolid hydrocarbons obtained from petroleum. It may contain a stabilizer. Petrolatum differs from automobile grease only in purity. The solid and liquid hydrocarbons making up this intermediate may contain impurities which are unsaturated. These will oxidize and become rancid. To prevent rancidity, some vitamin E is generally added in the processing. Petrolatum is used as an ointment base, emollient, and protective.

(f) White petrolatum (white petroleum jelly; petrolatum album). This substance is nothing more than yellow petrolatum which has been decolorized. It, too, is used as an ointment base and protective. It is also employed in the cosmetic industry.

(g) Mineral oil (heavy liquid petrolatum; liquid paraffin; white mineral oil). This is a viscous, clear liquid, containing hydrocarbon chains in the range of 18 to 24 carbon atoms. It is frequently used as a laxative because it acts as an intestinal lubricant. Since it is generally taken every day to promote regularity and soften the stool, and because it dissolves oil-soluble vitamins and allows them to be excreted, this preparation should only be administered at bedtime when it will not interfere with the assimilation of foods.

(h) Light liquid petrolatum (light liquid paraffin; light mineral oil). Light liquid petrolatum is not intended for internal use. It is the main ingredient in baby oils which may also contain rose oil for its pleasant scent and lanolin for its softening action. It is also used in the cosmetic industry. In the past, many nose drops and sprays used light mineral oil as a base, mainly because the ingredients were soluble in it. These are no longer widely used because the oil slicks down the hair-like structure (cilia) in the nostrils and allows bacteria to pass freely into the lungs. There is also the danger of children aspirating the oil into the lungs and developing lipoid (fatty) pneumonia.

5. Derivatives of the aliphatic hydrocarbons. By substituting chemically an element such as chlorine, or a radical such as hydroxyl, OH, for one or more of the hydrogen atoms of a hydrocarbon, hydrocarbon derivatives are achieved. Many of these substitution products are important in med-

icine. Notice in the following graphic formulas how elements have been substituted for hydrogen in methane to arrive at some important medicinal products.

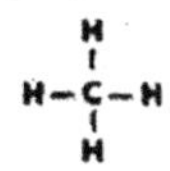

Methane

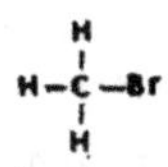

Methyl Bromide

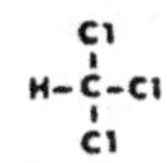

Chloroform

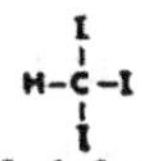

Iodoform

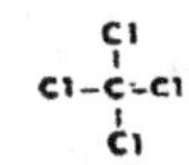

Carbon Tetrachloride

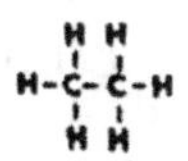

Ethane

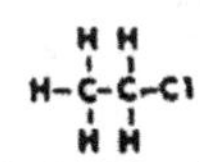

Ethyl Chloride

a. Ethyl chloride, CH_3CH_2Cl. Local anesthetic spray.

b. Butyl chloride (n-butyl chloride) CH_3 CH_2 CH_2 CH_2 Cl. An anthelmintic agent.

c. Carbon tetrachloride CCl_4 (tetrachloromethane). Solvent, anthelmintic, fire extinguishing agent.

d. Chloroform, $CHCl_3$. General anesthetic, carminative, solvent for extraction of alkaloids, irritant in liniments, and sedative expectorant in cough mixtures.

e. Trichloroethylene (Trilene).

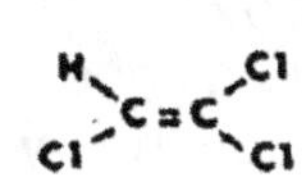

Trilene is an inhalation-type anesthetic.

f. Halothane (Fluothane) $CF_3CBrClH$. An inhalation anesthetic.

g. Iodoform (triiodomethane) CHI_3. An antibacterial used to impregnate gauze packing and dressings.

6. Aliphatic alcohols. Among the many important oxygen-containing compounds in the field of organic chemistry are the alcohols.

a. Structure. The general structure of the aliphatic alcohols can be represented by the formula R-OH; R being the hydrocarbon chain, and OH the alcohol group. Up to this point, you have been taught that an OH group signifies an alkali or base. In organic chemistry, the OH takes on a different meaning and lends far different characteristics and properties to the compound containing it. It is important that you thoroughly understand at this point that the OH group is now characteristic of the alcohol. It is this group which gives the compound its chemical properties as well as its therapeutic effects. Alcohols may contain one or more OH groups.

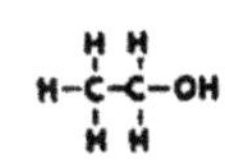

Ethyl Alcohol

b. Placement of alcohol group. Alcohols containing one hydroxyl group are called monohydric or monohydroxy alcohols, and those containing two or more OH groups are polyhydric or polyhydroxy alcohols. The placement of the alcohol group on the hydrocarbon chain greatly affects the nature of the compound. The alcohol groups may attach to a primary carbon atom (a carbon atom attached to only one other carbon), a secondary carbon atom (a carbon atom attached to two other carbons), or a tertiary carbon atom (a carbon atom attached to three other carbons). The alcohol formed when the hydroxyl group attaches to a primary carbon atom is a primary (1°) alcohol; to a secondary carbon atom, a secondary (2°) alcohol, and so on. In the graphic formulas below are shown the primary, secondary, and tertiary carbon atoms and the alcohol which results from attachment to each.

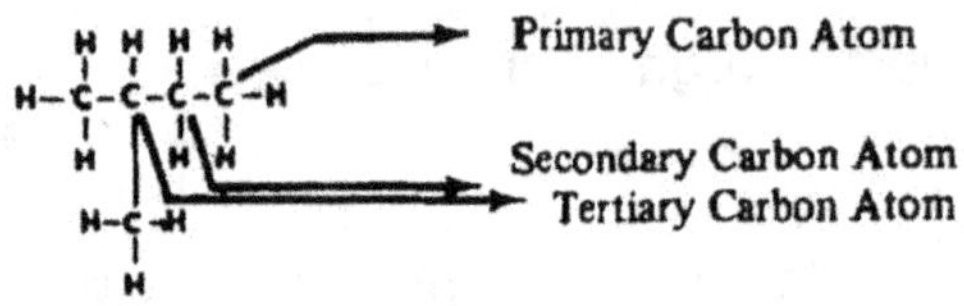

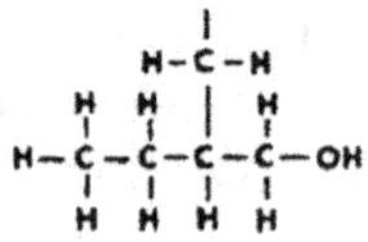

Primary (1°)
Alcohol

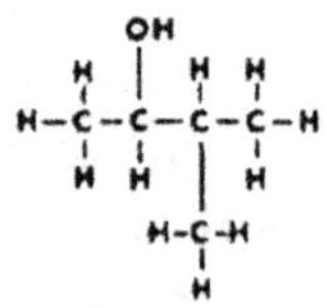

Secondary (2°)
Alcohol

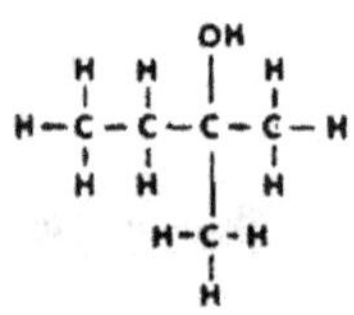

Tertiary (3°)
Alcohol

c. *General formulas for alcohols.*

- Primary Alcohol $R-CH_2OH$
- Secondary Alcohol 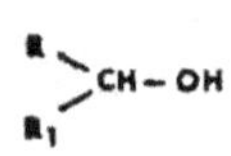
- Tertiary Alcohol 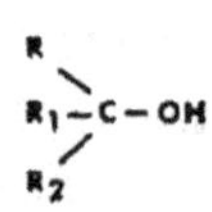

d. *Properties.* The following general properties can be stated for alcohols:

(1) Most monohydric alcohols are lighter than water; that is, they have specific gravities less than 1.000.

(2) Normal aliphatic alcohols are liquids up to 11 carbons in the chain and solids after 13.

(3) Addition of more OH groups increases the specific gravity and they become heavier than water. Alcohols also become sweeter as more OH groups are added to them. Sugar is a polyhydric alcohol.

(4) The alcohols are chemically neutral, that is, neither basic nor acidic. They do resemble bases in that they react with acids to form salts.

(5) Alcohols are miscible with water, but as the length of the chain increases, the solubility decreases. Solubility increases, however, as the number of hydroxy groups increases.

e. *Nomenclature.*

(1) Common name system. The common names of the alcohols are formed by taking the name of the radical and adding the word ìalcohol.î Thus, CH_3OH, containing a methyl radical, is called methyl alcohol. C_2H_5OH, containing an ethyl radical, is called ethyl alcohol. The common name system is satisfactory up to five carbon atoms in the radical. Beyond that it becomes too complicated for general use.

(2) International Union of Chemists (IUC) system. The IUC has established a system for naming the alcohols which is far superior to the common name method. This system is based upon ending the name with ìol.î Taking the stem from the longest continuous carbon chain which contains the OH radical, the ìeî is dropped and ìolî is added. Refer back to the nomenclature for the alkanes. By the IUC method, methyl alcohol becomes methanol and ethyl alcohol becomes ethanol.

f. *Occurrence.* Alcohols occur in nature as such (glycerin and mannitol) and with other radicals attached (glucose). Esterified alcohols are widely distributed in nature as volatile oils, fixed oils, fats, and waxes.

g. *Preparation.*

(1) Primary alcohols. Primary alcohols are prepared by the hydrolysis of the corresponding alkyl halide (halogen derivative) as in

$$C_2H_5Br + HOH \xrightarrow{NaOH} NaBr + HOH + C_2H_5OH$$

(2) Secondary alcohols. Secondary alcohols are prepared by the hydration of alkenes, by the reduction of ketones, or by the fermentation of sugars.

(3) Tertiary alcohols. Tertiary alcohols are made by the hydration of alkenes.

h. Reactions. The following are typical reactions which alcohols undergo:

(1) Hydrogen replaced by a metal to form salts.

$$2ROH+2Na \rightarrow H_2+2RONa$$

(2) Reaction with acids to form esters.

$$ROH+H_2SO_4 \rightarrow ROSO_3H+HOH$$

(3) Replacement of the hydroxyl group by a halogen.

$$ROH+HCl \xrightarrow{ZnCl_2} HOH+RCl$$

(4) Oxidation to form an aldehyde and a molecule of water.

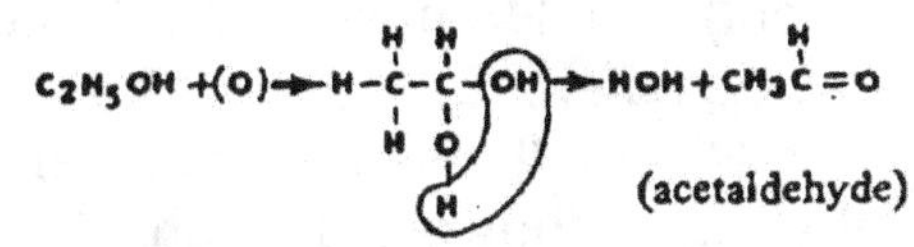

i. Alcohols used in pharmacy.

(1) Methyl alcohol (methanol; wood alcohol) CH_3 OH. Because it was manufactured by the destructive distillation of wood, methanol was given the common name of wood alcohol. Today, it is primarily synthesized directly from carbon monoxide and hydrogen. Extremely poisonous both internally and externally, this alcohol is used in pharmacy only as a solvent, a denaturing agent, a fuel for alcohol lamps, and as a starting point for the synthesis of other organic compounds.

(2) Alcohol [ethanol, ethyl alcohol, spiritus vini rectificatus (SVR)] C_2H_5OH. Alcohol is manufactured by the process of fermentation, an enzymatic decomposition of carbohydrates. When alcohol is called for in a prescription or formula, this is the alcohol to be used unless otherwise specified.

(a) Uses. Ethyl alcohol is found in beverages, and although large quantities are toxic, it is intended for internal administration as well as external. It is used as a vehicle for liquid medications, as a preservative, and as a rub. It is a starting point in the manufacture of ether.

(b) Composition. In its official form, alcohol is a mixture of 95 percent C_2H_5OH and 5 percent water by volume. It is 95 percent pure or 190 proof.

(3) Diluted alcohol (diluted ethanol). Diluted alcohol is a mixture of equal volumes of ethyl alcohol and distilled water. This mixture is accompanied by a rise in temperature and a contraction in the total volume. When 500 ml. of alcohol and 500 ml. of water are mixed, the resulting volume is NOT 1000 ml., but closer to 970 ml., a loss of approximately 3 percent. Diluted alcohol is useful as a solvent because it combines the solvent properties of both alcohol and water.

(4) Alcohol rubbing compound (rubbing alcohol). Rubbing alcohol is 70 percent absolute ethyl alcohol, and 30 percent water and denaturants. The denaturants make it unsuitable for drinking and consequently it need not be controlled on stock record cards. Rubbing alcohol is used externally only.

(5) Isopropyl alcohol (isopropanol; 2-propanol) $CH_3CH(OH)CH_3$. This alcohol, produced synthetically as a byproduct in the hydrocracking of petroleum, is described by the National Formulary as a pharmaceutical necessity. It is supplied in a 99-percent strength to be used either full strength or diluted as desired. It is most commonly used in a 70-percent concentration, for external use only.

(6) Denatured alcohol. Ethyl alcohol rendered unfit for human consumption is termed denatured alcohol. There are 50 or more formulas for accomplishing this denaturation. The additives may be poisonous or may be substances which promote vomiting on internal ingestion. It is used as a solvent and as a fuel in alcohol burners and lamps.

(7) Glycerin (glycerol).

Glycerin (glycerol).

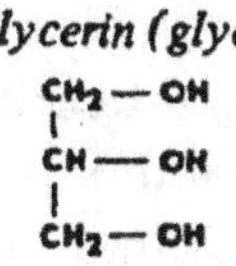

Glycerin is a clear, colorless, viscous liquid, sweet to the taste. As can be seen from the formula, it is a trihydric alcohol and is miscible with water in all proportions, as well as with other alcohols.

(a) Sources. Glycerin is a byproduct of the soap industry. A fat or oil reacted with an alkali such as sodium hydroxide yields a soap plus glycerin. It is also produced by the fermentation of sugar and chemically from propylene, a byproduct of the petroleum industry.

(b) Reactions. When glycerin is heated to a very high temperature, it is dehydrated to acrolein, a substance with a very irritating odor. The fumes resulting from the burning of animal or vegetable fats smell of acrolein. Glycerin is very easily oxidized and when combined with oxidizing agents such as permanganates may explode. This is an incompatibility for glycerin about which more will be said in chapter 8.

(c) Uses. Glycerin has many uses in medicinal preparations.

- Glycerin is a good solvent.
- Glycerin is slightly antiseptic and in high concentrations may be used to prevent microbial growth in some preparations.
- Glycerin is humectant and emollient; that is, in preparations for external use, it moistens and lubricates the skin.
- Glycerin is used in some internal preparations as a sweetening agent.
- Glycerin is the active ingredient in glycerin suppositories.
- Glycerin in combination with water can be used as a permanent or reusable refrigerant. Packed in hermetically sealed containers, teething rings, ice collars, or caps, it can be chilled or frozen repeatedly.

Ethylene glycol:

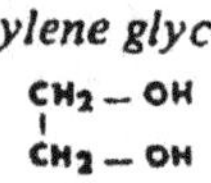

Ethylene glycol is a dihydric alcohol, toxic to the body. It is mainly used as a solvent in manufacturing procedures but must be carefully removed if the product is intended for internal use. Commercially, it is used as a permanent antifreeze.

(9) Propylene glycol (1, 2-propanediol).

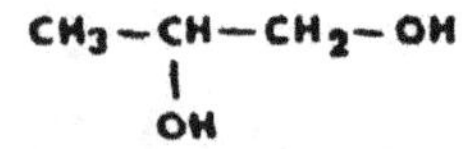

Propylene glycol is a relatively nontoxic substance and is often used as a substitute for glycerin. It is not quite as sweet as glycerin.

7. Ethers. Another class of oxygen derivatives of the hydrocarbons is the ethers. These are the dehydration products of two molecules of alcohol.

a. *Structure.* The general formula for an ether is ROR (the R represents an alkyl radical). The R's may be the same or they may be different.
If the R's are the same, the ether is a simple ether and if they are different, it is a mixed ether. Study the following examples:

CH_3-o-CH_3-4 ↔ Dimethyl ether, a simple ether

C_2H_5-o-$CH_2CH_2CH_3$ ↔ Ethyl n-propyl ether a mixed ether

b. *Graphic versus empirical formula.* We have previously stated that the graphic formula was preferable over the empirical formula, as it completely identified the substance. This can now be illustrated by the comparison of dimethyl ether and ethyl alcohol. The following are graphic formulas for these two different compounds:

Ethyl Alcohol　　Dimethyl Ether

These formulas show at once that the compounds are different. One is an alcohol, the other an ether. The empirical formula, however, for both these compounds is C_2H_6O. Given only the empirical formula and no other information, it would be impossible to determine which compound was being considered. Ethyl alcohol and dimethyl ether are structural isomers.

c. *Properties.* Except for the saturated hydrocarbons, ethers are one of the most chemically inert classes of organic compounds. They do react, however, with bromine and chlorine to form halogenated ethers. Because of this stability, ethers are fine solvents. Ethers are more volatile than their isomeric alcohol counterpart and they decrease in volatility, inflammability, and water solubility as the molecular weight increases. Ethers are miscible with all organic solvents and with the volatile and fixed oils.

d. Preparation. Alcohols dehydrated in the presence of sulfuric acid at a temperature of approximately 135° C. (etherifying temperature) react to form the corresponding ether. A mixture of alcohols will logically form a mixture of ethers. The following equations illustrate the reactions taking place in the preparation of ether.

$$C_2H_5OH \;+ H_2SO_4 \xrightarrow[\Delta]{} C_2H_5HSO_4 \;+ HON$$

Ethyl Alcohol	+ Sulfuric Acid	Ethyl Sulfuric Acid	+ Water

$$C_2H_5HSO_4 + C_2H_5\text{-}OH \rightarrow C_2H_5\text{-}O\text{-}C_2H_5 + H_2SO_4$$

Ethyl Sulfuric Acid	+ Ethyl Alcohol	Ethyl Ether	+ Sulfuric Acid

A modification of the preceding process uses as a starting point, ethylene which is reacted with sulfuric acid to produce ethylsulfuric acid, and then proceeds as above.

e. Important ethers.

(1) Ether (diethyl ether; ethyl ether) C_2H_5-O-C_2H_5. Ether contains 96-98 percent ethyl ether; the remainder is alcohol and water. It is widely used as a general inhalation anesthetic. Since ether is highly volatile and flammable, the monograph bears this official caution- "Ether is highly volatile and flammable. Its vapor, when mixed with air and ignited, may explode." When ether is exposed to air, toxic oxidation products may form. The USP contains an official caution note relative to this danger: "Ether to be used for anesthesia must be preserved in tight containers of not more than 3-kg. capacity, and is not to be used for anesthesia if it has been removed from the original container longer than 24 hours. Ether to be used for anesthesia may, however, be shipped in larger containers for repackaging in containers as directed above, provided the ether at the time of repackaging meets the requirements of the tests of this pharmacopeia."

(2) Ethyl oxide (solvent ether) C_2H_5-O-C_2H_5. This product is chemically the same as ether for anesthesia EXCEPT that it is not as pure and free of oxidation products. It bears the official caution- "Ethyl oxide must not be used for anesthesia. Ethyl oxide is highly flammable. Do not use where it may be ignited." This commercial grade of ether is used as a solvent and as a motor ether for priming the carburetors of gasoline and diesel engines.

(3) Vinyl ether (divinyl oxide) CH_2=CH-O-CH=CH_2. Vinyl ether has two points of unsaturation, one at each side of the oxygen atom. The CH_2=CH group is known as the vinyl radical. This is a quite popular inhalation anesthetic. Because of its volatility, it cannot be used in the tropics. Vinyl ether bears this caution- "Do not use Vinyl Ether for anesthesia if the original container has been opened longer than 48 hours."

8. Aldehydes. Aldehydes are the oxidation products *of primary* alcohols.

a. Structure. Aldehydes have the general structure of R-CHO or $R\text{-}\overset{\overset{C}{\|}}{C}\text{-}H$ and are recognizable by the carbonyl group (C=O) plus a hydrogen and either another hydrogen or an alkyl radical in the general formula.

b. Nomenclature. Although the IUC has set up a system for naming the aldehydes, as for other compounds, because of the widely accepted usage of common names in pharmacy and even by organic chemists, we will pass over the IUC method fleetingly and use the common names.

(1) IUC nomenclature. The IUC method for naming the aldehydes is to use the hydrocarbon base, as with compounds previously discussed and drop the *e* and add *al* in its place. Thus the name for the simplest aldehyde is methanal (IUC) or, by common name, formaldehyde.

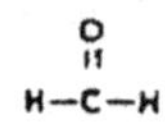

Formaldehyde (Methanal)

(2) Common names. The common names of the aldehydes are taken from the acid formed from the oxidation of that aldehyde. *For example,* oxidation of $H-\overset{O}{\overset{\|}{C}}-H$ yields formic acid and therefore it is named formaldehyde. Oxidation $CH_3-\overset{O}{\overset{\|}{C}}-H$ yields acetic acid, and thus it is named acetaldehyde. The same follows for propionaldehyde and butyraldehyde.

c. Properties. Formaldehyde, a gas with an extremely disagreeable odor, produces a painful choking sensation in the respiratory tract. Acetaldehydeìs odor is not quite so disagreeable. The lower liquid members of the aldehyde family have pungent odors and as they progress toward higher molecular weights, the odors become more agreeable and finally very pleasant. These high molecular weight aldehydes are the substances which lend the fragrance to plants. Often they are employed in the manufacture of perfumes. Octalaldehyde, for example, has the odor of rose or jasmine; nonylaldehyde, the odor of rose; and decylaldehyde, the odor of orange. The first two aldehydes in the series are water soluble. As the number of carbons in the chain increases, the water solubility falls off rapidly. They are soluble, however, in the organic solvents.

d. Reactions. Some of the more important reactions that aldehydes undergo are the following:

(1) Oxidation. Aldehydes may be readily oxidized to their corresponding acid (one with the same number of carbons). This, in fact, is a test for aldehydes.

(2) Addition. Because of the unsaturation at the carbonyl group, aldehydes readily undergo addition reactions. A great number of different additions can take place and the following illustrates one such reaction.

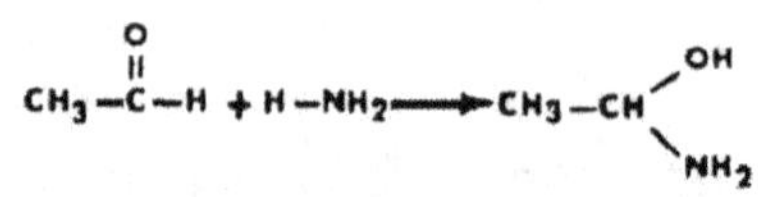

Acetaldehyde - ammonia

(3) Polymerization. A team of individual molecules of the same substance joining together without the formation of additional products is known as polymerization. Aldehydes tend to undergo this joining.

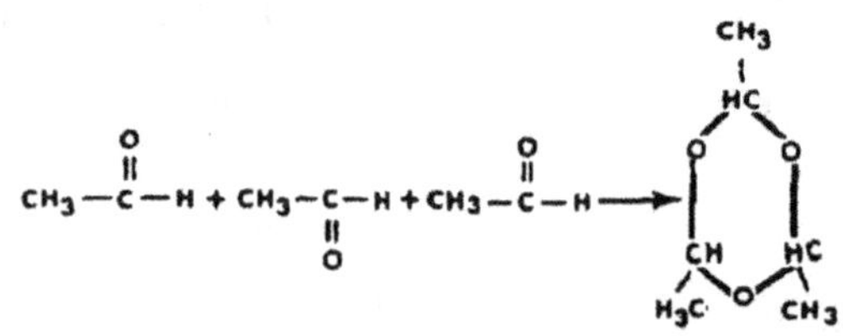

Paraldehyde

(4) Reduction. Since aldehydes are the oxidation products of primary alcohols, they can be reduced back to the corresponding primary alcohol.

$$RCHO \xrightarrow{2H} RCH_2OH$$

(5) Halogen replacement. Halogens may replace certain hydrogen atoms in the aldehyde molecule. This is illustrated in the following reaction.

$$3Cl_2 + CH_3CHO \rightarrow 3HCl + Cl_3CCHO$$

(Trichloroacetaldehyde)

This reaction is important because addition of water to the molecule of trichloroacetaldehyde gives an important pharmaceutical productchloral hydrate.

$$Cl_3CCHO + HOH \rightarrow Cl_3CCH(OH)_2$$

(Chloral hydrate)

(6) Condensation. The ìaldol condensation reactionî results in the addition

of an aldehyde to itself or to another aldehyde in the presence of a weak base. This reaction is extremely important in synthetic work and is a means of forming extremely complex molecules from those already existing in nature. An example of an aldol condensation reaction is

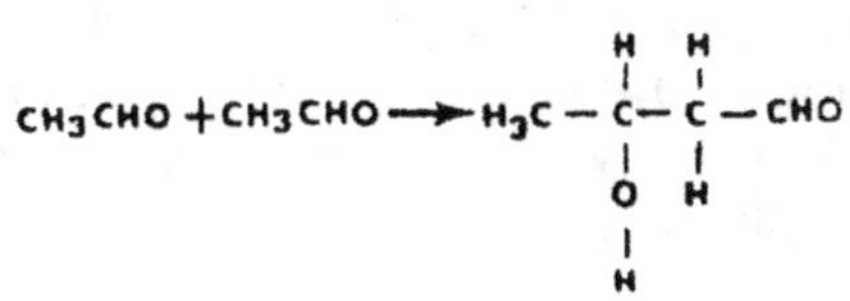

(an aldol)

(7) Silver mirror reaction. When a mixture of formaldehyde and ammoniacal silver nitrate is warmed, silver is deposited on the surface of the vessel in which the reaction is taking place. It is this reaction which is used in the mirror-making industry.

$$HCHO + 2AgNO_3 + NH_4OH \rightarrow HCOONH_4 + 2Ag + 2H_2O$$

e. Occurrence. The simpler aldehydes are not found to a significant extent in nature but some longer chain aldehydes are constituents in plant and flower oils.

f. Preparation. Aldehydes may be prepared from their corresponding primary alcohol by the processes of dehydrogenation or oxidation. Acetaldehyde has a special method of preparation from acetylene.

(1) Dehydrogenation.

$$CH_3OH \xrightarrow[200\text{-}350^0]{Cu} H_2 + H_2C{=}O$$

200-350°

(2) Oxidation.

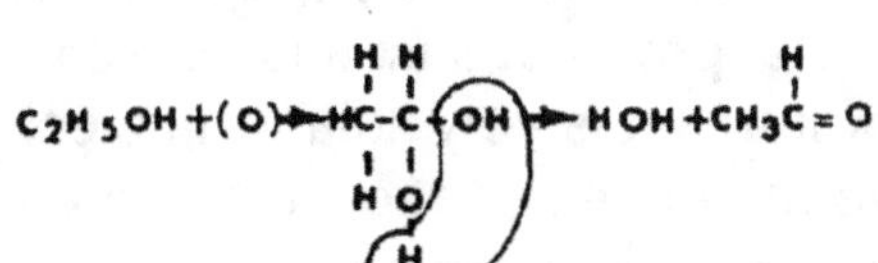

(acetaldehyde)

(3) Preparation of acetaldehyde from acetylene.

$$C_2H_2 + HOH \xrightarrow{Cat} CH_3CHO$$

The catalysts in this reaction are mercuric sulfate and sulfuric acid.

g. Important aldehydes.

(1) Formaldehyde solution. Formaldehyde solution, also known as Formalin, is a 37-percent solution of formaldehyde gas (HCHO) in water (w/w). Methyl alcohol is added to prevent polymerization. This solution is used full strength or diluted up to 1:10 for disinfection of inanimate objects. It is an ingredient in embalming fluids where it functions as a tissue preservative. Specimens are frequently preserved in formaldehyde solution.

(2) Paraldehyde.

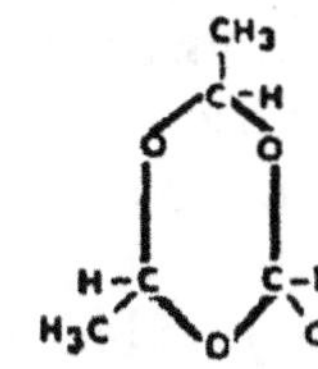

Paraldehyde is a clear, colorless liquid having a strong, characteristic, pungent odor. Some people seem to like the odor; others find it obnoxious. It is used as a sedative or hypnotic; its widest use is in the treatment of delirium tremens. It may be administered orally, rectally, or by injection. The USP states: "Paraldehyde is subject to oxidation to form acetic acid. Preserve in well filled, tight, light resistant containers holding not more than 30 ml., at a temperature not exceeding 25° C." Paraldehyde must not be used if it has a brownish color or the odor of acetic acid. Because of the oxidation to acetic acid any unused paraldehyde should be discarded 24 hours after the container has been opened.

(3) Chloral hydrate (chloral) $Cl_3CCH(OH)_2$. Chloral hydrate is a white or colorless crystal with a sweet and slightly acrid odor. This odor can also be classified as characteristic. It is used as a sedative and hypnotic.

9. Ketones. Ketones are to secondary alcohols what aldehydes are to primary alcohols. In other words, ketones are oxidation products of secondary alcohols.

a. Structure. Ketones are similar in structure to the aldehydes as represented below in their general formulas.

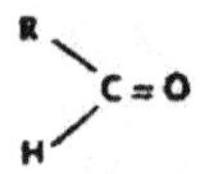

Aldehyde

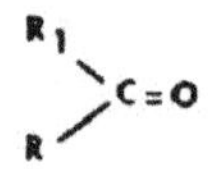

Ketone

The difference, as you can see, between an aldehyde and a ketone is an additional radical in place of the hydrogen on the aldehyde.

b. Properties. Acetone, the first member of the ketone series, is a clear, colorless liquid with an odor similar to nail polish. The higher members of the series are colorless liquids or solids.

c. Reactions. Due to the absence of the hydrogen, ketones are less reactive than the aldehydes. They undergo oxidation less readily and, unlike the aldehydes, ketones are not reducing agents. They may be oxidized by powerful oxidizing agents into acids with less carbons than the ketones themselves. This is due to the splitting between carbon atoms as illustrated in the following reaction:

$$CH_3\overset{O}{\overset{\|}{C}}CH_3 + 4(O) \longrightarrow$$
$$CO_2 + HOH + CH_3COOH \quad \text{(acetic acid)}$$

In other respects, the reactions of the ketones follow the same pattern as the aldehydes.

d. Nomenclature. Like the aldehydes, ketones are given both common and IUC names.

(1) Common name. The names of both groups attached to the carbonyl group are followed by the word "ketone." Thus-

$$CH_3-\overset{O}{\overset{\|}{C}}-CH_2-CH_3$$

is called methyl ethyl ketone.

(2) IUC name. As with other compounds, the IUC system bases its name for ketones on the hydrocarbon name of the longest chain containing the carbonyl group. The *e* is dropped from the hydrocarbon name and *one* is added in its place. The position of the carbonyl group is indicated by number. Thus-

$$CH_3-\overset{O}{\overset{\|}{C}}-CH_3 \quad \text{is Propanone}$$

$$CH_3-\overset{O}{\overset{\|}{C}}-CH_2-CH_3 \quad \text{is 2-Butanone}$$

e. Preparation. Just as oxidation of the corresponding primary alcohol yielded an aldehyde, oxidation of the corresponding secondary alcohol yields the ketone. Although there are other methods of preparation, for our purposes and needs this one will suffice.

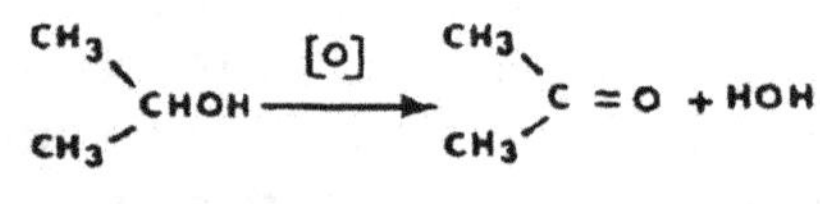

Isopropyl Alcohol Dimethylketone

f. Important ketones.

(1) Acetone (dimethyl ketone) CH_3COCH_3. Acetone is an excellent organic solvent, easily dissolving fats, resins, pyroxylin, and similar substances. It is widely used in organic syntheses, i.e., in the manufacture of chloroform, chlorobutanol, and ascorbic acid. Acetone is a colorless, extremely volatile and flammable liquid, having a characteristic odor. Acetone is readily miscible with water, alcohol, chloroform, ether, and most Volatile oils. Because of its extremely inflammable nature, the NF bears this official caution: "Acetone is very flammable. Do not use where it may be ignited."

(2) Camphor (2-camphanone) $C_{10}H_{16}O$. Camphor is a colorless crystal, granule, or mass with a very penetrating odor which probably accounts for its use in nasal preparations. It is not soluble in water, but is very soluble in alcohol, chloroform, and ether. It occurs naturally in turpentine oil and is synthetically produced from pinene. It is commonly referred to as gum camphor because of its gummy nature and lauryl camphor from the plant from which it is extracted.

(a) Uses. Camphor is a mild anesthetic, mild antiseptic, rubefacient (reddens the skin), circulatory and respiratory stimulant, and expectorant. It is mainly used in preparations for external applica-

tion for its rubefacient action and in some nasal solutions for its penetrating odor. A good deal of the therapeutic qualities of camphor may be psychological, due to its odor. Camphor is an ingredient in paregoric (Camphorated Tincture of Opium).

(b) Eutexia. When camphor is rubbed with chloral hydrate, thymol, menthol, phenol, and many other solids, the resulting mixture liquefies spontaneously. This mixture of two or more ingredients resulting in spontaneous liquefaction at room temperature is called a eutectic mixture.

(3) Rotenone, $C_{23}H_{22}O_6$. Rotenone is a ketone which is very toxic to insects and fish. It is used as an insecticide and as an agent to purge ponds and lakes of unwanted marine life. It is interesting to note that only one part in twenty million will kill goldfish in 3 hours. Oddly enough, rotenone is practically nontoxic to man.

10. Aliphatic monocarboxylic acids. Of the many types of organic acids, the two most important ones are carboxylic acids and their derivatives. Carboxylic acids may contain one or more carboxyl groups (COOH) and the number contained is signified by the prefixes mono, di, tri, or poly. The word carboxyl is derived from carbonyl and hydroxyl, showing that a carboxyl group is a combination of the two.

a. Structure. Monocarboxylic acids have the general formula of RCOOH, or graphically, $R-\overset{\overset{\displaystyle O}{\|}}{C}-OH$ An example of a true monocarboxylic acid, illustrating the general formula, is that of acetic acid, graphically shown below.

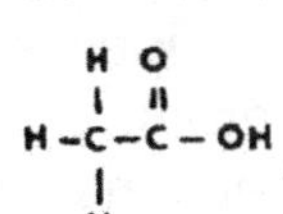

b. Properties. The monocarboxylic acids are colorless. The first nine normal members of the series are liquids; higher members are solids. The first three members have painful, stinging odors; the succeeding members to C_{10} have foul, rancid odors; those above C_{10} are odorless, or nearly so. The solubility of these acids ranges from completely water soluble (C_1 to C_3), decreasing rapidly from C_4 upward, until those over C_{12} are, for all intents and purposes, insoluble in water. The solid acids are greasy and wax-like to the touch and because many of them are actually prepared from fats, they are frequently called the "fatty acids." Acetic acid, when frozen, appears ice-like and so acquires the name ìglacialî acetic acid. The organic acids ionize only slightly in solution and consequently are weak acids.

c. Reactions. The monocarboxylic acids undergo a variety of reactions. They are altered either in the hydrocarbon chain to yield substituted acids, or at the carboxyl group to yield acid derivatives. Halogen acids, hydroxy acids, and amino acids are substituted acids, while salts, esters, and amides are acid derivatives.

d. Occurrence. Organic acids are widely distributed in nature both in the free and the combined form. They are found in resins, carbohydrate derivatives, proteins, salts, human tissues, and fats. The substance injected by many insects, including the ant, bee, and wasp, is formic acid.

e. Preparation. There are a variety of methods for preparation of the carboxylic acids, most of which have oxidation or hydrolysis as one of the steps involved.

(1) Oxidation. You have learned that the hydrocarbons can be oxidized to alcohols, further to aldehydes, and now the aldehydes can be even further oxidized to organic acids. Still further oxidation results in breaking up of the molecule into carbon dioxide and water. Notice the progressive oxidation stages in the reaction below.

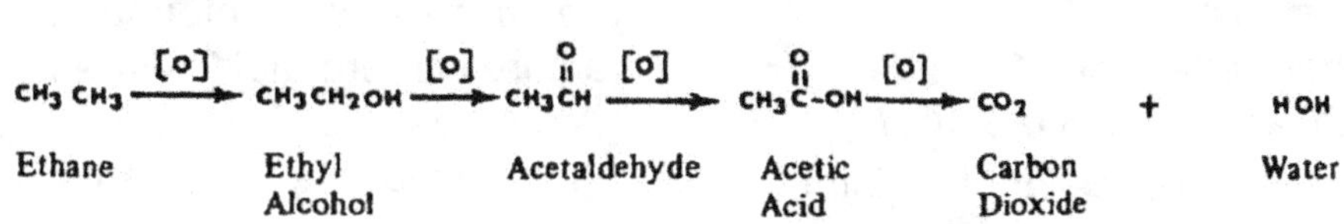

(2) *Hydrolysis.* Esters of the carboxylic acids on hydrolysis yield carboxylic acids.

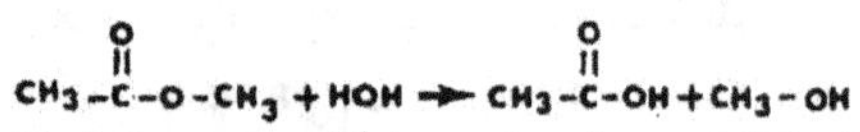

Methylacetate Water Acetic Acid Methanol

f. The important aliphatic monocarboxylic acids.

(1) *Acetic acid (ethanoic acid) CH_3COOH.*

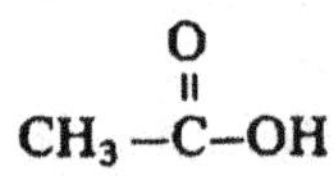

Acetic acid is a 36- to 37-percent solution of CH_3COOH by weight in water. It is a clear, colorless liquid with a strong, characteristic odor. It is miscible with water, alcohol, and glycerin. Acetic acid is used as a solvent and as the substance diluted to yield diluted acetic acid. It is mainly official because it is pharmaceutically essential for the compounding of aluminum subacetate solution. It is extremely important as a starting point in the synthesis of acetates, sulfa drugs, and acetanilid.

(2) *Diluted acetic acid.* This product is made by adding enough water to 158 ml. of acetic acid to make 1000 ml., yielding a 6-percent solution. Diluted acetic acid is bactericidal and spermatocidal in 1-percent concentrations and has been used as a wetting solution for surgical dressings, as well as a contraceptive and antibacterial douche.

(3) *Glacial acetic acid.* Glacial acetic acid is similar to, but more concentrated than, acetic acid. It is 99 percent by weight.

(4) *Oleic acid. $CH_3(CH_2)_7 CH = CH(CH_2)_7 COOH$.* Oleic acid, obtained from tallow (abdominal fat of the sheep or ox), may contain some of the other fatty acids such as linolenic and stearic acids also present in tallow. It is mainly used as a pharmaceutical necessity in the manufacture of oleates, medicinal soft soap, and benzyl benzoate lotion.

(5) *Undecylenic acid (10-undecenoic acid), $CH_2 = CH(CH_2)_8COOH$.* Undecylenic acid is an excellent fungistatic agent. It is used externally in a 1-percent to 10-percent concentration in ointments, liquids, and powders, to treat athleteís foot, ringworm, and similar infestations.

(6) *Stearic acid.* Stearic acid is a mixture of solid organic acids consisting mainly of stearic acid ($HC_{18}H_{35}O2$) and palmitic acid ($HC_{16}H_{31}O_2$). It is obtained from tallow. The chief use of stearic acid in pharmacy is in the preparation of sodium stearate, a solidifying agent in glycerin suppositories.

11. Salts of the monocarboxylic acids. Salts of organic acids occur from the reaction between an organic acid and a metal, or the salt of a weaker acid such as a carbonate, oxide, or hydroxide.

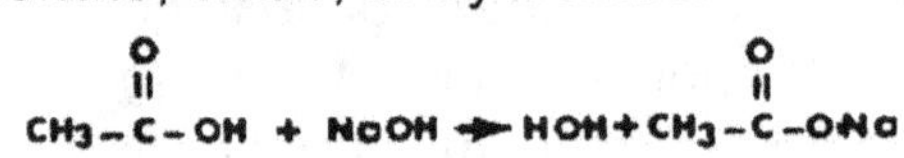

Acetic Acid Sodium Hydroxide Water Sodium Acetate

Although organic substances in general are not widely water soluble, the salts of organic acids are. Some of the more important salts of monocarboxylic acids are-

a. Potassium acetate, CH_3COOK. Potassium acetate is used as a systemic and urinary alkalizer.

b. Sodium acetate, CH_3COONa. Sodium acetate is used as a systemic and urinary alkalizer.

c. Zinc undecylenate $[CH_2=CH(CH_2)_8COO]_2 Zn$. Used alone and in combination with undecylenic acid and other substances, this salt is effective in the treatment of athleteís foot and other fungal infections. It may be found in the form of a 20-percent ointment, liquid, or powder for topical application. A commercially marketed preparation for the treatment of such infections combines zinc undecylenate and undecylenic acid.

d. Mercury oleate. This compound, containing the equivalent of 25-percent mercuric oxide, is intended for the manufacture of Mercurial Ointment which is used as a parasiticide. Many commercial patent remedies for the treatment of psoriasis contain oleate of mercury as their active ingredient. Siroil and Riasol are examples.

12. Esters. Esters are products formed from the reaction between an alcohol and either an acid, an acid chloride, or an acid anhydride. The hydrogen of the carboxyl group is replaced by a radical.

a. Structure. The general graphic formula for esters of the organic monocarboxylic acid is

$$R\overset{\overset{\displaystyle O}{\|}}{C}-OR_1$$

b. Properties. Esters may be either liquids or solids, all of which are colorless and essentially insoluble in water. The liquid members have strong and unusual odors, mostly quite pleasant.

c. Reactions. Esters are capable of many reactions, including hydrolysis, reduction, and reaction with ammonia to form amides. Examples of these reactions are enumerated below.

(1) Hydrolysis.

$$\underset{\text{ester}}{RCOOR_1} + \underset{\text{water}}{HOH} \rightarrow \underset{\text{acid}}{RCOOH} + \underset{\text{alcohol}}{R_1OH}$$

(2) Reduction.

$$\underset{\text{ester}}{RCOOR_1} \xrightarrow{4H} \underset{\text{alcohol}}{RCH_2OH} + \underset{\text{alcohol}}{R_1OH}$$

(3) Reaction with ammonia.

$$\underset{\text{ester}}{RCOOR_1} + \underset{\text{ammonia}}{HNH_2} \rightarrow \underset{\text{alcohol}}{R_1OH} + \underset{\text{amide}}{RCONH_2}$$

These reactions are important to pharmacy in producing compounds that otherwise are hard or impossible to obtain.

d. Occurrence. Esters occur in nature, widely distributed in fruits, flowers, and other parts of plants and animals. Esters are the forms in which the naturally occurring fatty acids exist. Esters impart the odor to many fruits and flowers. *For example,* amyl acetate has the odor of banana; amyl butyrate, the odor of apricot; octyl acetate, the odor of orange; and ethyl butyrate, the odor of pineapple.

e. Preparation.

(1) Reaction between alcohol and acid.

$$RCOOH+R_1OH \rightarrow HOH+RCOOR_1$$

This reaction progresses very slowly, but more rapid and better yields can be obtained by (2) below.

(2) Reaction between alcohol and acid anhydride.

$$(RCO)_2O+ROH \rightarrow RCOOH+RCOOR$$

(3) Reaction between alcohol and acid chloride.

$$RCOCl+ROH \rightarrow HCl+RCOOR$$

f. Uses. The uses of esters vary widely. Some are used in manufacture of insecticides, others in the making of perfumes and flavors, some as solvents, some in plastics, and still others in explosives and medicine.

g. Important esters. Most of the important esters will be discussed later in the chapter with other classes to which they are related. Three products are listed below which are esters of inorganic acids.

(1) Ethyl nitrite spirit (sweet spirit of nitre; spirit of nitrous ether). Ethyl nitrite spirit is a solution in alcohol containing 4 percent of C_2H_5ONO. It was once mainly used as a diuretic and diaphoretic but today is considered less reliable than other more recent agents.

(2) Amylnitrite, $CH_3CH(CH_3)CH_2CH_2ONO$. This very volatile liquid is inhaled in the treatment of attacks of angina pectoris. It is very flammable and should not be used where it is likely to be ignited.

(3) Glyceryl trinitrate tablets (nitroglycerin; Trinitrin). These tablets produce coronary artery dilation and are therefore useful in the treatment of attacks of angina pectoris.

13. Fats and fixed oils. Fats and fixed oils are much alike. Chemically, their structure is essentially the same in that both are glyceryl esters of fatty acids. The differentiation between a fat and an oil rests in the

physical state of the substance at normal temperatures. A solid glyceryl ester of a fatty acid is a fat and a liquid glyceryl ester of a fatty acid is a fixed oil.

a. Structure. The following formulas depict a molecule of glycerol, three molecules of fatty acid (stearic in this case), and finally the fat molecule, stearin, an ester of the two.

(1) Mixed esters. Stearin contains glycerolplus three molecules of stearic

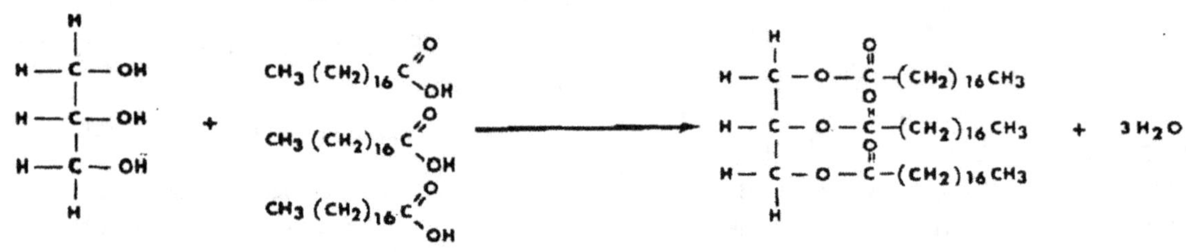

Glycerol — Stearic Acid (3 Molecules) — Stearin — Water

acid. It is quite possible that more than one fatty acid may join with a single molecule of glycerol to give a *mixed ester.* In fact, most of the naturally occurring fats and oils are mixtures of mixed esters of glycerol and fatty acids.

(2) Carbon chains. Most of the fats and fixed oils contain carbon chains of even numbers ranging from C10 to C16. The four most common fatty acids combined with glycerol to form the fats and fixed oils in nature are all chains with 18 carbon atoms. Stearic, oleic, linoleic, and linolenic acids all have 18 carbon atoms, but differ in saturation. Stearic acid has no double bonds; oleic has one; linoleic has two double bonds; and linolenic has three.

b. Properties. Previously we said that at normal temperatures fats are solids and oils are liquids. This is a rather vague description because what is an oil in torrid climates might well be a fat in the Arctic. Since the glycerol portion of the molecule is common to all, it is the fatty acid composition which determines the properties of the particular fat or oil. The chain may be either short or long, completely saturated, partially unsaturated, or completely unsaturated. Long chain (high molecular weight) fatty acids in the molecule tend to make it insoluble in water and solid. Short chains tend toward liquidity and water solubility. Partially or completely unsaturated chains are more likely to be oils; those which are nearly saturated will be fats.

c. Classes of fixed oils. The fixed oils are sometimes grouped into classes by the amount of saturation they possess. The characteristics of these groups are reflected in their names.

(1) Drying oils. These oils contain fatty acids with many double bonds (highly unsaturated). They easily combine with oxygen and quickly dry into a hard, resinous coat. These oils give paint its drying properties. This drying process is an exothermic reaction, that is, reaction giving off heat, and can lead to spontaneous combustion. Rags or other combustible material, soaked with these drying oils and confined, become warmer and warmer as the oils dry and heat is liberated. Finally, the cloth reaches its ignition temperature and a fire results. A good example of a drying oil is linseed oil.

(2) Semidrying oils. Corn oil is a good example of a semidrying oil. There is less unsaturation in these oils and they oxidize to a gummy, resinous mass but do not harden completely.

(3) Nondrying oils. The nondrying oils, on exposure to the atmosphere, remain sticky and do not dry; they have the least number of double bonds. Olive oil is nondrying.

d. Occurrence. As a general rule, it can be stated that fats occur in the animal kingdom and oils in the plant kingdom. There is some overlapping, but for the most part this is the case. The fats and fixed oils are gathered by expression, a procedure of compressing by hydrolic pressure the ground-up plant or animal tissue. Animal fats are often collected from the process of rendering in which the fatty tissue is heated until the fat melts and is collected.

e. Reactions. Fats and oils undergo definite chemical reactions and yield some very important products.

(1) Hydrolysis. Listed first, because it is of the most significance in nature, is the reaction of hydrolysis in which fats and oils react with water to form fatty acids and glycerol. When butter becomes rancid, the molecule has been broken down by hydrolysis to fatty acids, one of which is butyric acid. Butyric acid is the foul-smelling substance liberated in rancidity of butter and other fats and oils. Hydrolysis takes place slowly, unless in the presence of catalysts. Acids, bases, and certain digestive enzymes catalyze this reaction. When fats or oils are hydrolyzed in the presence of an alkali, the resulting products are glycerol and the metallic salt of the acid. The metallic salt of a fatty acid is a soap; this process then is termed saponification. More will be said about soaps and saponification later in the chapter.

(2) Oxidation. Short-chained acids, aldehydes, and ketones are produced when a fat or oil undergoes oxidation. In rancidity, this process is closely related to hydrolysis. Oxidation is hastened by light, heat, moisture, and metals.

(3) Hydrogenation. The unsaturated fats and oils may add hydrogen atoms at the point of unsaturation to become more nearly saturated. It is by this process that liquid cooking oils are solidified to yield a solid cooking fat that is more stable than lard or butter.

f. Uses. The fats and fixed oils are important to life and health from many standpoints. First, and probably foremost, they are essential foods (foods necessary to the proper function of the human body). Absence of fats and oils from the diet results in skin conditions, emaciation, and death. From the medical and pharmaceutical standpoint, fats and oils are used as laxatives, as bases for ointments and oleaginous preparations, as sources of vitamins, and in the manufacture of other pharmaceutically important preparations. The salts of several of the fatty acids are fungicidal. Other derivatives are soaps, detergents, and bactericides.

g. Pharmaceutically important fats and oils.

(1) Expressed almond oil (almond oil; sweet almond oil). Almond oil is not the flavorful part of constituent of almonds; therefore, the common name of sweet almond oil is misleading. Almond oil is an emollient, used in hand creams and lotions such as rose water ointment, and in the cosmetic industry.

(2) Castor oil (oleum ricini). This thick oil from the castor bean is an effective cathartic because of the liberation of ricinoleic acid in the intestine. This acid is irritating and produces catharsis. Castor oil is also used as a lubricating oil and a constitutent of collodion to make it flexible.

(3) Corn oil (oleum maydis). Corn oil is official mainly for its use as a vehicle for injections where the active ingredient is oil soluble. Many hormone injections which we will discuss later in the chapter are dissolved in corn oil for administration by injection. Corn oil is a good food substance. There are several patented products on the market which are emulsions of corn oil. These are used to supply extra calories to the debilitated and to those who wish to gain weight. Corn oil is also used as a liquid cooking substance and in the manufacture of soaps.

(4) Cottonseed oil (oleum gosypii seminis). This is another oil suitable for the vehicle in injections. It is taken internally as a cathartic, to increase caloric intake, and to decrease gastric secretion and motility. Cottonseed oil is used in the manufacture of soaps, glycerin, oleomargarine (and other lard substitutes), lubricating agents, and cosmetics. In the liquid form, it is

widely used as a cooking and salad oil. Hydrogenated into a solid state, it becomes similar to shortening.

(5) Linseed oil. Linseed oil, no longer official, is expressed from flaxseed. It is mainly used in the preparation of liniments. Flaxseed is a greasy seed which can be used to clean handmade gelatin capsules before dispensing. It is used in the form of meal, combined with water, as a poultice to draw pus from wounds. The commercial linseed oil purchased in hardware and paint stores has been boiled with lead oxide and is poisonous; it is not suitable for medicinal use.

(6) Olive oil (sweet oil). Olive oil is an emollient substance used in the manufacture of lotions, emulsions, ointments, liniments, and plasters. It has good food properties and can be used as a caloric booster. It is frequently used as a salad oil. Sweet oil, used as a mild eardrop in children for many years, is nothing more than olive oil. Its soothing effects to earaches are due to its emollient action and its ability to dissolve encrusted wax.

(7) Peanut oil (arachis oil; oleum arachis). Peanut oil is used mainly in the preparation of oil soluble substances for injection. It is also used in the manufacture of liniments and ointments. Peanut oil is a frequently used base in the preparation of oleaginous nose drops.

(8) Sesame oil (oleum sesami). Sesame oil is used in the manufacture of injections; in liniments, emulsions, oleomargarine, cosmetics; and as a food. Because it is more quickly saponifiable and does not rapidly turn rancid, sesame oil has replaced cottonseed oil in many products.

(9) Cod liver oil. As the name suggests, this fixed oil is extracted from the livers of codfish. It has a nigh nutrient value and supplies rich quantities of vitamins A and D. (Vitamins A and D are treated more thoroughly in chapter 9.) It is more widely used today in the veterinary field because animals seem to relish the fishy taste. Applied topically in the form of ointments, this oil has excellent emollient properties and is quite healing, especially to diaper rash. Whiteís A and D ointment contains vitamins A and D and has the same uses.

(10) Theobroma oil (cacao butter; cocoa butter). Despite the official name, theobroma oil is a fat. At room temperature, it is a brittle, waxy solid with a strong chocolate odor. At body temperature, it melts rapidly, becoming a loose liquid, and is therefore widely used as a base for suppositories. Cocoa butter is also used as an emollient when applied to the skin for inflammation. It is incorporated into many skin creams.

14. Waxes. The waxes, although closely related to the fats and oils, differ from them in that instead of glycerol, they are composed of high-molecular-weight monohydric alcohols in combination with fatty acids. The two more commonly occurring alcohols are lauryl and cetyl.

a. Occurrence. Waxes occur in the leaves of plants, are excreted by some insects, and are found in the head of the sperm whale.

b. Properties. Generally, waxes are harder substances than fats, having higher melting points and are brittle and less greasy.

c. Important official waxes.

(1) Anhydrous lanolin (wool fat; refined wool fat; adeps lanae). Wool fat is a fat-like wax extracted from the wool and/or skin of sheep. It resembles closely the natural human body oils. It contains cholesterol (a sterol) which gives it the property of being able to absorb large quantities of water (up to about one-third its own weight). For this reason it may be incorporated into ointment bases to allow absorption of aqueous solutions of ingredients. Because it has been found that many people are allergic to lanolin, this substance has been deleted from many preparations and has been replaced by a suitable amount of cholesterol.

(2) Lanolin (hydrous wool fat; adeps lanae hydrosus). Hydrous wool fat is

wool fat containing between 25- and 30-percent water. When water is added to anhydrous lanolin, the sticky, yellowish-brown, translucent mass becomes a yellow, creamy, opaque ointment. This substance, because it contains water, is used more for its emollient properties than for its water absorbent qualities. It does, however, possess the ability to absorb still more water. Be careful at this point to fix firmly in your mind the official and common names of these two closely related compounds and know the difference between them.

(3) Spermaceti (cetaceum). Spermaceti is a waxy substance obtained from the head of the sperm whale. This wax is used to thicken the consistency of ointments. It is used in both ointments and suppositories to elevate their melting points. There is little or no absorption of spermaceti through the skin. It is found in the formula for cold cream.

(4) Yellow wax (beeswax). As the common name implies, this substance is the purified wax obtained from the honeycomb of the bee. Like other waxes, this wax is used to raise melting points of ointments and stiffen their consistency. It is officially used in the preparation of yellow ointment.

(5) White wax (bleached beeswax; cera alba). This wax differs from yellow wax only in being bleached. It is officially used in the preparation of white ointment and is more widely employed in pharmacy than the yellow variety.

15. Sterols. Another group of lipid compounds is the sterols. These are high molecular weight cyclic alcoholsspecifically, tetracyclic, unsaturated, secondary alcohols. They are derived from the unsaponifiable portion of fats.

a. Classification. Depending upon their source, sterols are grouped into the following categories:

(1) Zoosterols (from animals).
(2) Phytosterols (from plants).
(3) Mycosterols (from fungi).

b. Official products.

(1) Cholesterol (cholesterin), $C_{27}H_{46}O$. Cholesterol is found in all animal tissue, mainly in nerve and brain tissues. This substance can be acquired by the body indirectly from the foods consumed, or directly by manufacture within the body. A great deal of research is being conducted at present to determine the relationship between cholesterol levels in the blood and heart disease. This would be an interesting area for outside reading. Pharmaceutically, cholesterol is of importance because of the water-absorbing qualities it imparts to ointments. The USP categorizes this substance as a pharmaceutical necessity for hydrophilic petrolatum.

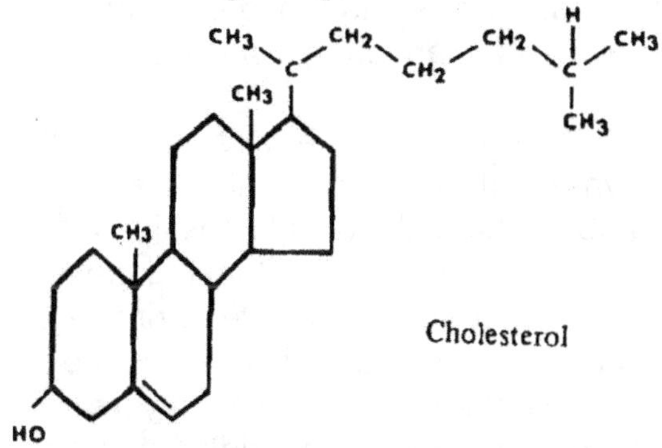

Cholesterol

(2) Hydrophilic petrolatum. This is a combination of stearyl alcohol, white wax, white petrolatum, and cholesterol. It is intended for use as a protective and water-absorbable ointment base.

16. Surface tension and surface active agents. Before discussing the surface active agents, or surfactants, as they are frequently called, it is necessary that you know what surface tension is and how it acts.

a. Surface tension. Surface tension is a property of liquids in which the exposed surface tends to contract to the smallest possible area. This property is attributable to the molecular forces of attraction within the liquid. You have seen surface tension at work if you have noticed the collection of droplets of water on a newly waxed automobile. The drops tend to pull themselves together into a spherical shape as if they were contained in a plastic film. It is surface tension which makes water spread out on a clean glass surface. In the first instance, the water and wax are immiscible substances, and there is no attraction of one for the other. Consequently, the cohesive properties of the water pull it together into a globule. There is, however, an affinity of water for clean, glass surfaces. The water spreads out, but the surface tension prevents the water film from being broken.

b. Surfactants (surface active agents). Surfactants are those substances intended to modify the surface tensions of liquids in contact with other liquids or solids. Try a couple of experiments first to show the effects of surface tension, and then the effect of a surfactant on this surface tension.

(1) Experiment one. In a bottle half full of water, add some mineral oil, replace the cap and shake the liquids briskly. Set the bottle down and watch. Shaking the liquids has caused them to mix temporarily, but because of their surface tensions they quickly separate into two distinct layers. Now repeat the procedure, adding a quantity of liquid detergent. This time, upon standing, the liquids do not separate as quickly. The surface tension has been modified by the detergent. The oil particles were able to be reduced to a much smaller size and the two liquids mixed. The resulting mixture is an emulsion. An emulsion can be defined on this basis as being a heterogeneous mixture of two or more immiscible liquids. Never confuse an emulsion with a solution.

(2) Experiment two. Soak a cloth in oil, allowing the oil to be well soaked into the rag. Wring it out and immerse it into a container of pure water. When you remove it from the water and allow the water to run off, it will be apparent that no water has soaked into the pores of the fiber. The oil has prevented the wetting of the material because of the surface tensions of the two liquids. The same oily cloth immersed in a solution of soapy water or water to which a detergent has been added will become wet, and if agitated in the solution for a time, the oil will be washed away. It is this principle of surface activation which allows greasy dishware to be washed clean in the kitchen.

c. Mixing immiscible liquids. There are many instances in pharmacy when it is necessary to mix two otherwise immiscible liquids. Emulsions, lotions, creams, and some of the ointments you will prepare in the pharmacy will employ a surfactant and a special mixing procedure to allow you to accomplish proper incorporation.

d. Classes of surfactants. Surface active agents can be divided into three classes: cationic (positively charged ion is responsible for the action), anionic (negatively charged ion is responsible for the action), and non-ionic (the whole molecule is active).

(1) Cationic surfactants. The activity of the cationic surfactants is due to the positive ion in colloidal solution. Most frequently used members of this group are the quaternary ammonium compounds and pyridinium salts. Examples of these types of compounds are shown with the individual agents in *(a)* below. For more detail about each, refer to chapter 9. These cationic agents are unusual in that they display, besides their surface active properties, strong germicidal ability and make extremely useful antiseptics. Sometimes they are keratolytic and have the ability to penetrate dead skin.

(a) Important cationic surfactants.

1. Benzalkonium chloride solution (Zephiran Chloride solution).

2. Benzalkonium chloride tincture (Zephiran Chloride tincture).

3. Benzethonium Chloride solution (Phemerol chloride solution).

4. Cetylpyridinium chloride (Ceepryn Chloride).

(b) Incompatibilities. These products, as well as the other cationic surfactants, are incompatible with soap and other anionic surfactants. Soap inactivates

the cationic surfactants and destroys their antibacterial properties.

(c) Properties. Most of these preparations are odorless, colorless, nonirritating, and, in germicidal concentrations, nontoxic. They are very stable, nonvolatile compounds and may be safely boiled or autoclaved.

(2) Anionic surfactants. Anionic surfactants owe their action to the negatively charged portion of the molecule. These agents are incompatible with the cationic surfactants. This class of surface active agents includes the soaps and detergents.

(a) Soaps. Soaps, if you recall, are the metallic salts of long-chain fatty acids. In the process of saponification, a metallic hydroxide is reacted with the fat, yielding the metallic salt of the fatty acid (soap) and glycerol. Depending upon the metallic hydroxide used in their manufacture, soaps may be either water soluble or oil soluble. We learned previously that group 1 metals and ammonium form water-soluble soaps, and that the group 2 metals (Ca, Mg) form oil-soluble (water-insoluble) soaps. Further, soaps may be considered either hard or soft, hard soaps being those with sodium as the base and soft soaps those with potassium as the base.

1. Action. Soaps are effective because of their emulsifying ability. The water-soluble soaps produce oil in water (o/w) emulsions; that is, emulsions in which oil is the internal (dispersed) phase and water is the external phase. In oil-in-water emulsions, the oil globules are broken down into very small particles and are dispersed throughout the water. In water-in-oil (w/o) emulsions, the reverse is true; the water is the internal phase and is surrounded by the oil. Oil-soluble soaps tend to produce water in oil emulsions. Emulsions will be considered in detail in "Manufacturing and Dispensing."

2. Important soaps.

• *Hard soap.* Hard soap has the following common names: sapo duris; soap; castile soap. It is a sodium soap. Hard soap is used to render resins soluble and modify harsh actions of certain drugs. As such, it is a common ingredient in pill masses, liniments, and dentifrices. The NF categorizes this preparation as a pharmaceutical necessity for the manufacture of other official preparations.

• *Medicinal soft soap (green soap; sapo mollis medicinalis; soft soap).* Medicinal soft soap is a potassium soap, made by saponification of a suitable vegetable oil (excluding coconut and palm kernel) without removal of the glycerin formed. Although the common name would lead you to believe this soap has a green color, this is no longer true. Long ago, the product was actually green in color due to the chlorophyll contained in the raw vegetable oil. Today, using pure ingredients, the soap has an amber color, but retains the historic common name. Medicinal soft soap is used in the preparation of medicinal soft soap liniment commonly known as tincture of green soap. This tincture is an alcoholic solution which is very effective as a detergent for cleansing both animate and inanimate objects. It is sometimes employed as a shampoo for scalp conditions.

• *Sodium stearate.* The sodium salt of stearic acid, consisting mainly of sodium stearate and sodium palmitate, is a chemically pure soap. Sodium stearate is a pharmaceutical necessity in the preparation of glycerin suppositories. Inserted rectally, these suppositories cause irritation to the colon and produce evacuation. Some people still refer to these suppositories as "soap sticks."

(b) Synthetic anionic surfactants. Aside from the soaps, there is an ever-increasing variety of related anionic compounds which exhibit similar properties. In the past few years, great strides have been made in this field. The official preparations in this type are:

1. Dioctylsodium sulfosuccinate, $C_{20}H_{37}NaO_7S$. This product is referred to by the abbreviation DOSS, and is marketed under various trade names. It is neither antibacterial nor detergent in action. It is a wetting agent (reduces surface tension and allows the substance to become wetted by the liquid it contacts). This property has been well utilized by using DOSS as a nonlaxative fecal softener to prevent constipation. By wetting the fecal matter, the bowel is more easily evacuated at regular intervals and without straining. This is very important to the hemorrhoid patient as well as the pregnant patient.

2. Sodium lauryl sulfate. Sodium lauryl sulfate is a true surface active agent and thus a very efficient detergent. Besides being frequently used in household scrubbing and dishwasher products, it is used in such pharmaceutical preparations as toothpastes and shampoos.

(3) The non-ionic surfactants. These surfactants consist of hydrophilic (water-loving) and lipophilic (oil-loving) portions which do not ionize in water. They may consist of high molecular weight alcohols, such as cetyl alcohol, and other substituted long-chain compounds. Although these non-ionic surfactants have not yet widely invaded the detergent field, there is little doubt that, in the near future, developments in this area will lead to better products. Falling into this group are the "spans" and "tweens," two series of solubilizing agents which allow oil and water to mix. These products have their best use in preparations where a flavoring oil tends to precipitate out of a hydroalcoholic solution, such as is the case in phenobarbital elixir and elixir of terpin hydrate with codeine. These spans and tweens will be further explained in "Manufacturing."

17. Dicarboxylic acids and similar compounds. Previously, we discussed the monocarboxylic acids and their derivatives. Polycarboxylic acids, especially the dicarboxylic acids with a normal chain of carbon atoms, are also important. Some of these compounds, naturally occurring and discovered centuries ago, are of pharmaceutical importance. Rather than going into the properties and reactions of the broad group of compounds, many of which are of no particular importance to us, well enumerate the official substances and say a few important things about each. The compounds in this area with which you should be familiar are:

a. Oxalic acid, $C_2H_2O_4$. Oxalic acid is the simplest of the dicarboxylic acids, having the formula HOOCCOOH. It is standard in analytical work, a stain remover for rust and iron tannate inks, and an anticoagulant for blood specimens. Being poisonous and caustic in concentrated solution, this preparation is NEVER used as an anticoagulant in vivo, that is, in the living body. Its uses are strictly for use in vitro (in glass).

b. Phosgene, $COCl_2$. Phosgene or carbonyl chloride is a carbonic acid derivative, but is discussed here because its derivatives are more like those of the dicarboxylic acids. Phosgene is a clear, colorless gas, formed by the union of chlorine and carbon monoxide (and compounds yielding these substances). It has a suffocating odor and is highly poisonous. It is classified as a lung irritant among the chemical warfare agents. Phosgene is of importance to the pharmacist only because it is a starting point in the synthesis of urea and the barbiturates.

c. Tartaric acid.

HOCHOOH
|
HOCHCOOH

The chief use of tartaric acid in pharmacy is in the manufacture of effervescent salts. It also imparts a tangy flavor to fruits and drinks.

d. Potassium bitartrate (cream of tartar), KOOCCH(OH)CH(OH)COOH. Besides being used in the preparation of other tartrates and tartaric acid, cream of tartar is a laxative, an ingredient in baking soda (mixed with bicarbonate-on addition . of water, CO_2 is liberated).

e. Potassium sodium tartrate (Rochelle salt), KOOCH(OH)-CH(OH)-COONa $4H_2O$. Rochelle salt is a saline cathartic, a pharmaceutical necessity, and an ingredient in compound effervescent powders.

f. Antimony potassium tartrate (tartar emetic), KO O C - C H OH-CHOH-COO (SbO) $1/2H_2O$. This substance has been used medicinally for its expectorant and emetic action; however, because of the toxicity of antimony, it is now generally reserved for treatment of parasite infections and tropical diseases, such as schistosomiasis, leishmaniasis, and filariasis.

g. Citric acid, $CH_2(COOH)C(OH)$-$(COOH)CH_2COOH$. Sometimes called salt of lemon because it is a natural ingredient in citrus fruits, citric acid is a saturated tricarboxylic acid. It is this substance which imparts the tart flavor to citrus fruits and the beverages using their flavors. Citric acid has the ability to mask undesirable tastes of certain drugs. It is also used in the preparation of citrate of magnesia, a saline cathartic preparation, as well as in effervescent salts.

18. Concepts and terminology of cyclic structures. In the preceding pages, we have been concerned almost exclusively with aliphatic compounds. For clarity and ease of presentation, it was necessary to treat a couple of ring compounds along with the aliphatics. From this point on, the great majority of the compounds presented will be cyclic. Regardless of the wordscyclic compound, ring, closed chainthe structure referred to is distinguished by a nucleus containing no terminal atoms; that is, each element in the structure is joined (bonded) to another member of the ring in an unbroken "fence-like" shape. All ring structures have three or more atoms in the ring.

a. Classification by atoms in the chain. If the atoms in the cycle are all alike, we have an *isocyclic* or *homocyclic* compound. And if these atoms are all carbon atoms, as they often are, the structure is *carbocyclic.* Any ring which includes more than one kind of atom is *heterocyclic.* Some examples should make this clearer.

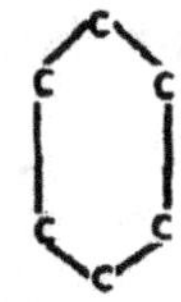

Homocyclic (Carbocyclic)

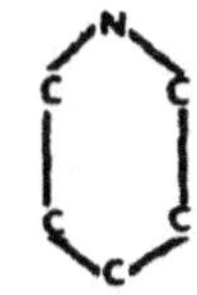

Heterocyclic

b. Classification by number of atoms in the ring. Aside from classifying cyclic compounds into isocyclic or heterocyclic, we also describe them by the number of atoms in the ring. This classification gives us useful information. When talking about a cyclic structure with three atoms in a closed ring, we speak of a three-member ring; four atoms in the cycle is a four-member ring; and so forth. The description, ìa three-member, carbocyclic ring,î then is very illustrative, telling us that there are three carbon atoms in a closed chain structure. Study the following abbreviated graphic formulas as illustrative of these fundamental principles.

(1) Three-member rings.

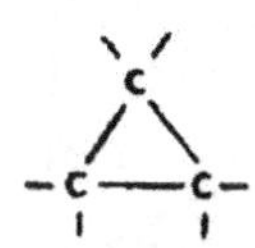

Carbocyclic

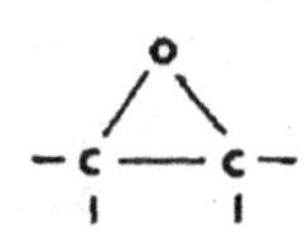

Heterocyclic

(2) Four-member rings.

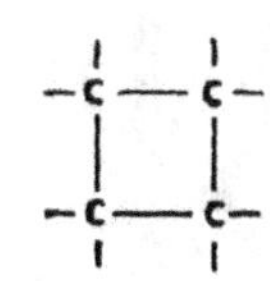

Carbocyclic

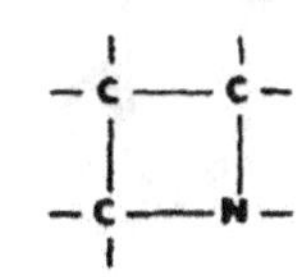

Heterocyclic

(3) Five-member rings.

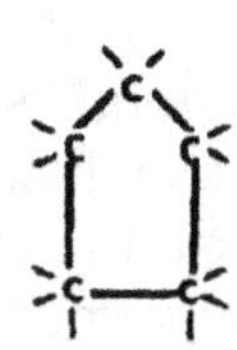

Carbocyclic

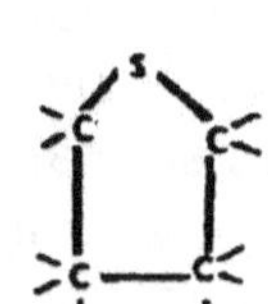

Heterocyclic

(4) Six-member rings.

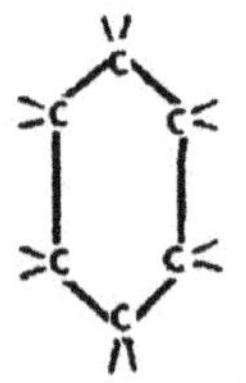

Carbocyclic

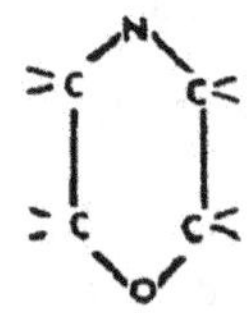

Heterocyclic

c. Alicyclic and aromatic subclasses of carbocyclic structures.

(1) Alicyclic. Alicyclic structures are by far the most common of the carbocyclic structures. They may be saturated, having single bonds as in those formulas shown before, or they may be unsaturated to varying degrees, as represented by the following formulas.

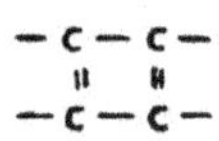

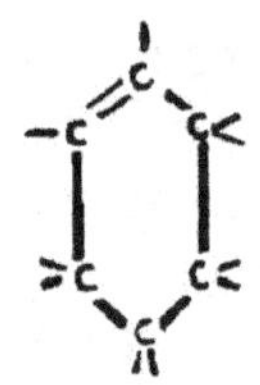

(2) Aromatic. The aromatic compounds are those carbocyclics having six carbon atoms with three double and three single bonds alternated around the cycle. In order to be truly aromatic, all these specifications must be met. In the following graphic formula, benzene, an aromatic compound, is represented.

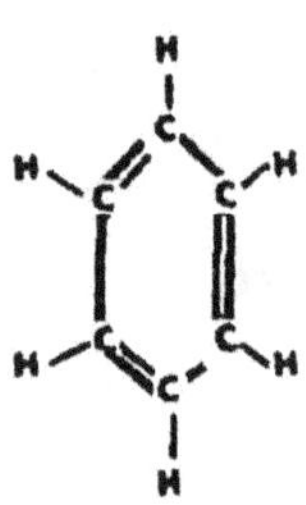

Benzene

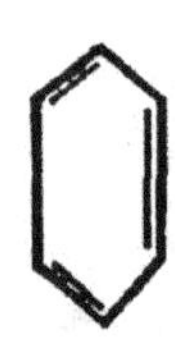

Benzene (simplified formula)

The word "aromatic" in our terminology of cyclic structures can cause considerable trouble if you do not understand its meaning. When aromatic is used in conjunction with organic chemistry, it refers to the specific structure of a group of compounds, NOT to odor!

d. Substitution and isomerism. Benzene, the simplest of the aromatic compounds, can undergo substitution. Because it is the simplest, we will use it as our illustrative device to explain substitution and isomerism.

(1) Monosubstitution. When a single hydrogen is replaced by an element or radical, it is termed monosubstitution. Regardless of which hydrogen is replaced, there is only one possible productxbenzene (where x equals the substituted radical). Replacement of a hydrogen by a chlorine atom produces chlorobenzene.

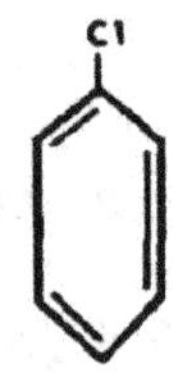

Chlorobenzene

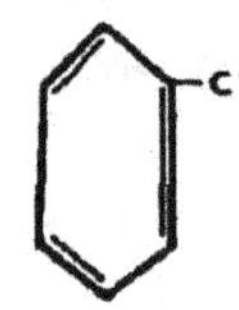

Chlorobenzene

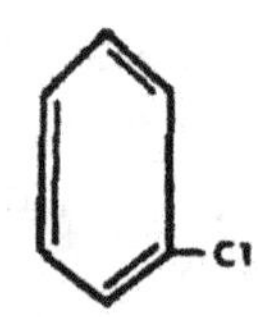

Chlorobenzene

(2) Disubstitution. When two hydrogens are replaced by chlorine, there are three possible isomers, depending upon the positions on the molecule the chlorine assumes. Thus we have

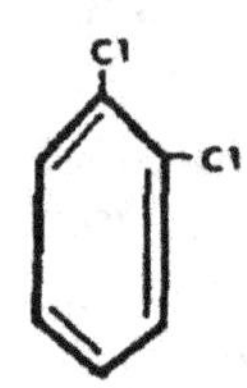

Ortho-Dichlorobenzene

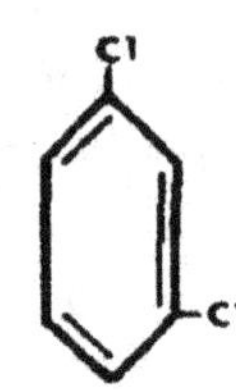

Meta-Dichlorobenzene

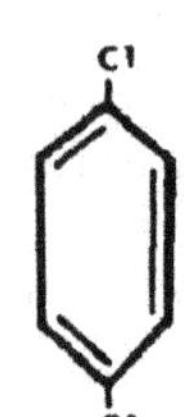

Para-Dichlorobenzene

"Ortho" means "straight line," and as you can see in the structure of ortho-dichlorobenzene, the substitution is in a straight line. "Meta" means "beyond," and in meta-dichlorobenzene, the substitution is beyond or separated by a single carbon. ìParaî means ìoppositeî and in paradichlorobenzene, the chlorine is substituted on carbons at opposite ends of the benzene ring.

(a) Numbering the benzene ring. The benzene ring is numbered in clockwise direction, giving the attached radicals the lowest possible numbers.

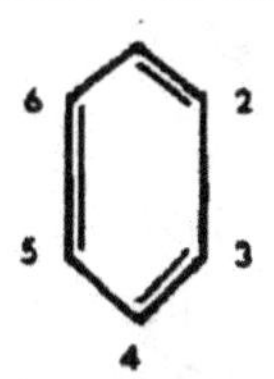

(b) Ortho-dichlorobenzene. Substitution at the 1 and 2 positions yields orthodichlorbenzene (1, 2-dichlorobenzene) which is more commonly written o-dichlorobenzene. It is a liquid used as a solvent and degreasing agent.

(c) Meta-dichlorobenzene. Substitution at the 1 and 3 positions yields meta-dichlorobenzene (1, 3-dichlorobenzene) which is more commonly written m-dichlorobenzene. It is also a liquid which is used as a deodorant in latrines.

(d) Para-dichlorobenzene. Substitution at the 1 and 4 positions yields para-dichlorobenzene (1,4-dichlorobenzene) which is more commonly written p-dichlorobenzene. It is a crystalline solid used almost exclusively for its ability to kill moths.

(3) Trisubstitution. As with the disubstituted rings, it is possible to have three different configurations with trisubstitution. The following illustrations should serve as adequate explanation of these configurations.

You should keep in mind that other representative illustrations, although placed in different positions than shown, will fall into one of the three groups simply by rotation of the molecule.

(4) Tetrasubstitution. Tetrasubstitution is handled in exactly the same manner as trisubstitution. The only difference is that the prefix ìtetraî replaces ìtri.î Thus, four chlorine atoms positioned at the 1, 2, 3, and 5 carbons will be 1, 2, 3, 5-tetrachlorobenzene.

(5) Other types of isomerism. As we progress further into the subject and come to specific instances, other types of isomerism will be illustrated. For the time being, it will serve to mention that isomers are not limited to structural isomers, but also include others such as tautomers, stereoisomers, geometric isomers, optical isomers, and diastereoisomers.

e. Basic structures. Certain basic structures will repeatedly show themselves throughout the field of organic chemistry. Since you should be able to recognize the basic portions of various molecules, you should know the structures of the following:

(1) Benzene (benzol), C_6H_6. Benzene is a clear liquid with extremely flammable vapors. It is miscible with alcohol, ether, acetone, chloroform, and oils, but immiscible with water. Therefore, it is a good solvent for fats, resins, and alkaloids. Benzene is very toxic. One teaspoon is lethal orally. In contact with the skin, toxic quantities may be absorbed. Toxicity becomes apparent in patients after prolonged breathing of only one part per mil-

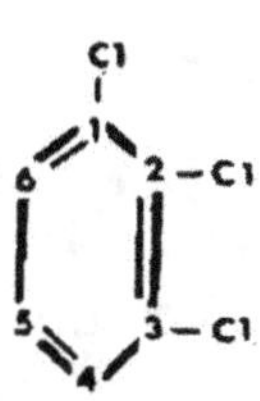

1, 2, 3-trichlorobenzene
(adjacent trichlorobenzene)

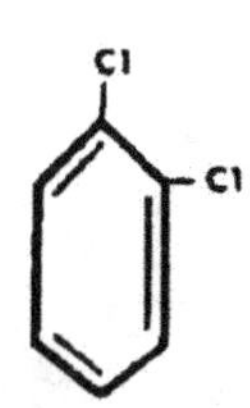

1, 2, 4-trichlorobenzene
(unsymmetrical trichlorobenzene)

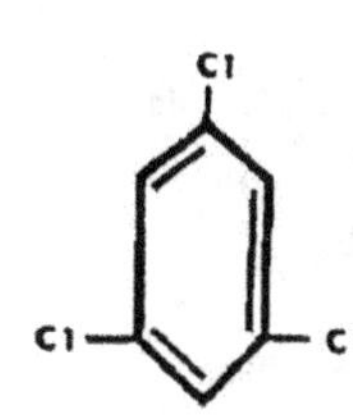

1, 3, 5-trichlorobenzene
(symmetrical trichlorobenzene)

lion. It has been used medicinally but because of its toxicity and doubtful value, its use, other than as a solvent and starting point in syntheses, is questioned by authorities. It has, however, been used as an antispasmodic, antiseptic, parasiticide, and as an agent against trichinosis and leukemia.

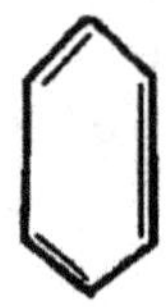

Benzene

(2) Toluene, C_7H_8. Toluene is similar in solvent properties to benzene which it also resembles in color and odor. It is an important solvent and is of great use in the synthesis of many medicinals, industrial chemicals, and dyes. Toluene is a coal tar derivative.

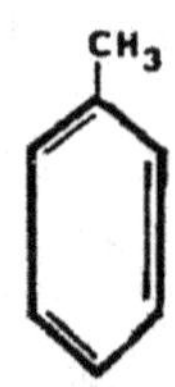

Toluene
(Methylbenzene)

(3) Xylene, C_8H_{10}. Xylene, another derivative of coal tar, is a mixture of the ortho, meta, and para isomers with the meta isomer predominating. It resembles benzene and toluene in its properties. It is used as a solvent, in the synthesis of dyes and other organic substances, and as a cleaning agent for microscope slides. When used as a solvent for Canadian balsam, an oil immersion substance is formed.

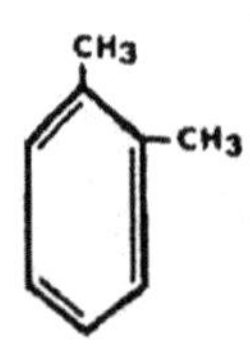

Xylene

(4) Naphthalene, $C_{10}H_8$. Also called tar camphor, napththalene is also obtained from coal tar. It is sold in flakes or balls for use as a moth repellent. It has some value as an antiseptic and anthelmintic. More important, however, is the role of naphthalene as an intermediate in the manufacture of organic preparations.

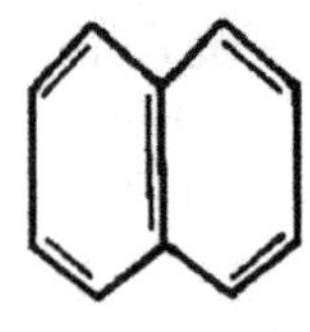

Naphthalene

(5) Anthracene, $C_{14}H_{10}$.
Anthracene is a solid obtained from coal tar. It is soluble in the usual organic solvents; less soluble in ether and alcohol than benzene, toluene, xylene, and naphthalene; and insoluble in water. Anthracene is of great importance because of its use in the manufacture of more complex organic compounds, particularly anthraquinone.

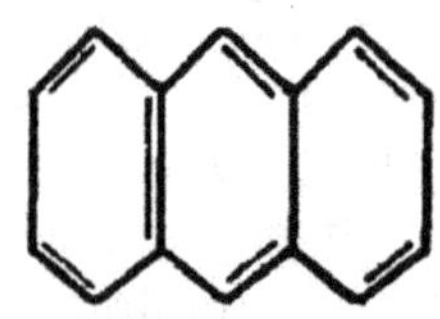

Anthracene

(6) Phenanthrene, $C_{14}H_{10}$ Phenanthrene, a structural isomer of anthracene, has properties similar to anthracene. It is pharmaceutically important because, when reduced, it resembles very closely some of the analgesic alkaloids, the sterols, bile acids, and sex hormones.

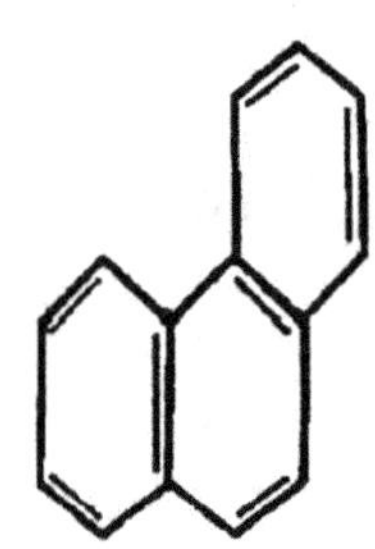

Phenanthrene
(isomer of anthracene)

19. Phenols and related compounds. Up to this point, the presence of a hydroxy group (OH) on a compound has signified that the compound was an alcohol. A hydroxy group attached to an aromatic

ring, however, is not an alcohol, but a *phenol.* Phenols, then, are hydroxy derivatives of aromatic rings. Because of the structural similarity of the phenols to the alcohols, many of their properties are similar.

a. Properties. Phenols which contain only the hydroxy group or groups are colorless or white crystals. Those formed from benzene or toluene are soluble in alcohol and to some degree are soluble in water. If the substance is even slightly ionizable, it will exhibit acidity and react with bases. For this reason, phenols are generally incompatible with alkalis. Most phenols are antiseptic and slightly caustic. The medicinal properties of coal tars and wood tar products are attributed to the phenols present in those substances. Phenols, like alcohols, can be esterified, and a large number of useful medicinal agents are esterified phenols.

b. Occurrence and preparation. Some phenols are obtained from the dry distillation of hard wood and coal. Others, particularly some of the very complex molecules, are extracted from plants and animals. Still others are synthesized.

c. Germicidal action and phenol coefficient. Since most of the phenols have germicidal action, a system for rating the efficiency of phenols in germicidal ability has been devised, using as a basis the germicidal action of phenol. The germicidal efficiency of each of the phenols is given a number rating relative to phenol. This number is the phenol coefficient.

d. Pharmaceutically important phenols and their derivatives.

(1) Phenol (carbolic acid), C_6H_5OH.

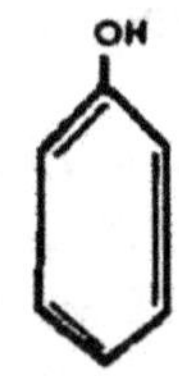

Phenol is a colorless-to-pink, needle-like crystal with a characteristic, antiseptic odor. When heated, the vapors are flammable.

(a) Solubility. Phenol is very soluble in alcohol, ether, chloroform, glycerin, and fixed and volatile oils. It is soluble 1:15 in water. When 90 Gm. of phenol are liquefied by the addition of 10 ml. of water, a permanent liquid results. The addition of more water causes the phenol to recrystallize.

(b) Relationship to acids. Although phenol is called carbolic acid, its only similarity to acids is its ability to neutralize bases. It is much more closely related to alcohol. Both the crystal and the liquefied forms are caustic to organic matter; they are protoplasmic poisons. Unlike acids and bases, phenolis caustic action is not restricted to surface tissue. Left in contact, it is not neutralized but continues to damage deeper tissue. Because of this unusual behavior and the fact that nerve endings are inactivated, deep and severe burns can occur before the victim is aware of it.

(c) Incompatibilities. Phenol is incompatible with camphor, menthol, thymol, phenacetin, and many other compounds, and forms eutectic mixtures with them. When two solids at room temperature are mixed and a liquid results spontaneously, the mixture is said to be eutectic. To illustrate this phenomenon to yourself, pour out equal quantities of phenol crystals and camphor on an ointment slab. With a rubber spatula, rub the two substances together. At first, it will become sticky; after a relatively short period, it will liquefy completely.

(d) Uses. Although officially classified in the USP as an antipruritic, it is further employed as a caustic, disinfectant,

antiseptic, preservative, and local anesthetic.

(2) Liquefied phenol (liquefied carbolic acid). This substance contains not less than 88 percent C_6H_6O. An official note in the USP states: "When phenol is to be mixed with a fixed oil, mineral oil or white petrolatum, use crystalline Phenol, not Liquefied Phenol." Liquefied phenol is categorized officially as a caustic to be applied locally in suitable dilution, and then removed with alcohol, but it is used more frequently in a number of preparations for various dermatologic conditions.

(3) Phenolated calamine lotion (compound calamine lotion). In a 1-percent concentration in calamine lotion, the phenol adds a slight anesthetic effect and helps relieve itching.

(4) Dihydroxybenzene, $C_6H_4(OH)_2$ Dihydroxybenzene which occurs in three isomeric forms-ortho, meta, and para-is pharmaceutically important only in its meta isomer. Meta-dihydroxybenzene is official in the USP under the name Resorcinol, common name, resorcin. It is a white, crystalline powder which acquires a pinkish tint on exposure to light and air. It has a characteristic odor. Resorcinol is soluble in alcohol, water, glycerin, and ether. To illustrate the added solubility of the extra hydroxy group over phenol (with one), phenol is 1:15 water soluble, whereas Resorcinol is soluble 1:1. Resorcinol is antiseptic and antifungal and is very effective against parasitic skin diseases such as eczema and ringworm, and other dermatitides such as psoriasis and seborrhea. It is applied in the form of lotions, pastes, and creams in strengths ranging from 1 to 20 percent; 5 percent is the most widely used concentration.

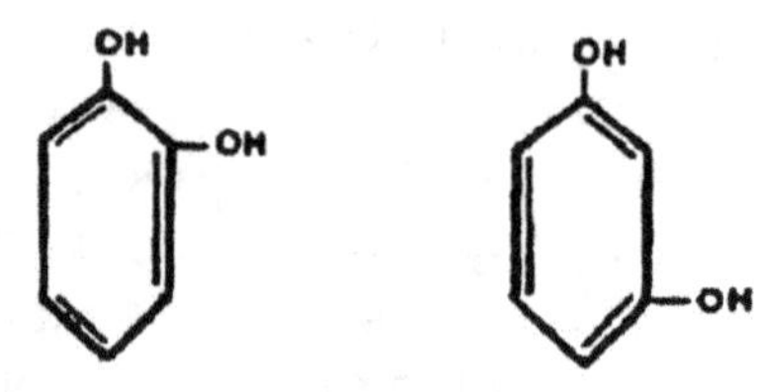

o-dihydroxybenzene (catechol) m-dihydroxybenzene (resorcinol)

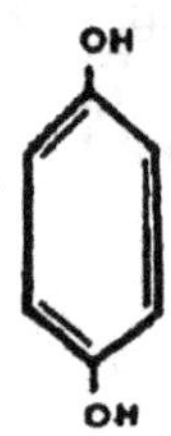

p-dihydroxybenzene (hydroquinone)

(5) Resorcinol monoacetate (resorcin acetate). By esterifying resorcin with acetic acid, the following reaction occurs to form resorcinol monoacetate.

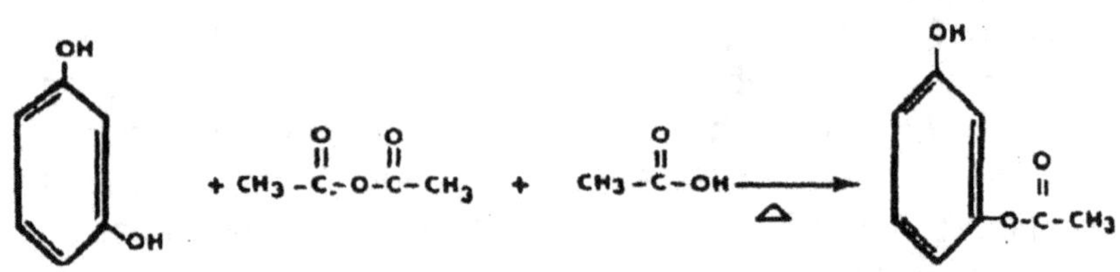

Resorcin Acetic Anhydride Acetic Acid Resorcinol Monoacetate

A common, although not official, name for this medication is Euresol. It is an amber-colored, thick liquid, soluble in alcohol and sparingly soluble in water. Euresol is an antibacterial and antifungal, as well as a local irritant. Although it is used also for psoriasis and eczema, its most common use is in scalp preparations for alopecia (hair loss or baldness). Since alopecia has several causes, you should deduce that resorcinol monoacetate will only be effective in those types caused by a bacterial or fungal infection.

(6) Anthralin (1, 8, 9-anthratriol; 1, 8-dihydroxyanthranol)

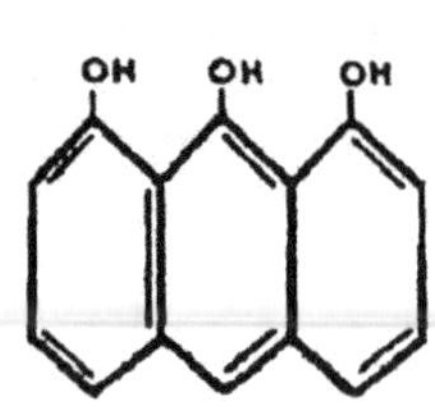

Anthralin is a yellowish-brown, water-insoluble powder, used in the manufacture of skin preparations, particularly anthralin ointment. Anthralin is a local irritant and antieczematic agent. At one time, chrysarobin was a widely used substance, but anthralin has replaced chrysarobin because it is somewhat less irritating and causes less skin discoloration.

(7) Danthron (Dorbane).

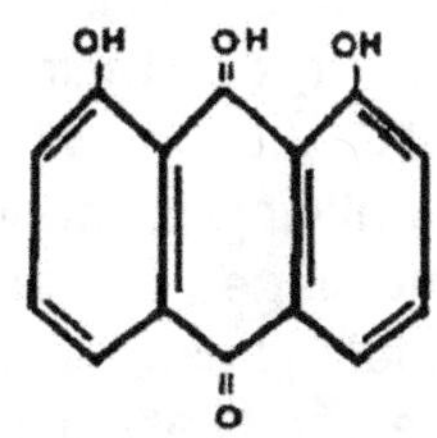

Danthron is a cathartic which appears as a pink dye in alkaline urine. It is most important as an intermediate in the manufacture of dyes and in veterinary medicine. Its use in human medicine is infrequent, probably because of the demoralizing effect on the patient upon seeing red-colored urine.

(8) Eugenol.

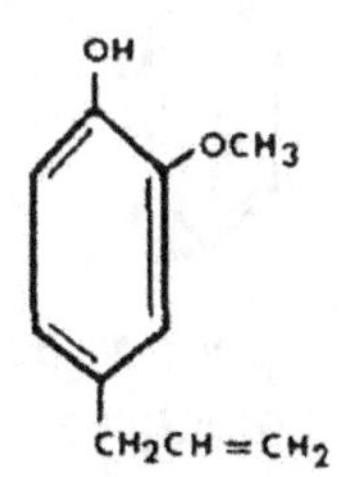

Eugenol is the main constituent in clove oil and, in fact, it is eugenol that is old as artificial oil of cloves. Eugenol occurs naturally in cinnamon oil, sassafras, bay leaves, and pimenta oil. The USP classifies eugenol as a dental obtundant (dulls sensibility to pain) for toothaches; it is applied either on a pledget of cotton or mixed with zinc oxide to form a temporary filling. The basic material used for the synthesis of vanillin is eugenol.

(9) Glyceryl guaiacolate. This stimulating expectorant is incorporated into cough preparations such as Robitussin. It is much easier to tolerate than the plain guaiacol which was previously used.

(10) Hexachlorophene.

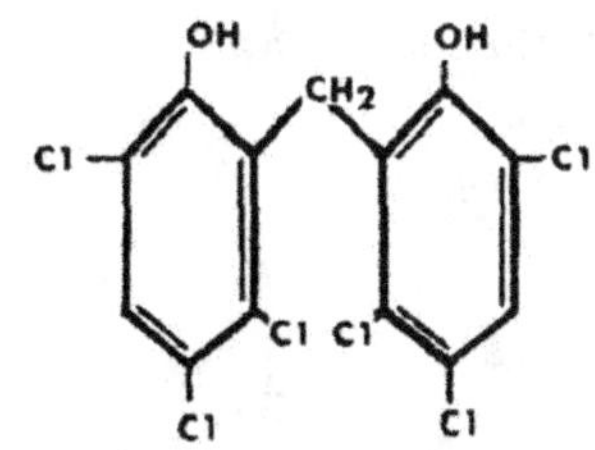

Hexachlorophene is an anti-infective agent. It is incorporated into soaps and surgical scrubs to reduce the bacterial flora. For proper activity it must be left on the skin as a residue to prevent bacterial growth. The protective film is removed when other cleansing agents are used and the bacteriostatic effect is lost. Damage to the nervous system is possible if soaps containing large amounts of hexachlorophene are used improperly over long periods of time. It is now under restricted use.

(11) Hexylresorcinol.

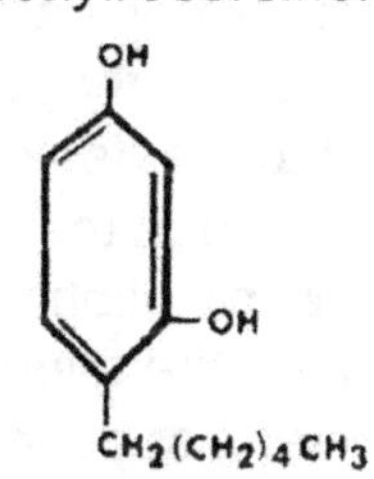

Hexylresorcinol is used in a 1:1000 dilution as an effective antiseptic. It has the advantage of being odorless and nonstaining. It is effective in the treatment internally of many worm infestations. Although relatively nontoxic, it is extremely irritating to the mucous membranes and may cause ulcerations if the capsule containing it is broken in the mouth. Hexylresorcinol is manufactured in the form of a coated pill which resists rupturing, even when chewed.

(12) Thymol.

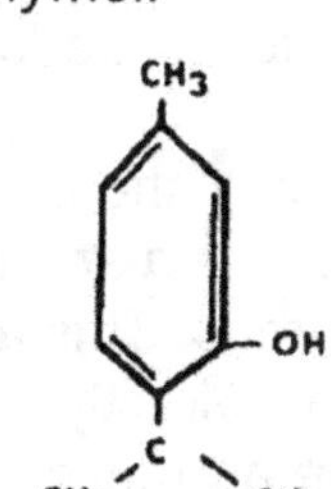

Thymol is an antiseptic, but its action is of short duration. Thymol is mixed with other substances such as camphor and menthol in mouthwashes. These preparations taste nice, but have little effect in sterilizing the field of application.

(13) Cresol.

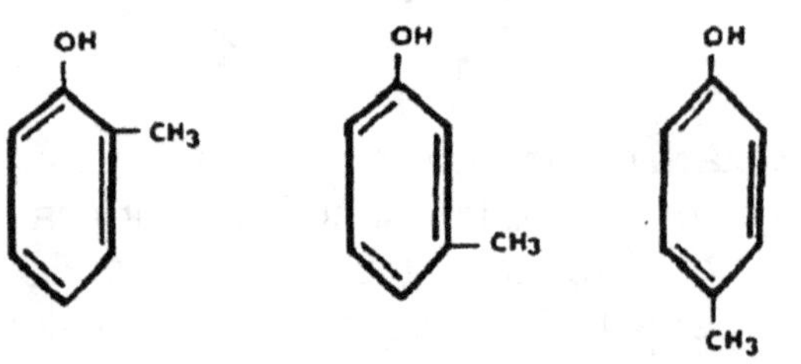

Ortho Meta Para

Cresol is a mixture of o-, m-, and p-cresols obtained from coal tar, containing not more than 5-percent phenol. Cresol is similar to phenol in antiseptic properties and is used as a preservative for injectable solutions.

e. *Aromatic alcohols and their derivatives.* The aromatic alcohols differ structurally from the phenols in that the hydroxyl group is attached to a side chain of the aromatic ring, rather than to the ring itself. The alcohols resemble the aliphatic alcohols in many respects. Like the aliphatics, they may exist as primary, secondary, and tertiary alcohols. The pharmaceutically important aromatic alcohols include:

(1) Benzyl alcohol (phenylcarbinol).

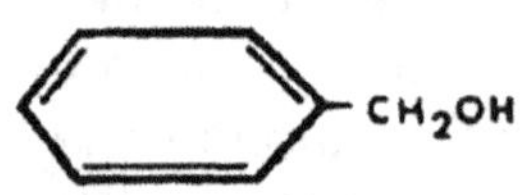

The main action of benzyl alcohol is as a local anesthetic by injection or by application to mucous membranes. It also functions as a bacteriostatic agent in certain injectables.

(2) Benzyl benzoate, C_6H_5-CO-O-CH_2-C_6H_5. Benzyl benzoate is used as a scabacide in the form of a lotion.

20. Aromatic acids and their derivatives. Aromatic acids contain an aromatic ring and a carboxyl group. This acid group may be attached either directly to the ring or to a side chain. The aromatic acids are important mainly because of the physiologically active agents produced by their esterification. Among these are analgesics, antispasmodics, antiseptics, and local anesthetics. The pharmaceutically important aromatic acids and their derivatives include

a. Benzole acid, C_6H_5COOH.

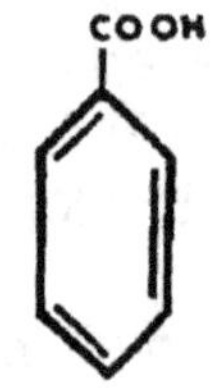

Benzoic acid occurs free in nature and esterified in balsams. It is quite soluble in alcohol but only about 3:1000 in water. It is used in external antiseptic preparations and as a preservative in mucilages and suspensions. Sodium benzoate is used as a food preservative. Derivatives and salts of benzoic acid are important pharmaceutically and these will be considered in later portions of this chapter under "anesthetic amines, amides. and vitamins."

b. Salicylic acid (O-hydroxybenzoic acid).

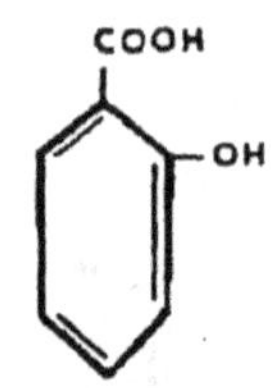

Salicylic acid is a phenol, as well as an aromatic acid, but is much less caustic than phenol. It has antiseptic and germicidal properties, and in stronger concentrations it acts as a keratolytic.

(1) Uses. Not used internally because of its irritating nature, salicylic acid is mainly employed in external preparations for the treatment of warts, corns, fungus infections, and some eczemas. Tissue cells swell, soften, and peel off after repeated or prolonged contact with salicylic acid.

(2) Whitfield's ointment Whitfield's ointment, used topically as a fungicide, is a combination of benzoic and salicylic acids in polyethylene glycol ointment.

c. Methylparaben; propylparaben. Two different but very closely related derivatives of benzoic acid are the parabens. These substances are used singly or in combination as preservatives in many pharmaceutical preparations and cosmetics. Combining the two produces a synergistic effect; that is, the antiseptic effect of the combination is greater than the total effect of the individual components.

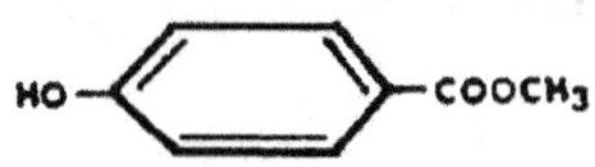

Methylparaben
(Methyl p-Hydroxybenzoate)

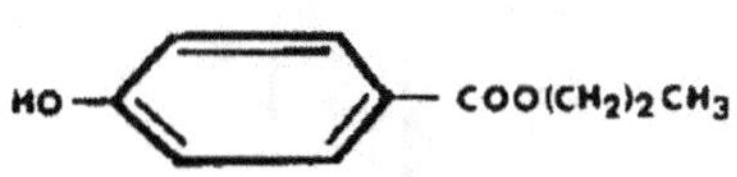

Propylparaben
(Propyl p-Hydroxybenzoate)

d. Sodium salicylatc.

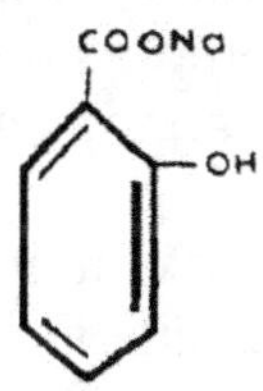

Sodium salicylate is widely employed as an analgesic and antipyretic.

e. Methyl salicylate (oil of wintergreen)

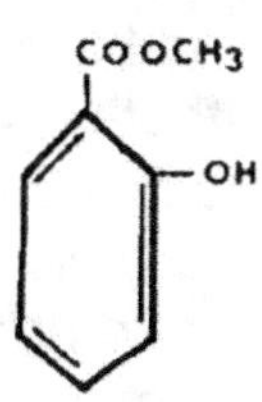

Methyl salicylate is used as a flavoring agent and as a counterirritant.

f. Phenyl salicylate (Salol).

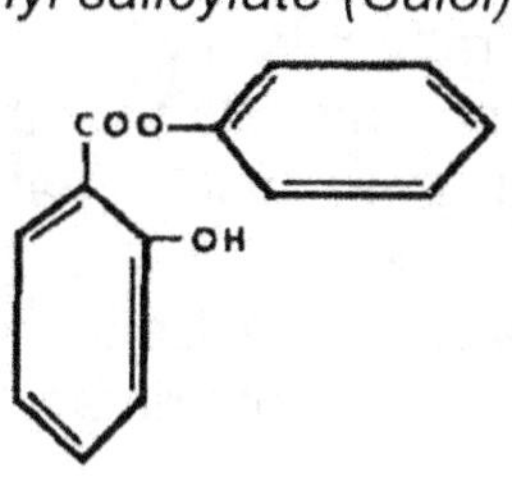

Phenyl salicylate is used as an extemporaneous enteric coating for tablets and capsules. This substance is not soluble in the acid media of the stomach but rapidly dissolves in the alkaline intestine. No more than necessary should be used for coating the tablets, as salol breaks down into phenol and salicylic acid in the body.

g. Aspirin (acetylsalicylic acid, ASA).

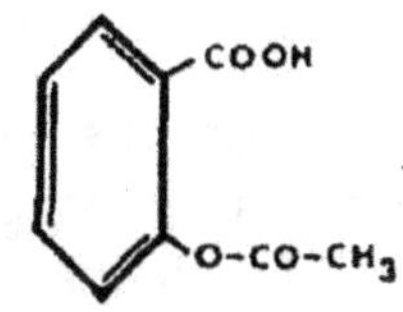

Like the other salicylates we have discussed, aspirin is analygesic and antipyretic and has some value in relieving pain of almost any origin. Aspirin is not soluble in water: it must bo administered as a tablet, capsule, or suppository. It may be solubilized to some extent, but the solutions are not stable and hydrolyzc within a few days to salicylic and acetic acids. Hydrolyzed aspirin has a strong odor of acetic aeid and tablets may display crystals of salicylic acid on their surface: they should not be used.

21. Aromatic halogenated compounds and similar structures. At the beginning of our discussion of cyclic structures, we illustrated some substitution possibilities of benzene, showing specifically chlorine mono, di, tri, and tetra substitution. In all these cases, the halogenation was directly on the benzene ring. It is also possible to halogenate a side chain; this was described in the aliphatic portion of this chapter. Since we have already discussed the reactions, let us look at some specific compounds resulting from halogenation of cyclic structures.

a. Gamma benzene hexachloride (benzene hexachloride; 1, 2, 3, 4, 5. 6-hexachlorocyclohexane; Lindane) $C_6Cl_6H_6$.

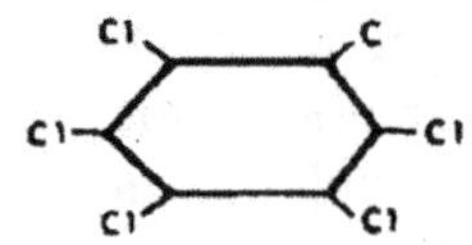

Gamma benzene hexachloride is the gamma isomer of hexachlorocyclohexane. It exists as a white crystalline powder with a musty odor. It is used as an insecticide and in the treatment of scabies and lice of the head, pubic area, and feet.

b. Chlordane. Chlordane is a nearly odorless liquid used as an insecticide. It is equal to DDT in its effectiveness as an insecticide and is superior to many other insecticides. It is used particularly against cockroaches, ants, grasshoppers, and some animal parasites. It is of no medical value to humans.

c. Halazone tablets (p-dichlorosulfamoylbenzoic acid).

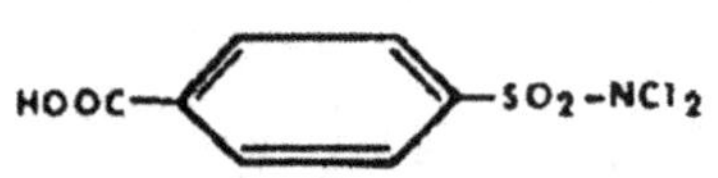

Halazone tablets, containing 4 mg. of active ingredient, produce a concentration of 2-5 parts per million when dissolved in a quart of water. Water which has been treated with halazone tablets and allowed to stand for 30 minutes is safe for drinking although it may not taste pleasant. This is an adequate and convenient method for the extemporaneous purification of water for drinking purposes when your water supply is contaminated or its potability is doubtful.

d. Merbromin (Mercurochrome).

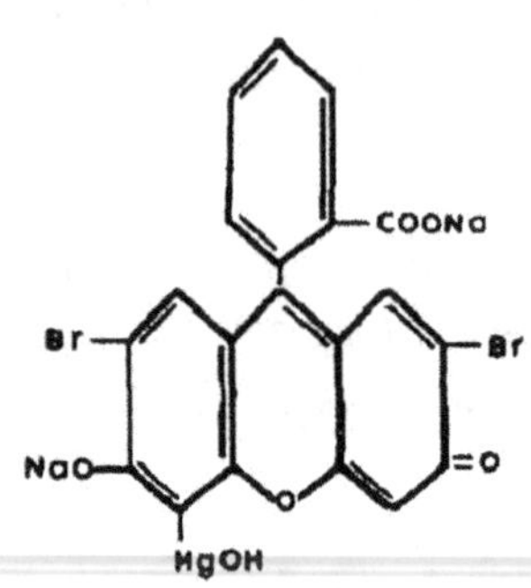

Merbromin is a weak antiseptic and acts as a bacteriostatic agent. It owes most of its activity to the mercury and, in tinctures, to the alcohol present.

e. Povidone-iodine (Betadine). By tying iodine into a very complex molecule (povidone), its sting is almost eliminated and the duration of its action is increased. Although basically not as effective as iodine, its sustained action and absence of sting are desirable qualities, and in minor cuts and abrasions it is a suitable antiseptic. It is also an effective throat gargle and douche.

f. Diiodohydroxyquin (Floraquin).

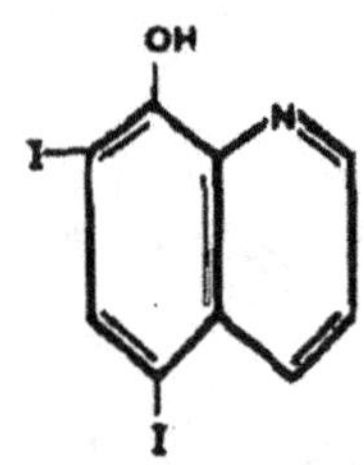

Diiodohydroxyquin is used in the treatment of intestinal amebiasis and certain fungal infections. It is administered as an enteric coated tablet and also applied topically.

g. Iodochlorhydroxyquin (Vioform). This compound is similar in structure and activity to diiodohydroxyquin.

22. Amines and amides (the nitrogen-containing compounds). In this broad class of substances arc the alkaloids, antihistamines, sulfa drugs, barbiturates, analgesics, and local anesthetics. The majority of the medications prescribed in todayís medicine are of the amine-amide group. No differentiation will be made here between amine derivatives or amide derivatives. It is important that you remember they are related, but different: and they all contain nitrogen. For further simplification, these products will be covered in groups with related action, rather than with related structure. The pharmacology of these compounds is treated in detail in chapter 9.

a. General structure. Below are shown the general structures of primary, secondary, and tertiary amines, and primary amides. We are limiting our coverage to primary amides because only they are of medical significance.

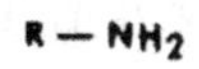

Primary Amine

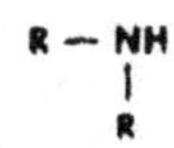

Secondary Amine

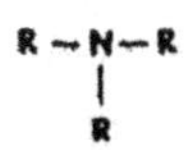

Tertiary Amine

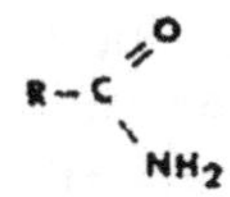

Primary Amide

b. The analgesic amines and amides. Agents which alleviate pain are termed analgesics. They are covered in chapter 9. Below are two members of this group; notice the similarities and differences in these compounds. Use this section in conjunction with your study of their pharmacology.

c. Local anesthetic amines and amides. Loss of feeling and sensation to a

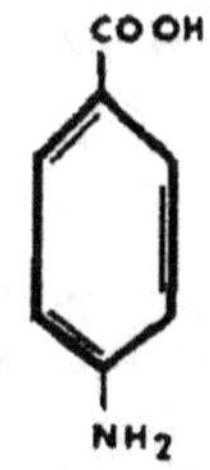

p-Aminobenzoic Acid

NOTE

By itself, p-aminobenzoic acid has no anesthetic properties. Its derivatives, however, do. Many of the important local anesthetics are closely related chemically to p-aminobenzoic acid.

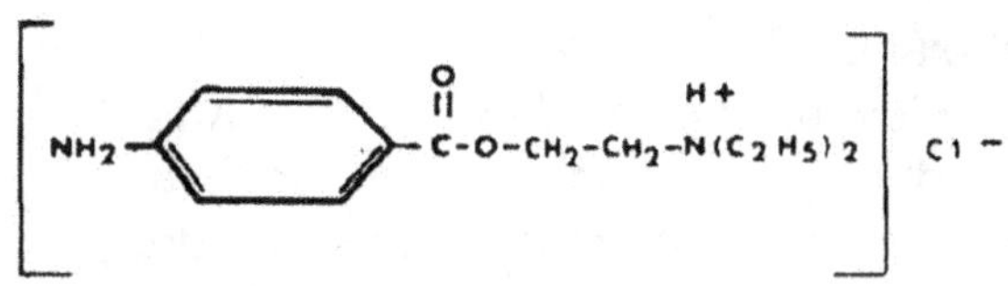

Procaine Hydrochloride (Procaine; Novocaine)

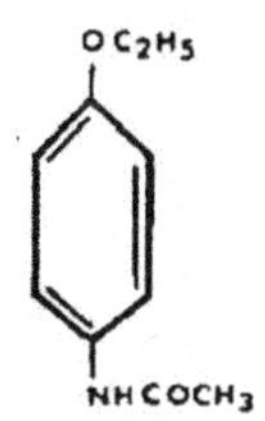

Phenacetin (Acetophenetidin)

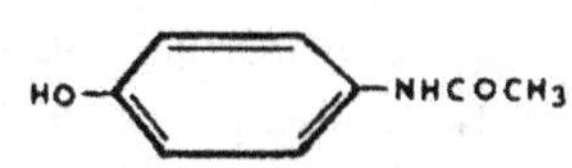

Acetaminophen (Tylenol)

localized portion of the body is known as local anesthesia. Such action may be caused by freezing, protoplasmic poisoning, or specific action on a nerve ending to prevent impulses from passing. Below are the names and structures of drugs that block nerve impulses.

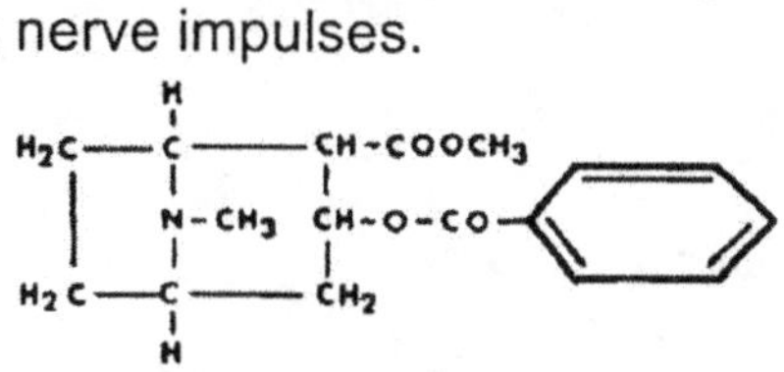

Cocaine

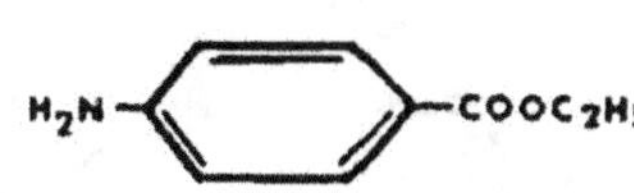

Ethylaminobenzoate (Benzocaine)

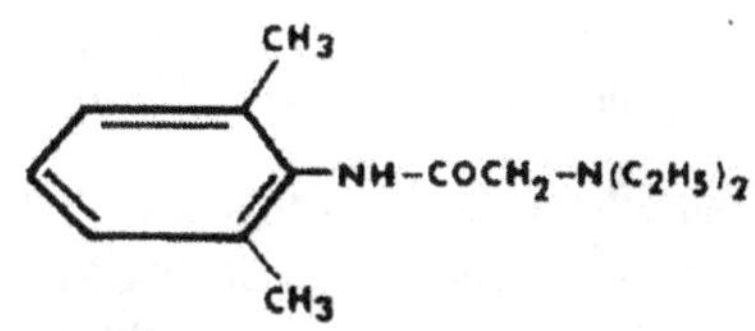

Lidocaine (Xylocaine)

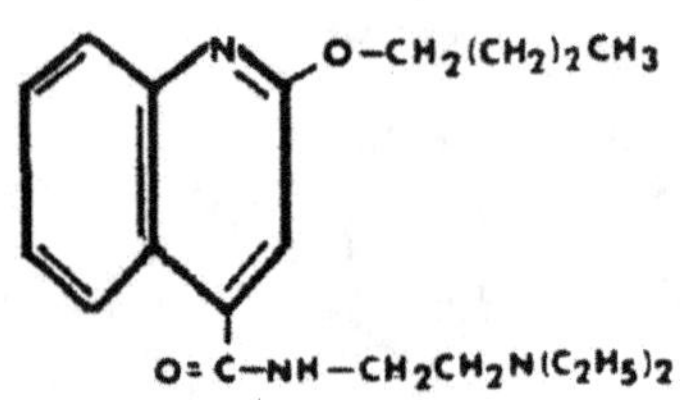

Dibucaine (Nupercaine)

d. Sedative and hypnotic amines and amides. Hypnotic, soporific, and somnifacient are synonymous terms, all referring to agents which produce sleep. Sleep may be produced by this class of drugs when there is no specific stimulus such as pain, coughing, or severe itch preventing it. Sedative drugs have a quieting effect. They produce relaxation, lessen excitement, and generally slow motor activity without producing sleep. Hypnotic and sedative properties are generally inherent in the same drug. Small doses produce sedation; larger doses produce hypnosis.

(1) Barbiturates. The barbiturates are a class of compounds called ureides, very closely related to amines and amides, and the most widely used sedatives and hypnotics. This class encompasses hundreds of compounds. The parent structure, barbituric acid or malonylurea, is formed by the combination of malonic acid and urea. As shown in the formulas below, barbituric acid exists as a mixture of two forms, the ìketoî form and the ìenolî form.

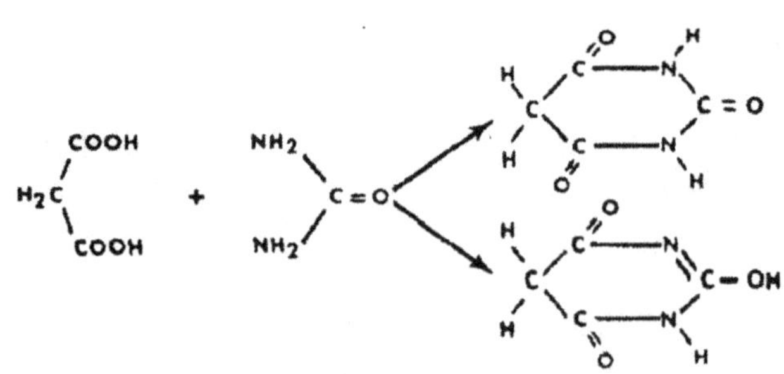

Keto Form

Enol Form

Malonic Acid Urea Malonylurea (Barbituric Acid)

(a) Barbituric acid. Barbituric acid itself is not active as a hypnotic or sedative. These properties are acquired through substitution of the hydrogens attached to the carbon atom. When organic groups are substituted for these hydrogens, the compounds become sedative and hypnotic. By replacing the hydrogen of the hydroxyl group in the enol form with sodium or potassium, soluble salts are produced. These soluble salts are important in the making of internal liquid preparations and injectables.

(b) Classes. Classes have been selected on the relative duration of action. The classes are: long-acting, intermediate-acting, short-acting, and ultra-short acting. Chapter 9 gives descriptions of these classes and detailed information about the individual agents.

(c) Long-acting barbiturates. The long-acting barbiturates are mainly used as sedatives. The more important members of this group are-

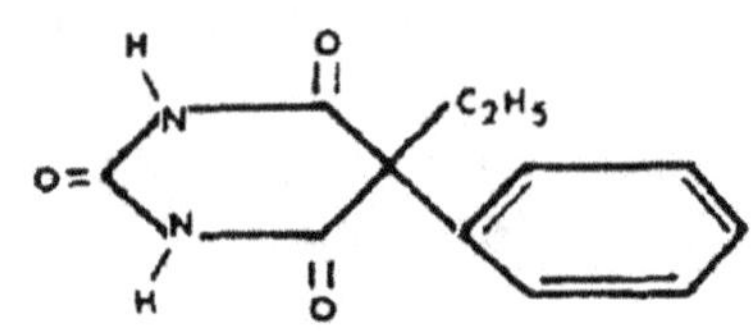

Phenobarbital (Luminal)

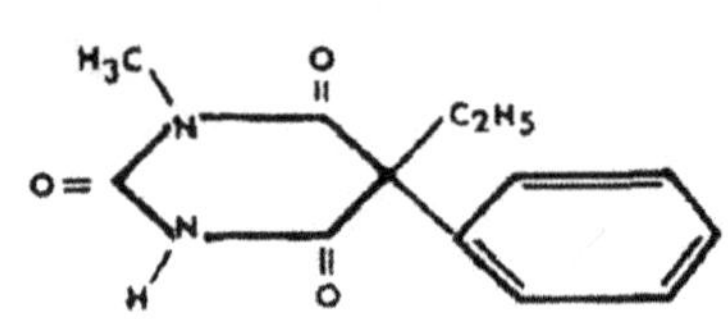

Mephobarbital (Mebaral)

(d) Intermediate-acting barbiturates.

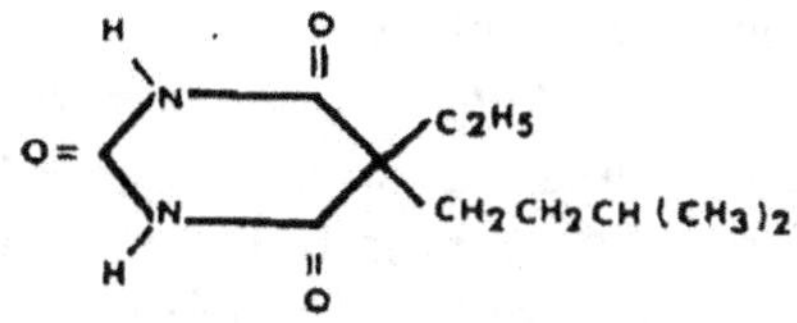

Amobarbital (Amytal)

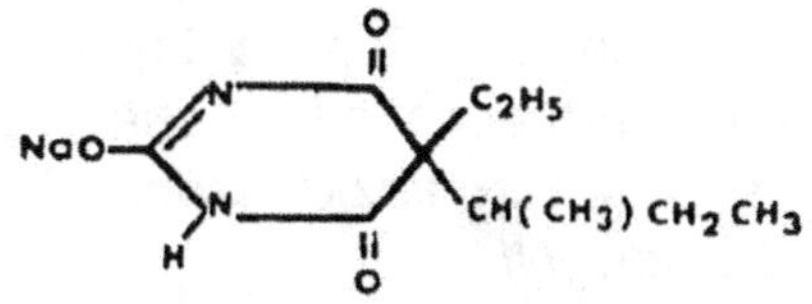

Butabarbital Sodium (Butisol)

(e) Short-acting barbiturates. The short-acting barbiturates are almost exclusively applied for their hypnotic rather than their sedative effects. Combinations of the short-acting and intermediate-acting are popular.

1. Pentobarbital sodium (Nembutal).

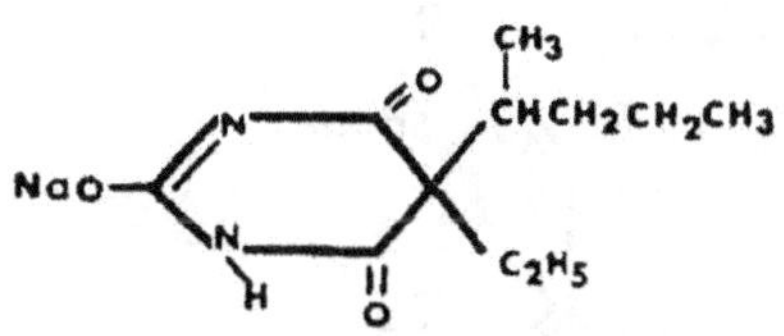

2. *Secobarbital (Seconal).*

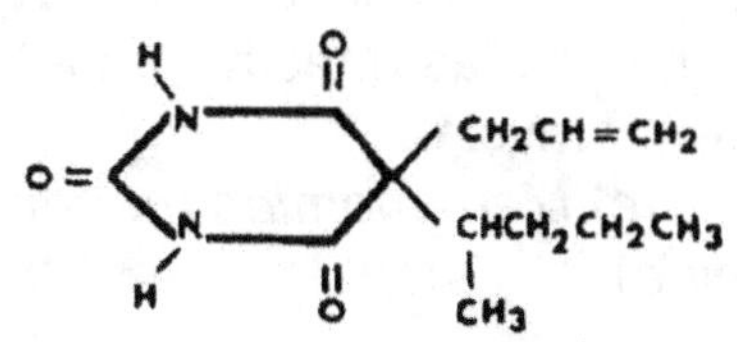

(f) Ultra short-acting barbiturates.

1. Thiopental sodium (Pentothal sodium).

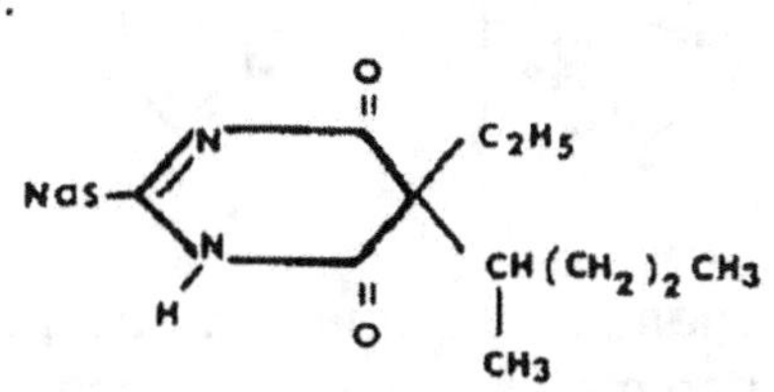

Here, for the first time in the barbiturate class of drugs, we find a sulfur atom in the molecule, and hence this barbiturate is called a thiobarbiturate (thio = sulfur).

2. Thiamylal sodium (Surital sodium).

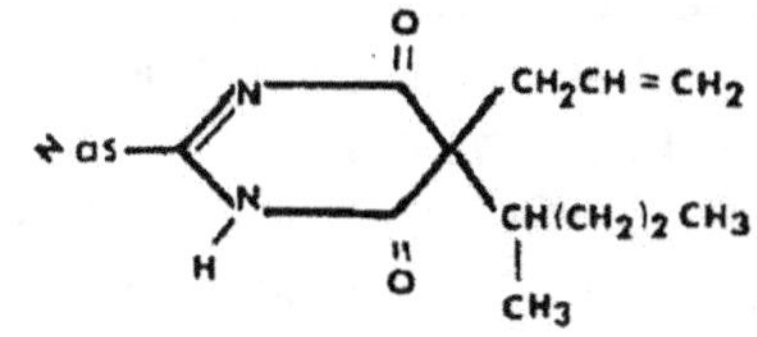

3. Hexobarbital sodium (Evipal sodium)

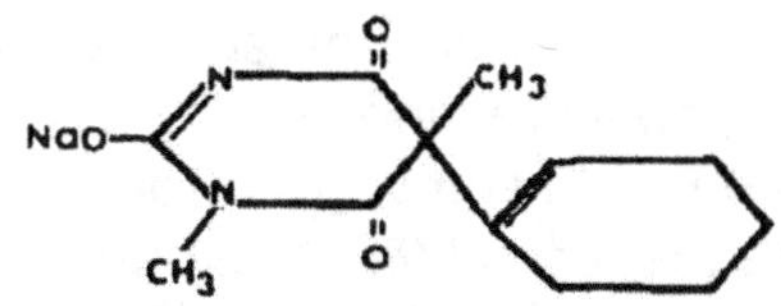

Notice in the molecular structure that an atom of oxygen replaces the sulfur. Certain authorities say that the substitution of oxygen for sulfur produces a safer drug.

(2) Other ureides. The hydantoins are ureides and are also central nervous system depressants but with selective activity. They depress the area of the brain where epileptic seizures originate but do not depress other areas. Epilepsy is a disease caused by unusual electric brain impulses. Generally, epilepsy is of four types, the two most important of which are grand mal and petit mal. Diphenylhydantoin (Dilantin), is the most widely used of this group.

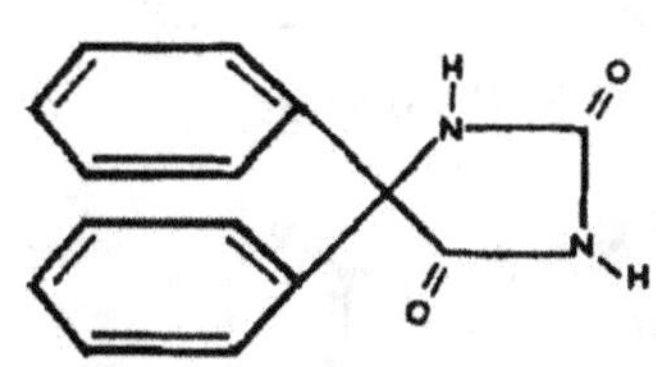

Diphenylhydantoin

e. Antimicrobial amines and amides. In 1908 a compound, p-aminobenzenesulfonamide, was synthesized. But it was not discovered until almost 30 years later that it had medicinal value. In 1935, a red dye discovered three years earlier was found to have wonderful curative powers. This compound was named Prontosil. Shortly thereafter it was determined that Prontosil was effective because of the p-aminobenzenesulfonamide portion of its molecule. Since then over 3300 sulfonamides have been used clinically. Other agents, unrelated to the sulfa drugs, have been discovered which display antimicrobial properties of the sulfa drugs.

(1) Sulfonamides.

(a) General formula. The general formula for the sulfonamides is-

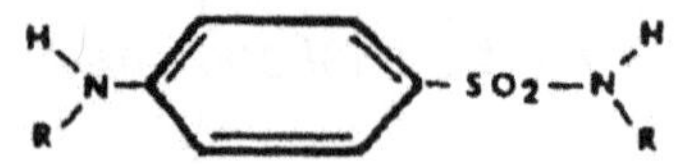

As we proceed from one specific sulfa to another, observe the very slight changes in this formula. In some, a hydrogen may replace the radical (R). In others, ring structures or aliphatic side chains may be the radical. Each of the sulfas, however, is very closely related to the rest.

(b) Important sulfonamides.

1. Sulfanilamide.

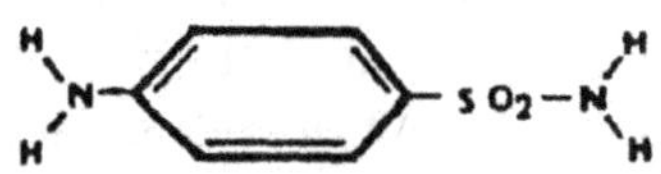

Learn the formula for sulfanilamide, for all the other sulfas are related to it. Although sulfanilamide itself has fallen into disuse in human medicine because of its toxicity, it is important as the parent compound of the other sulfonamides.

2. Sulfadiazine.

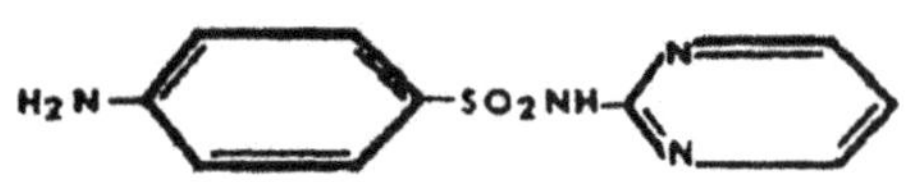

3. Sulfisoxazole.

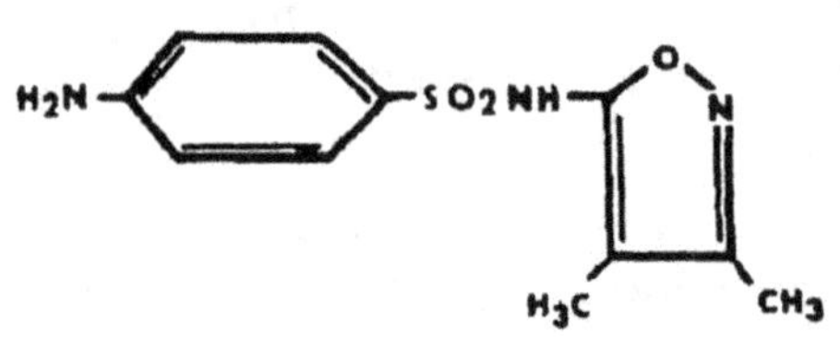

A big breakthrough in sulfonamide therapy came with the discovery of sulfisoxazole. It is safer than the others and is effective in urinary tract infections.

(c) Incompatibilities. Most of the incompatibilities encountered with the sulfa drugs are of an acid-base nature. Aqueous solutions of the sodium salts of sulfonamides have a pH between 9 and 10. They precipitate on exposure to air because they absorb CO_2. Sulfonamides are precipitated from solution by mineral acid salts of the local anesthetics (Procaine HCl, Tetracaine HCl), the sympathomimetic amines (cphedrine HCl), and by many other substances yielding an acid pH.

(2) Antimicrobial agents not related to the sulfonamides. Other than the nitrofurans, each member of this group is so widely different from the next that we will treat each member individually without any generalizations. Chapter 9 will give descriptions and actions of these agents.

(a) Isoniazid / isonicotinic acid hydrazide(INH)/.

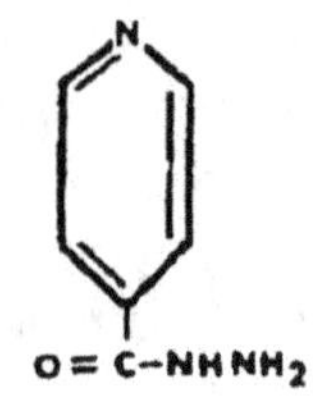

This potent and selective drug is a specific in the treatment of tuberculosis.

(b) Aminosalicylic acid [p-aminosalicylic acid (PAS)].

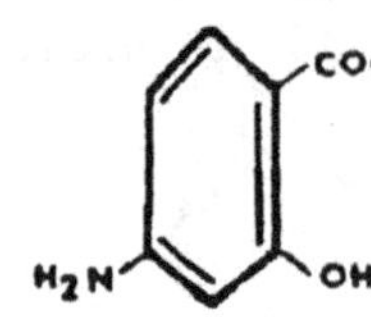

PAS is another antibacterial with selective action against the tubercle bacillus. When used alone, it is not as effective as either isoniazid or streptomycin.

(c) Methenamine mandelate (Mandelamine).

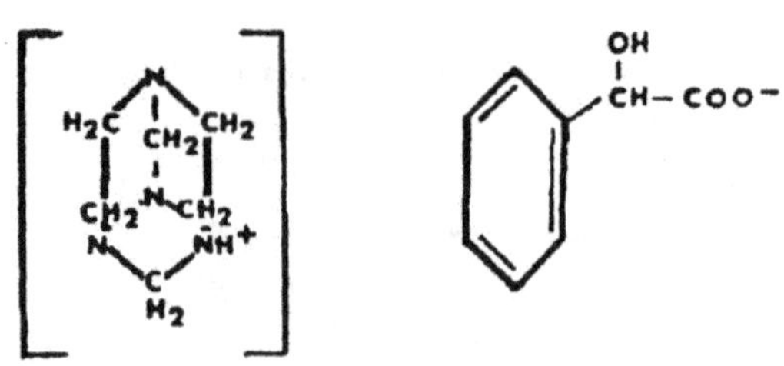

Methenamine is a urinary antiseptic. Because methenamine is effective in an acid pH (6 or below), it is generally administered in combination with mandelic acid or sodium acid phosphate. Thus methenamine mandelate is an efficient combination.

(d) Nitrofurans.

1. Nitrofurazono (Furacin).

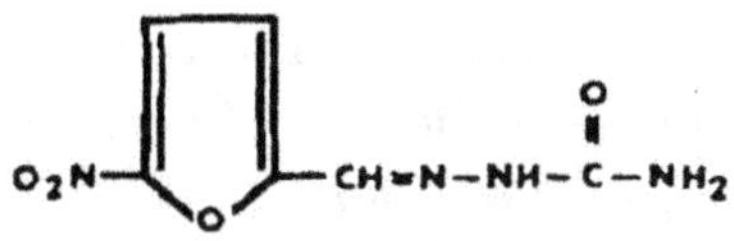

Nitrofurazone is a *local* antibacterial agent applied in the form of solutions or ointments.

2. *Furazolidone (Furoxone).*

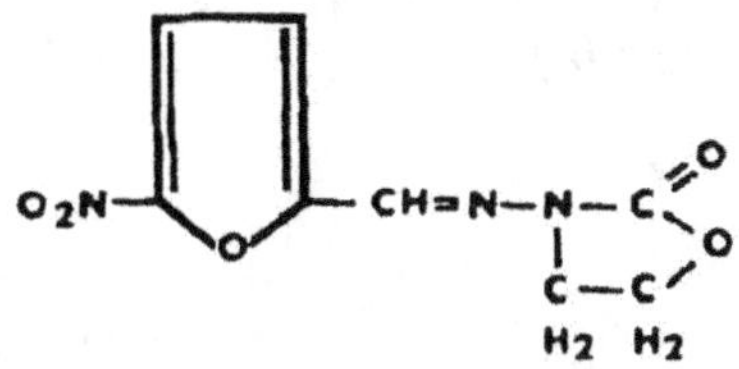

Furazolidone is an anti-infective agent employed for local activity in the intestinal tract and vagina.

3. *Nitrofurantoin (Furadantin, Macrodantin).*

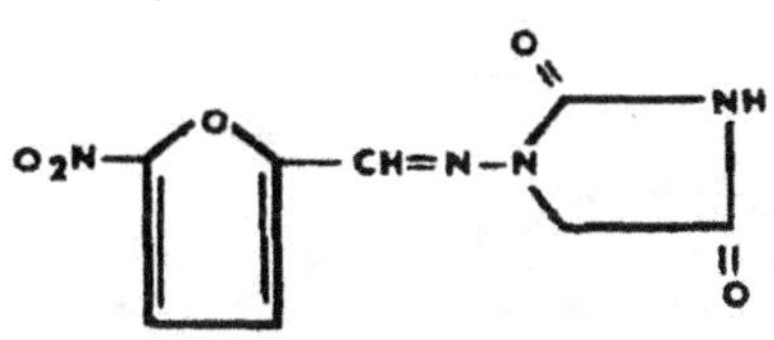

Nitrofurantoin is an anti-infective which is generally limited in therapeutic usage to infections of the urinary tract.

f. Antihistamines. Generally speaking, all the antihistamines are alike in action, differing only in potency and dosage. A few, however, have antinauseant properties, and may be agents of choice for motion sickness. A more detailed discussion of the antihistamines is covered in chapter 9. The most widely used antihistamine preparations are-

(1) Diphenhydramine hydrochloride (Benadryl HCl).

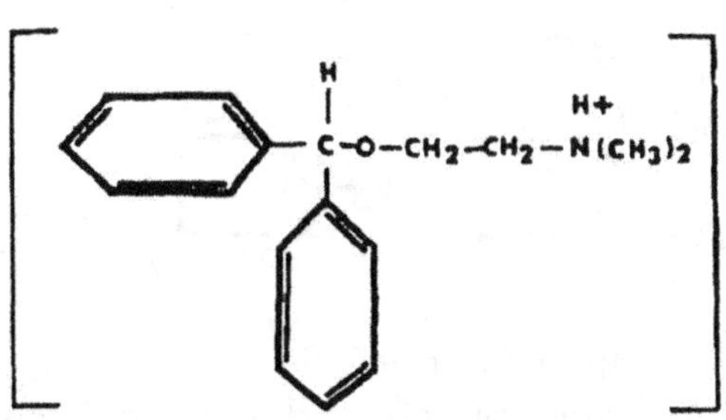

Diphenhydramine hydrochloride is a general antihistamine.

(2) Tripelennamine hydrochloride [Pyribenzamine HCl (PBZ)].

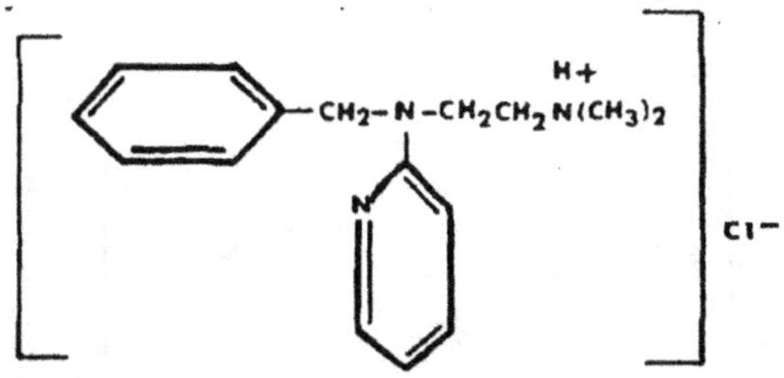

Tripelennamine is a general antihistamine.

(3) Chlorpheniramine maleate (Chlor-Trimeton maleate; Teldrin).

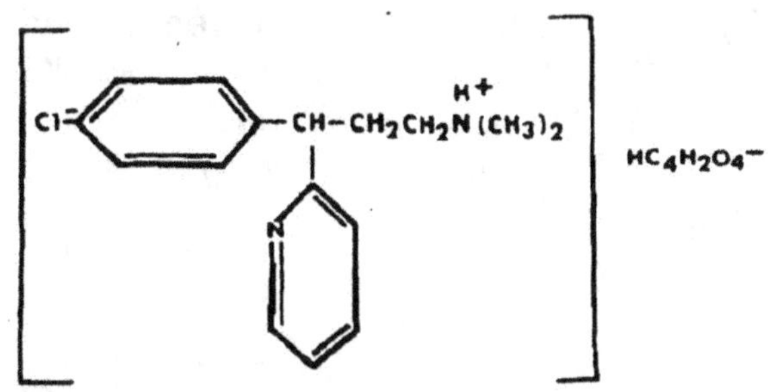

Chlorpheniramine maleate is a general antihistamine.

(4) Promethazine hydrochloride (Phenergan).

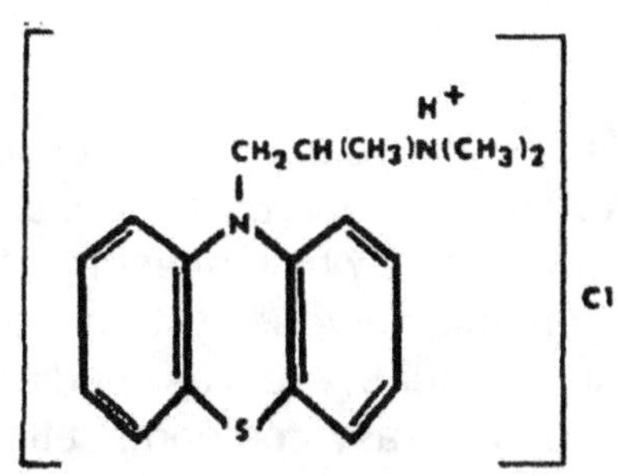

Promethazine is used as a general antihistamine and sedative in cough preparations.

(5) Dimenhydrinate (Dramamine).

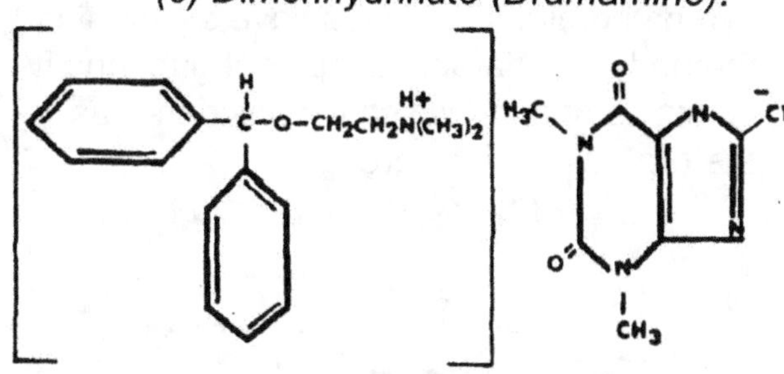

Dimenhydrinate is a combination of diphenhydramine(Benadryl) and 8-chlorotheophylline. Dimenhydrinate does not have very good antihistamine properties, but is antinauseant in action. It is mainly used for its antimotion sickness effects.

(6) Cyclizine hydrochloride (Marezine *HCl*).

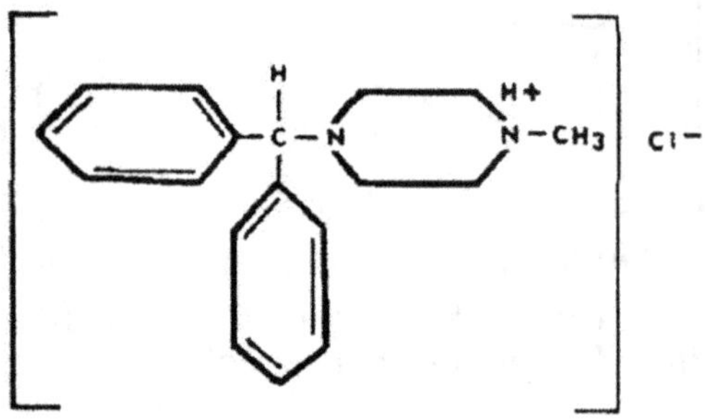

Cyclizine is effective in the prevention and relief of the dizziness, nausea, and vomiting associated with motion sickness.

(7) Meclizine hydrochloride (Bonine).

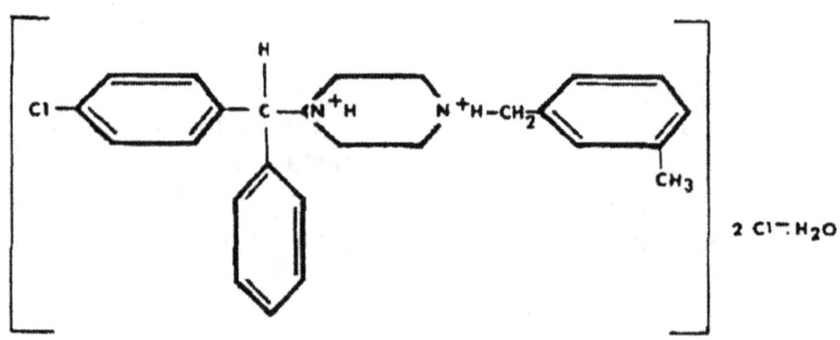

Meclizine is effective in motion sickness.

g. Autonomic nervous system amines and amides. Drugs which affect the action of the autonomic nervous system (covered in detail in chapter 9) are classified as sympathomimetic, parasympathomimetic, sympatholytic, or parasympatholytic, depending upon their action.

(1) Sympathomimetic amines. The sympathomimetic amines have actions in the body comparable to epinephrine, and it is this compound which is considered as the prototype of the group.

(a) Epinephrine (Adrenalin).

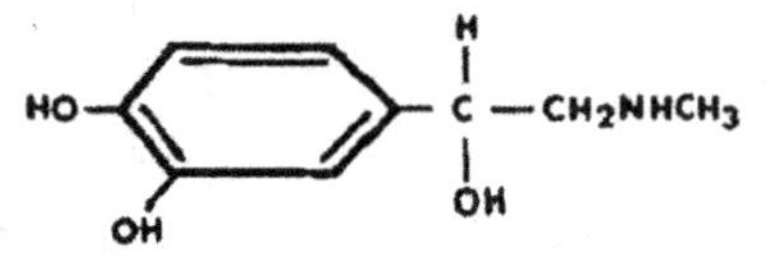

In the presence of oxidizing agents and sunlight, epinephrine decomposes, first turning pink and then showing a brown sediment. Preparations which are brown in color or contain a precipitate should not be used.

(b) Ephedrine.

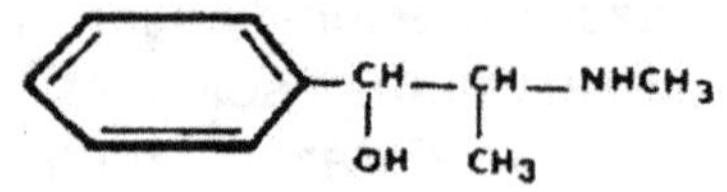

(c) Amphetamine sulfate (Benzedrine sulfate).

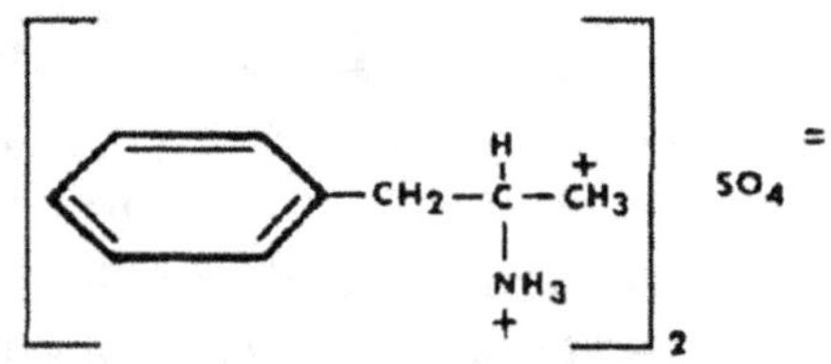

(d) Phenylephrine hydrochloride (Neo-Synephrine hydrochloride).

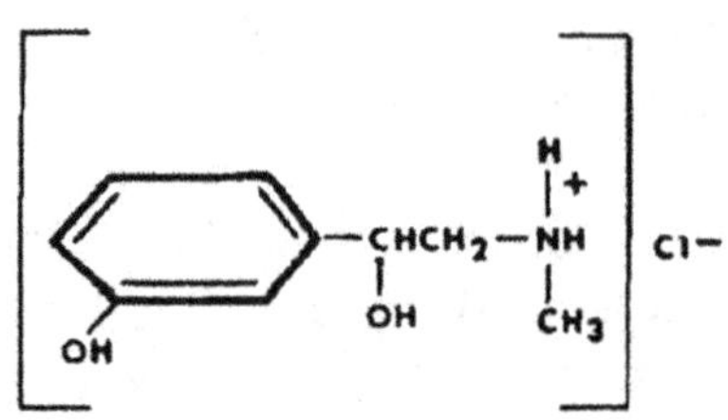

Phenylephrine is used as a decongestant in nose drops.

(e) Naphazoline hydrochloride (Privine HCl).

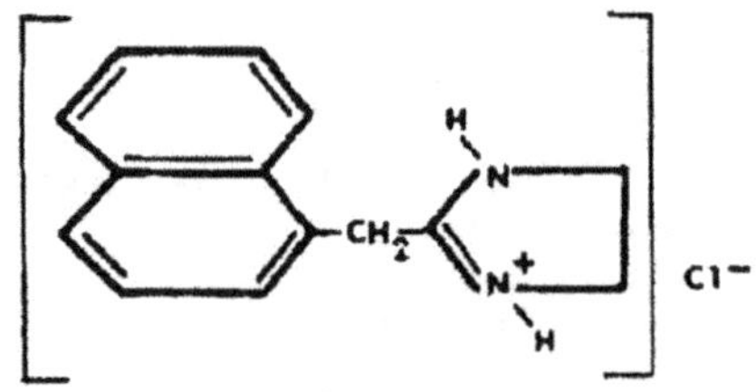

Although they differ greatly in structure, naphazoline, epinephrine, and phenylephrine have similar vasoconstrictor properties.

(2) Parasympathomimetic amines. Acetylcholine is the natural parasympathctic amine occurring in the body. Since it is almost immediately inactivated in the body by cholinesterase, it is of no therapeutic significance. Pilocarpine shares many of the actions of acetylcholine, as does bethanechol.

(a) Acetylcholine

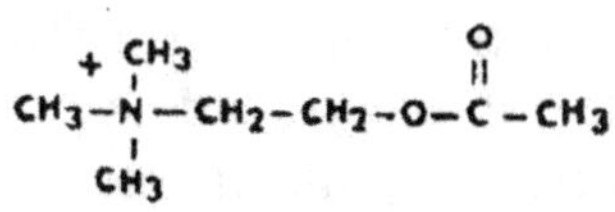

(b) Pilocarpine hydrochloride.

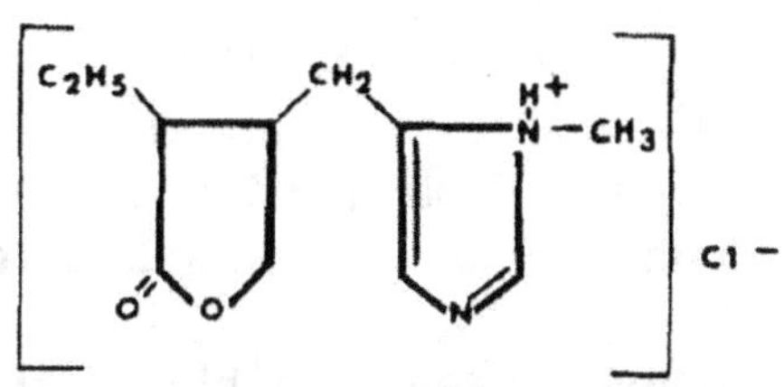

(c) Bethanechol chloride (Urecholine)

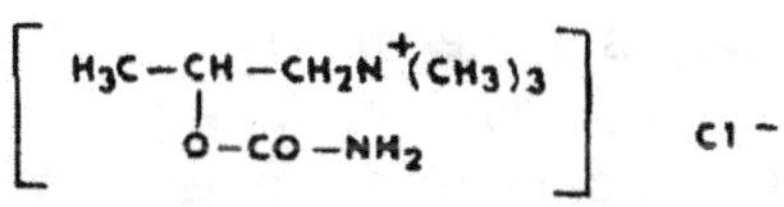

(3) Sympatholytic agents. The sympatholytic agents block the action of the sympathetic stimuli by their presence at the nerve receptor.

(a) Phenoxybenzamine hydrochloride (Dibenzyline HCl).

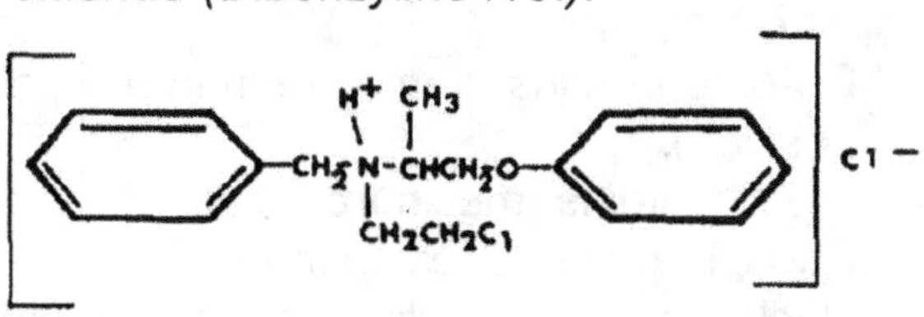

(b) Phentolamine hydrochloride (Regitine HCl).

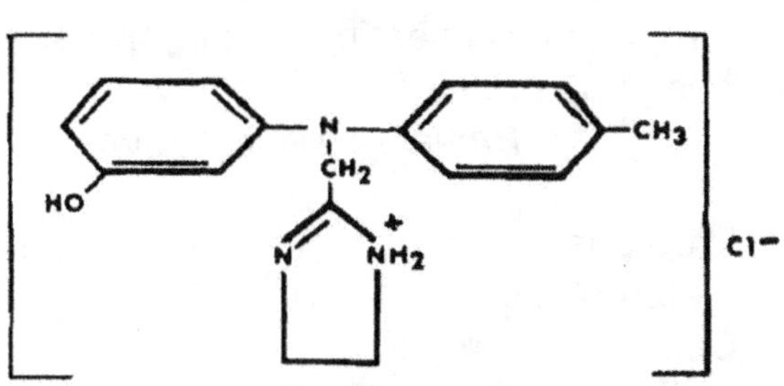

(4) Parasympatholytic agents. These agents cause actions opposite to the parasympathomimetic drugs previously discussed. The two prototypes are atropine and propantheline.

(a) Atropine.

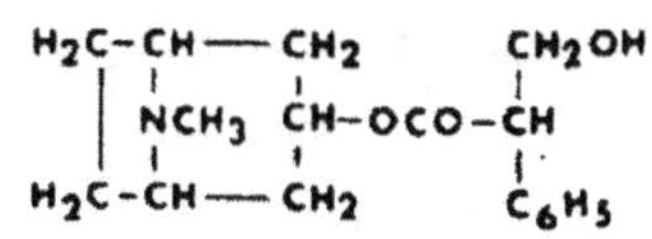

(b) Propantheline bromide (Pro-Banthine).

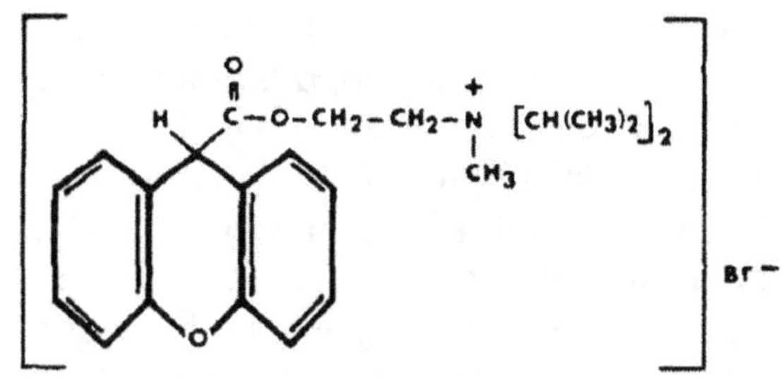

23. Amino acids, peptides, and proteins.

a. Amino acids. Amino acids are difunctional organic compounds containing an amino group and a carboxylic acid.

(1) General formula. The general formula for the amino acids is

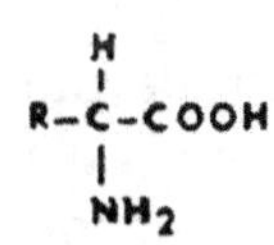

(2) Glycine. Glycine, the simplest of the amino acids, conforms to the general formula

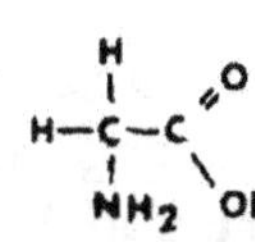

(3) Essential amino acids. Twenty-one different amino acids are found in the body and all are necessary for proper body function. Most amino acids can be manufactured in the body; however, ten are not. These amino acids must be included in the diet and are known as ìessential amino acids.î

Threonine	Phenylalanine
Methionine	Tryptophan
Lysine	Histidine
Arginine	Leucine
Valine	Isoleucine

b. Peptides. Two or more amino acids may combine to form a peptide and water.

During digestion, amino acids are liberated from complex protein structures and condense together to form polypeptides. The formula below shows a typical dipeptide with the molecule of water before it is eliminated.

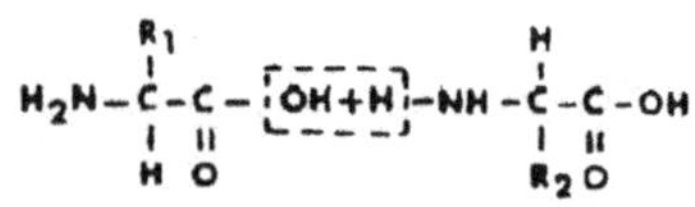

c. Proteins. Proteins are polymers of amino acids. They are important food substances. Proteins are extremely high molecular weight (10,000 to 1 million) polypeptides. In the following formula for a very small part of a protein molecule, you should be able to distinguish the individual amino acids making up the complex structure.

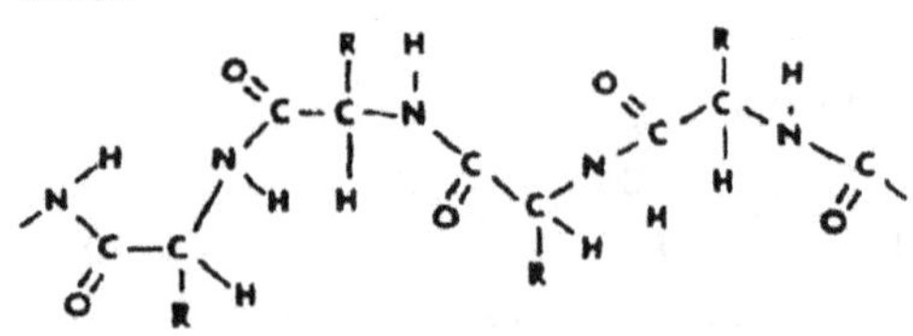

(1) Properties. Unlike many organic materials, particularly those of high molecular weight, a considerable number of the proteins are soluble in water and insoluble in the general organic solvents. All proteins contain carbon, hydrogen, oxygen, and nitrogen; many contain sulfur and phosphorus.

(2) Precipitation and salting-out. Precipitation and salting-out are similar in that both result in a substance coming out of the solution. Salting-out, however, is a particular kind of precipitation in which the substance is thrown out of solution because another has been dissolved. Protein precipitants and substances causing salting-out include alcohol, acetone, neutral salts, heavy metal salts, and some acids. In some instances, addition of excess solvent will cause a redissolution of the protein; in other instances, the precipitation is not reversible.

(3) Coagulation. Irreversible precipitation of proteins is known as coagulation. This reaction is preceded by denaturation in which some of the bonds of the protein are ruptured, forming an insoluable substance. We have previously described the coagulation of proteins in inorganic chemistry with the experiment of a heavy metal salt introduced into egg white. Frying or boiling an egg demonstrates the effect of heat on proteins.

(4) Classification. The classification of proteins is based upon their solubility and upon the results of their hydrolysis. Proteins cannot be isolated as pure individual compounds with distinct properties, so a really satisfactory chemical classification is impossible.

(a) Simple proteins. These are the proteins which yield only alpha amino acids or derivatives of alpha amino acids when broken down into simpler compounds. In this class fall:

- Albumins (egg albumin, blood serum albumin).
- Globulins (serum globulin of blood).
- Glutelins (glutenin in wheat). Prolamines (gliadin from wheat).
- Albuminoids (elastin in tendons; keratin in hair; collagen in connective tissue).
- Histones (histone from the thymus gland).
- Protamines (salmin in salmon sperm).

(b) Conjugated pro teins. These are combinations of simple proteins and other nonprotein groups.

- Chromoproteins (hemoglobin in red corpuscles).
- Glycoproteins (mucin from saliva).
- Phosphoproteins (casin in milk).
- Nucleoproteins (nuclein from cell nuclei).
- Lipoproteins (lecithin + protein).

(c) Derived proteins. These are proteins produced by chemical action on naturally occurring proteins.

1. Primary protein derivatives:

- Proteans.
- Metaproteins.
- Coagulated proteins.

2. Secondary protein derivatives:

- Proteoses.
- Peptones.

- Peptides.

(5) The importance of proteins. Proteins supply the specific amino acids important to life and health which cannot be manufactured in the body. They are essential to growth and repair of tissues. Industrially, proteins are used in the manufacture and processing of leather, gelatin, glue, ice cream, cheese, textiles, and plastics.

(6) Pharmaceutically important amino acids and proteins.

(a) Fibrinogen (Human Fibrinogen) is a blood plasma clotting factor.

(b) Gelatin, obtained from the skin, connective tissue, and bones of animals, is a pharmaceutical necessity for capsules, emulsions, and suppositories, as well as a nutritive substance.

(c) Gelfoam, a sterile, pliable, nonantigenic surgical sponge prepared from gelatin. is used by itself or saturated with thrombin, as a hemostat.

(d) Glutamic acid hydrochloride is a gastric acidifier which is used in conditions where insufficient or no acid is naturally secreted, as in the achlorhydria of pernicious anemia.

(e) Infant formulas. The prepared liquid and powdered formulas used for feeding infants during their first few months of life are mainly protein portions of milk.

(f) Methionine (Meonine) is a sulfur-containing amino acid used in the prevention and treatment of liver damage.

(g) Protamine sulfate is an antidote for an overdose of heparin (an anticoagulant).

(h) Protein hydrolysates are solutions of amino acids and short chain peptides. They are used as nutritive agents where oral intake of proteins is limited. They are generally administered IV and only in severely ill patients.

(i) Others. Many other official products contain proteins but are placed in their more specific categories. Such compounds are enzymes, some hormones, biologicals, surgical sutures, and mild silver protein.

24. Volatile oils. The volatile or essential oils are found in various plant organs and tissues. Generally, they are the odorous and taste-bearing principles of the plants in which they occur. Volatile oils may contain hydrocarbons, alcohols, acids, esters, aldehydes, ketones, phenols, lactones, nitrogen compounds, and sulfur compounds.

a. Properties. Volatile oils differ widely in taste, smell, composition, density, and boiling range.

- Pure oils are colorless, becoming varicolored on exposure to air.
- The most distinctive property of the individual oil is its odor.
- The taste of volatile oils varies from sweet to mild, pungent, hot, acrid, caustic, or burning.
- The majority of the volatile oils are lighter than water; their specific gravity varies from about 0.8 to 1.17.
- Most of the oils are optically active (dextro or levorotatory).
- Most oils are not water soluble, but on contact with water they dramatically flavor and scent it. They are soluble in alcohol, ether, chloroform, oils, fats, and resins.
- Because of their volatility, these oils should be stored in well-filled, tightly stoppered amber bottles, away from light and heat.

b. Preparation. Volatile oils are generally obtained from plants through distillation, steam distillation, expression, or extraction. These four processes are explained in chapter 6.

c. Important pharmaceutical volatile oils and preparations.

(1) Oils used almost exclusively for their flavoring ability are

- Lavender oil
- Peppermint oil
- Spearmint oil
- Cinnamon oil
- Rose oil
- Lemon oil
- Orange oil
- Anise oil

- Sassafras oil
- Cherry juice
- Raspberry juice
- Caraway oil
- Fennel oil
- Cardamon oil

(2) Other oils. Other oils are used as carminatives, germicides, diuretics, perfumes, condiments, stimulants (local), astringents, preservatives, antiseptics, toothache drops, expectorants, and inhalants for bronchial infections.

25. Carbohydrates. We have discussed in the preceding parts of this chapter two types of food substances, the fats and oils, and the proteins. The third food substance, the carbohydrates, is at least as important as the others.

a. Composition. Chemically, the carbohydrates are polyhydroxy aldehydes or ketones, or organic compounds which on hydrolysis yield polyhydroxyaldehydes or ketones. They are definite chemical compounds, not merely hydrated forms of carbon. Widely distributed in nature, they are obtained from the plant kingdom and used by the animal kingdom.

b. Classification. The diagrammatic breakdown of the carbohydrate class of compounds shown in figure 1 will be helpful to you in understanding the relative position of the various subclasses involved. The diagrammatic breakdown of the carbohydrate family illustrates that it is subdivided first into two broad categories, the sugars and the nonsugars. The sugars are sweet and water soluble.

(1) Monosaccharides. Within the subclass of sugars is a group which contains three

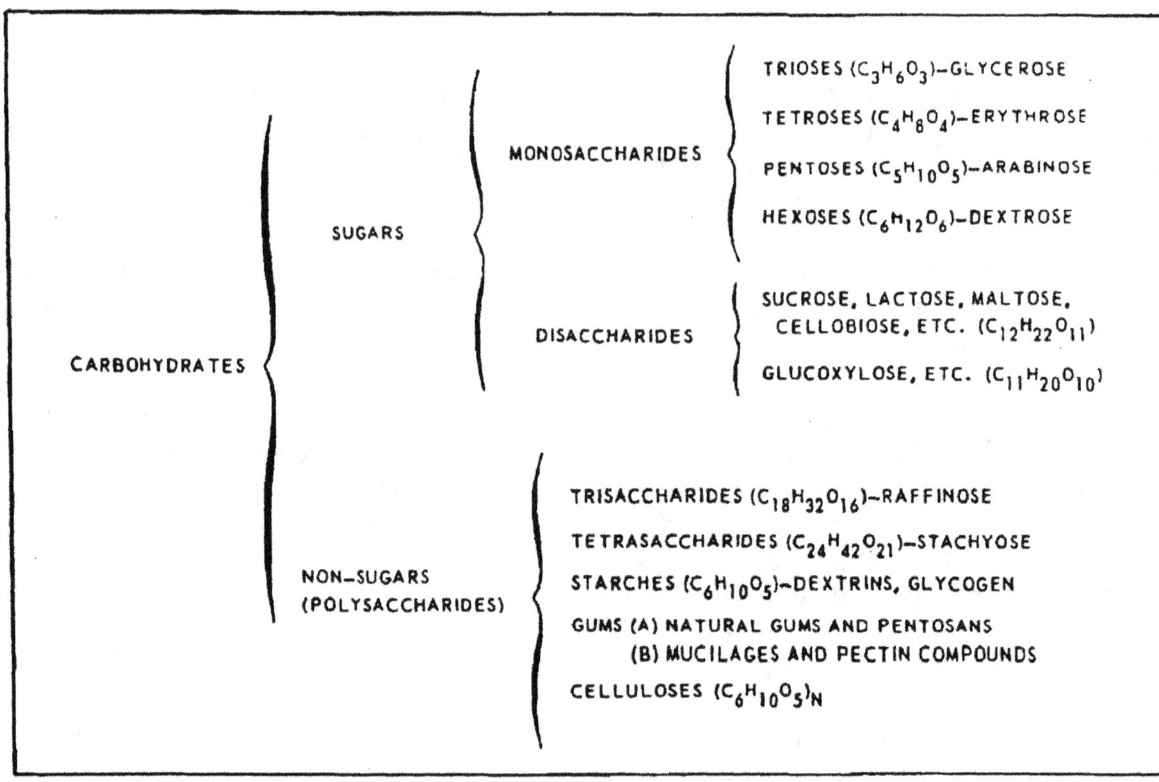

Figure 1. Diagrammatic breakdown of the carbohydrates.

or more carbons and cannot be hydrolyzed. These are the monosaccharides. These sugars are naturally occurring.

(2) Disaccharides. Sugars which are made up of two molecules of monosaccnarides are called disaccharides. Upon hydrolysis, these disaccharides are broken down into the two separate monosaccnarides of which they are composed.

(3) Polysaccharides. The more complex carbohydrates, which on hydrolysis are broken down into three, four, or more monosaccharide units, are the polysaccharides.

c. Stereoisomerism. Stereoisomerism is a long and complex idea involving many different types of isomers. It will serve our purposes adequately to explain that Stereoisomerism is due to spatial rather than structural arrangement and that the two most common forms of Stereoisomerism are geometric and optical.

(1). Geometric isomerism. Isomers are formed because some factor, such as double bond, prevents free rotation of the atoms within the molecule. The isomers formed by geometric isomerism are termed cis- and trans- and the difference is shown below in the diagrams of the two geometric forms of butenedioic acid.

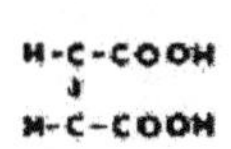

cis-form

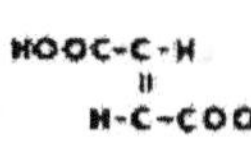

trans-form

The double bond illustrated holds the atoms from rotating, and thus there are two distinctly different geometric possibilities.

(2) Optical isomerism. In optical isomerism, the isomers differ in their ability to rotate polarized light, due to asymmetrical structure or crystalline structure.

(a) Asymmetric atom. An asymmetric atom (in our study it will always be a carbon atom) is one which has four different atoms or radicals attached to it. Glyceraldehyde has one asymmetric carbon atom. This carbon has attached to it a hydrogen, a hydroxyl group, an aldehyde group, and an alcohol group.

(b) Minor images. Hold your hands up in front of you with the palms turned in. What you see are two identical five-fingered extremities. They are identical in every respect except that they are mirror images of each other. The isomers formed in optical isomerism are similarly mirror images of each other.

(c) Polarized light. A film or crystal that allows only light vibrating in one direction to pass is a polarizer. The lenses of Polaroid sunglasses are an example. Light vibrating in every direction approaches the lens, but only light vibrating in one plane passes; the remainder is stopped by the lens. A second polarizer placed crosswise to the first will exclude the light passed by the first. The illustration in figure 2 shows light being polarized.

(d) Optical rotation. When polarized light is passed through a solution of an optically active substance, it will be diverted either to the left or to the right. A substance which rotates the light to the right is called the dextro (d-) or (+) isomer. That which rotates the light to the left is the levo- (1-) or (-) isomer. A mixture of 50 percent each of the d- and l-isomers will produce no rotation. Such a mixture is called a racemic mixture.

(e) Enantiomorphs. Looking again at glyceraldehyde, you see that there are two optical isomers, each the mirror image of the other. Such isomers are called enantiomorphs (from the Greek meaning ìopposite formî).

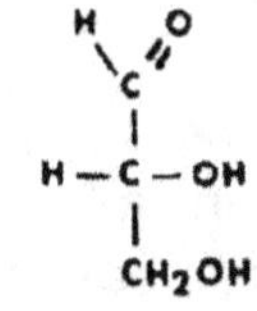

d-glyceraldehyde

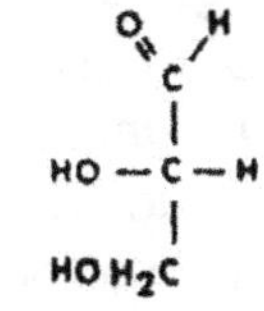

l-glyceraldehyde

(f) Nomenclature. In naming optical isomers, we wish to know two things: the spatial arrangement of the

atoms (configuration) and the direction of optical rotation. If the OH group nearest the end opposite the carbonyl group is on the right, it has the D configuration. If on the left, it has the L configuration.

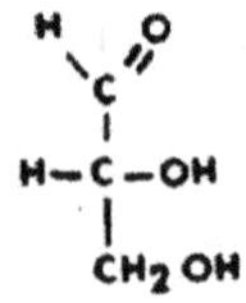

Glyceraldehyde

d. Monosaccharides. The simplest carbohydrates are the monosaccharides. They cannot be broken down by hydrolysis. Monosaccharides are classified according to the number of carbon atoms they contain. If a monosaccharide contains five carbon atoms it is known as a pentose; one containing six carbons is a hexose. These are the most common types of monosaccharides. Carbohydrates are further classified as aldoses or ketoses to indicate whether they are aldehydes or ketones.

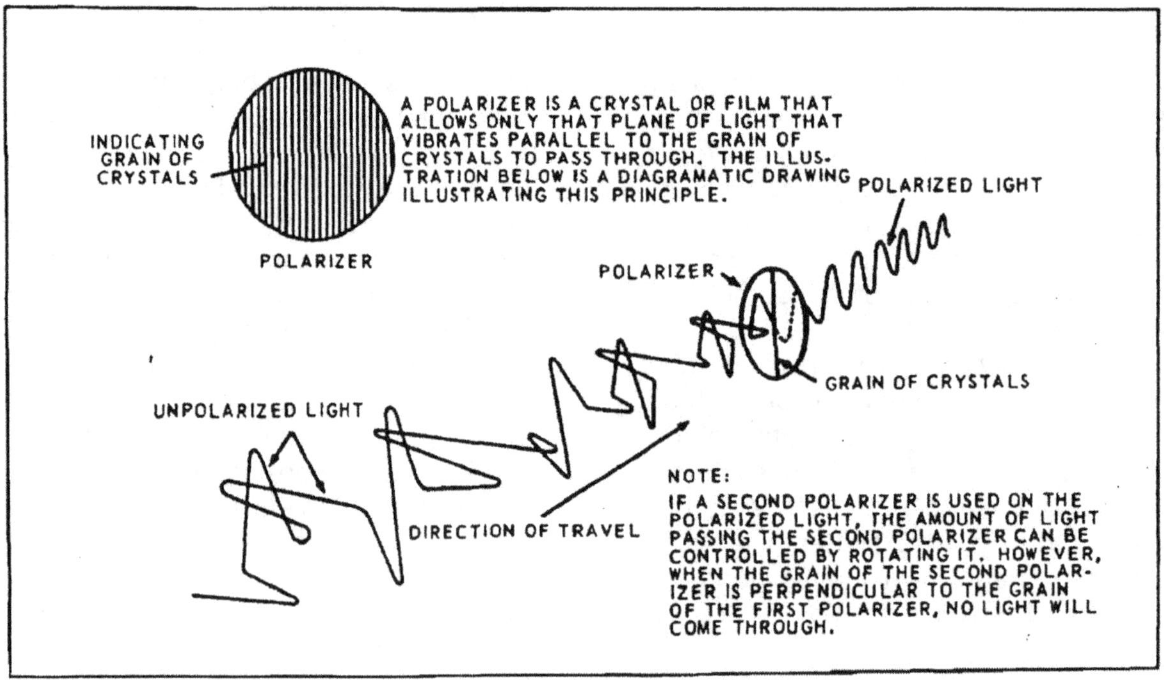

Figure 2. principle of polarization.

Under this system, the compound above becomes D-(+) glyceraldehyde. The OH on the carbon farthest from the carbonyl group is on the right side, thus the D-. By experiment, this compound is found to rotate the light to the right, thus the (+). If the compound were to rotate the light to the left, it would have been called D-(-) glyceraldehyde.

(g) Number of enantiomorphs. Each asymmetric carbon atom can yield two enantiomorphs, and as the number of asymmetric carbons increases, the number of isomers increases. The possible number of enantiomorphs for a compound is 2^x, in which the x stands for the number of asymmetrical carbons.

The most common monosaccharide, glucose, is an aldohexose, a six-carbon sugar containing an aldehyde group.

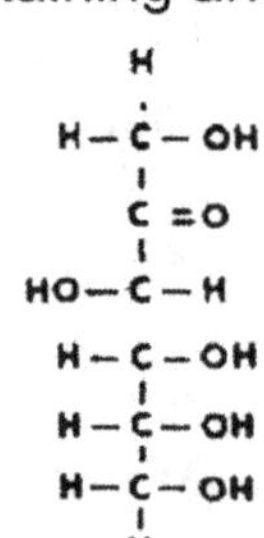

D-Fructose, a ketohexose

(1) Glucose. In photosynthesis, plants take carbon dioxide and water, in the presence of sunlight, and manufacture glucose. As a byproduct of this reaction, oxygen is liberated into the atmosphere.

Energy + $6CO_2$ + $6H_2 OC_6 H_{12}O_6$ + $6O_2$ ↑
In man and animals, the reverse takes place; glucose is broken down into carbon dioxide and water, and in the process usable energy is liberated.

(a) Formula.

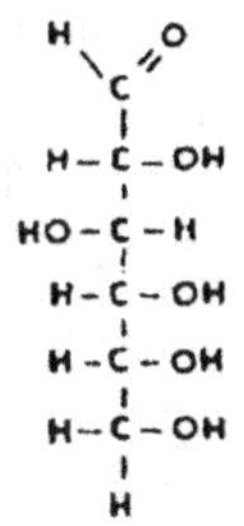

D (+) Glucose

(b) Occurrence and preparation. Glucose, which is also known as dextrose, is widely distributed in nature, and made commercially by the breakdown of starch. It is the carbohydrate used by the body tissues and is the sugar most commonly found in blood and other body fluid. In sugar diabetes (diabetes mellitus), it is dextrose that appears in large quantities in the blood and urine.

(c) Uses. Glucose is used as a food substance and a sweetening agent. Patients who, for one reason or another, cannot be fed by the normal oral route are given intravenous feedings of sterile glucose solution.

(d) Preparations.

- Dextrose (D-glucose; grape sugar) a sweetish granular crystalline substance, is the principal source of energy in the human body. It is stored in the liver in the form of glycogen. Dextrose may be either hydrous or anhydrous; the containerís label must specify the type.
- Dextrose injection is a sterile solution of dextrose intended for intravenous administration. It may be used, depending upon the purpose, in concentrations ranging from 5 to 50 percent. The 5-percent solution is isotonic with the blood and is intended as a blood volume replenisher. Higher concentrations are intended as nutrients and diuretics. Bacteriostatic agents are not allowed in this preparation because it is given in large quantities which could provide the patient with excessive doses of the bacteriostatic agent at the same time. Because of the absence of any bacteriostatic agent, this preparation must be meticulously sterilized and that portion which is not immediately used when the container is opened should be discarded. Units showing any sign of turbidity should not be used.
- Dextrose and sodium chloride injection is a nutrient and fluid and electrolyte replenisher.

(2) Fructose (levulose).

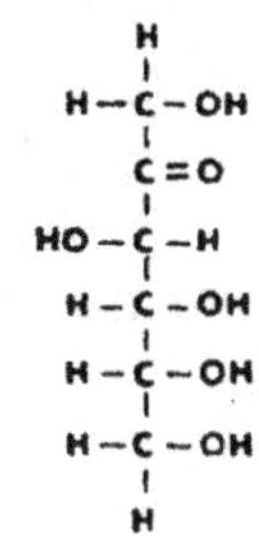

Fructose is a monosaccharide and the only official ketone sugar. It is levorotatory.

(a) Occurrence. Fructose occurs naturally, chemically united with glucose in our common table sugar and in honey. It is the sweetest sugar known.

(b) Uses. Fructose is commonly employed as a nutrient and sweetening agent.

(c) Preparations.

- Fructose injection is used as a parenteral nutrient, as it is more rapidly metabolized than dextrose. Fructose can be injected in concentrations twice as strong as dextrose without ill effects. It is especially useful in nutrition pr hydration of diabetics as they can tolerate fructose almost normally.
- Fructose and sodium chloride injection is used either as a nutrient or as an electrolyte replenisher for patients in bad states of nutrition.

e. Disaccharides. Chemically, disaccharides are ìdouble sugars,î that is, two molecules of monosaccharides linked chemically.

(1) Sucrose (saccharum; sugar: cane sugar; beet sugar). Sucrose is a combination of the monosaccharide units, glucose and fructose. It is commercially

obtained from sugar cane, sugar beet, and sorghum. Upon hydrolysis, sucrose yields a mixture of glucose and fructose; the combination is frequently referred to as invert sugar. Invert sugar is sweeter, more easily digested, and more rapidly assimilated than sucrose. Sucrose is a nutrient and is subject to contamination by molds and bacteria. In very high concentrations, as in syrup, the osmotic pressure is so high that it acts as bactericide by dehydrating the organisms which it contacts. Pharmaceutically, sucrose is of major importance in the preparation of syrup which is an 85-percent solution of sugar in water. Syrup is used as a sweet vehicle.

(3) Relative sweetness. In discussing the sugars, we have indicated that they vary in sweetness. It may be interesting for you to note the relative sweetness of some of the sugars. The formulation below shows the relative sweetness of several of the sugars compared to sucrose, which has been given the arbitrary value of 100.

Fructose.. 173
Invert sugar................................ 123
Sucrose 100
Glucose 74
Maltose... 32
Galactose 32
Lactose... 16

Glucose Portion

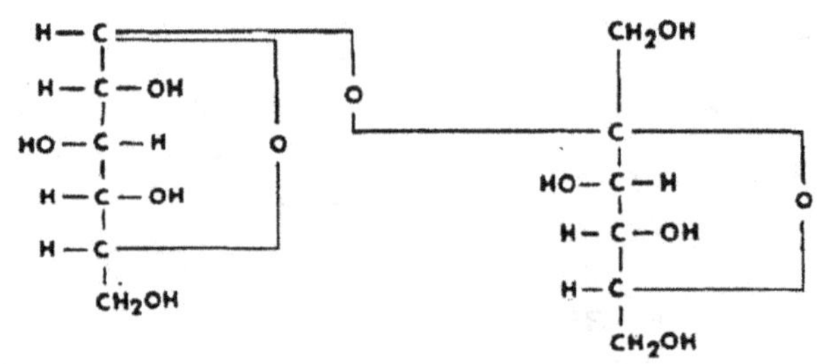

Fructose Portion

(2) Lactose (saccharum lactis; milk sugar). Lactose is the disaccharide most commonly found in both human and cow's milk and is commonly called milk sugar. Upon hydrolysis it breaks down into the two monosaccharides, glucose and galactose. Though not as sweet tasting as some of the other sugars, lactose is easily digested and is a common ingredient in baby formulas. Milk sugar is used in pharmacy as a diluting agent in most capsules, tablets, and hypodermic tablets. Specially refined, beta-lactose is more soluble than ordinary lactose and is preferred, especially for the hypodermic tablets. Lactose is often an ingredient in the nutrient medium used in the culture of the *Penicillium notatum* organism.

f. Polysaccharides. At the beginning of our discussion of the carbohydrate family, we subdivided carbohydrates into sugars and nonsugars; the sugars were further subdivided into monosaccharides and disaccharides, which we have already discussed. The nonsugars, or polysaccharides, are actually broken down into starches, gums, and celluloses. Rather than going into discussion of the nonsugars by class, we will merely mention and state some facts about the more important substances and agents which will fall into this category of nonsugars.

(1) Starch (amylum; corn starch):

(a) Occurrence. Starch is naturally occurring in plants such as corn, potatoes, rice. tapioca, and wheat. Plants store

Glucose Portion 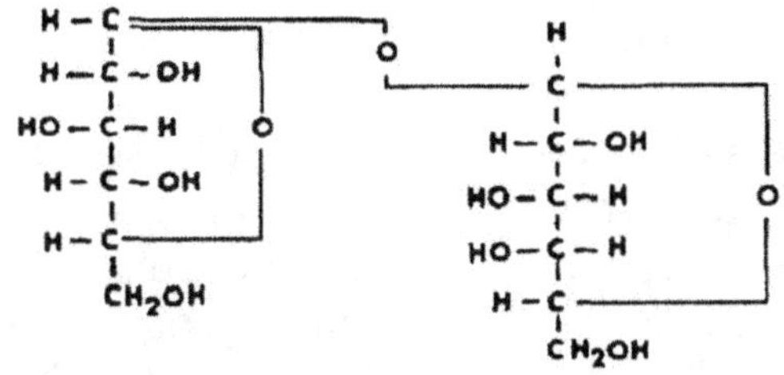 Galactose Portion

starch for the same reason animals store glycogen, that is, as a reserve source of energy. Glycogen is often called animal starch. Starch occurs as small granules which, under microscope, reveal a very distinct shape which varies with the source from which it is obtained.

(b) Properties. Starch is not soluble in cold water, but in boiling water it forms a milky solution or paste. When heated alone, starch breaks down into gummy dextrins. In theironing of clothes treated with starch, the dextrins formed give the material a stiff, shiny finish. Dextrins in water solution are used as adhesives. Iodine is a test for starch, yielding a bright blue color.

(c) Uses. Starch is categorized as a pharmaceutical necessity and is an ingredient in many official preparations. It is a good absorbent, filling agent, dusting powder, and tablet disintegrator. On contact with the liquids in the stomach, the starch grains absorb the moisture, swell, and physically disintegrate the tablet.

(2) Cotton. Cotton is a complex polysaccharide of natural origin. It is not soluble or digestible, and is of no food value. It is the most widely used surgical absorbent. It is official in the USP and must meet very specific requirements. Official cotton must be free of impurities, have no fatty matter, must be bleached white, and be sterilized in its final container. It must meet strenuous standards for fiber length, and water absorbability. There are specific instructions for its storage and labeling.

(3) Acacia (gum arable). Acacia may be in the form of flakes or powder and is used in the pharmacy as a suspending or emulsifying agent and as a demulcent. Acacia is soluble in water, producing a colloidal solution known as a mucilage. Such solutions are incompatible with high alcoholic solutions and other organic solvents.

(4) Pectin. Pectin is a purified carbohydrate from citrus fruit and apple pulp. It is a coarse or fine powder and slightly yellowish in color. It dissolves in about 20 times its weight in water and forms a thick colloidal solution. Pectin is not digested in the human alimentary canal and forms a thick protective coating on the intestinal wall. In combination with kaolin, it is usually efficacious in symptomatic treatment of diarrhea. Pectin is used commercially as a jelling agent in making jellies and has further pharmaceutical application as an emulsion stabilizer.

(5) Agar (agar-agar). Agar, when dissolved in water, forms a gel which can absorb five or more times its weight of water. The gel is used as a culture medium for bacteria and as a stabilizer in emulsions.

(6) Tragacanth. Tragacanth absorbs water and swells to form a soft adhesive mucilage which is used in the base for sterile lubricants and nasal jellies. It is also used as an adhesive in pills and troches; as a suspending agent; as an adjuvant to emulsifiers to retard creaming and to increase consistency; and as a soothing application or demulcent.

(7) Plantago seed (psyllium seed). Plantago seed is indigestible and mucilaginous and acts as a mild cathartic. Metamucil makes use of the actions of the plantugo seed.

(8) Methylcellulose (Methocel). Methylcellulose, a neutral, odorless, tasteless, and inert substance, is a synthetic substitute for gums and mucilages. It is used as a dispersing, thickening, emulsify-

ing, and coating agent, and as a bulk laxative. It is used in eye drops, nose drops, creams, lotions, burn preparations, and in cosmetics and dentifrices. Tablets of methylcellulose taken internally with water produce a normal, non-straining bowel evacuation for chronic constipation. Its bulking ability is also of value in satisfying the empty feeling of diet patients.

26. Glycosides. Glycosides are organic compounds consisting of a combination of sugars with nonsugar molecules. The pharmaceutically important glycosides are naturally occurring in plants and are only rarely found in animals.

a. Structure. Upon hydrolysis, the glycosides break down into one or more sugar molecules and one or more nonsugar molecules. The nonsugar portion is termed the aglycone. The most commonly occurring sugar found in glycoside molecules is glucose, and those compounds containing glucose are called glucosides. Glycosides, including glucosides, may be alpha or beta, and as shown in the graphic formulas below, the alpha form is that in which the OR group (OCH_3 in this case) is on the same side as the OH of the second carbon atom.

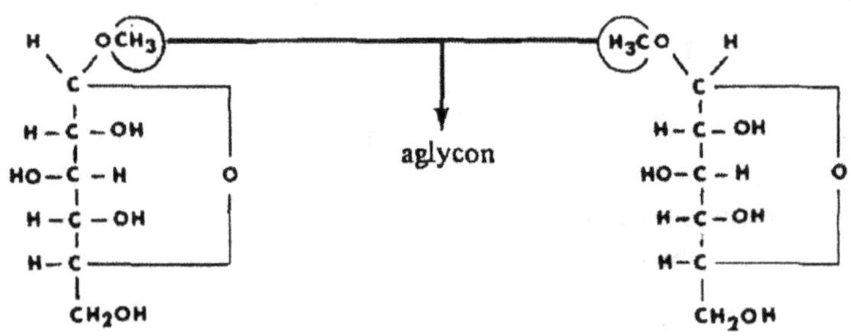

a–Methylglucoside *β–Methylglucoside*

b. Properties. Generally, the glycosides are colorless or white, optically active, alcohol or dilute-alcohol soluble extracts. They may be classified by a number of methods, based upon chemical grouping, occurrence, or therapeutic application.

c. Classes of glycosides. The two most important classes of glycosides, pharmaceutically, are the cardiac and the cathartic glycosides.

(1) Cardiac glycosides. Often referred to as the digitaloid drugs, the cardiac glycosides are not all glycosides, nor are they all derived from digitalis. However, the aglycone portions of the molecules are all very similar chemically and the actions are almost identical except for the onset and duration of action. These medications strengthen the contraction of heart muscle and are sometimes called cardiotonic drugs. Their main application is in the treatment of congestive heart failure. Digitalis is the prototype of this class.

(a) Digitalis (foxglove; digitalis leaf). Digitalis is the dried leaf of *Digitalis purpurea.* It is biologically standardized, one USP unit being the smallest quantity necessary to kill a pigeon. One hundred mg. of the powder equals one unit. After exhaustive investigation, scientists agree that the most important constituents of digitalis are digitoxin, gitoxin, digoxin, and lanatoside C.

(b) Digitoxin (Crystodigin; Purodigin).

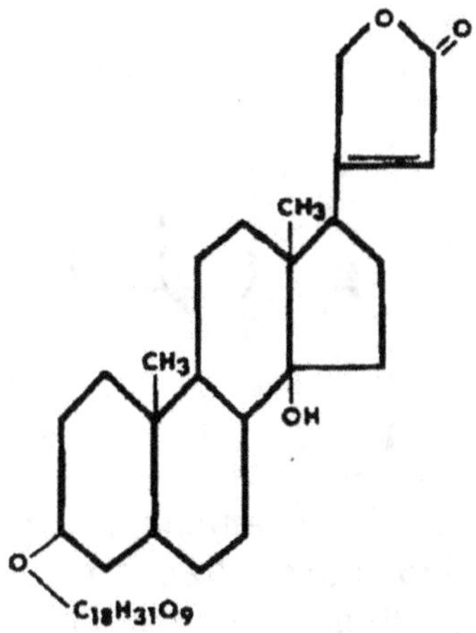

Digitoxin is the primary active glycoside in official digitalis and its action is similar to that of digitalis.

(c) Digoxin (Lanoxin).

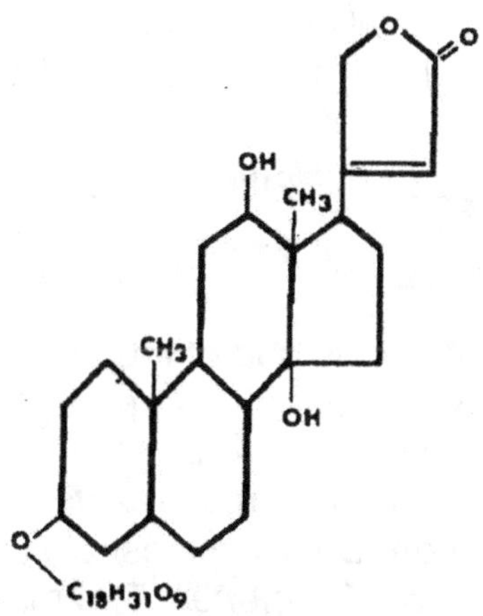

Digoxin is the cardiac glycoside from the leaves of *Digitalis lanata.* Its action, although of less duration, is similar to digitalis.

(d) Lanatoside C(Cedilanid).

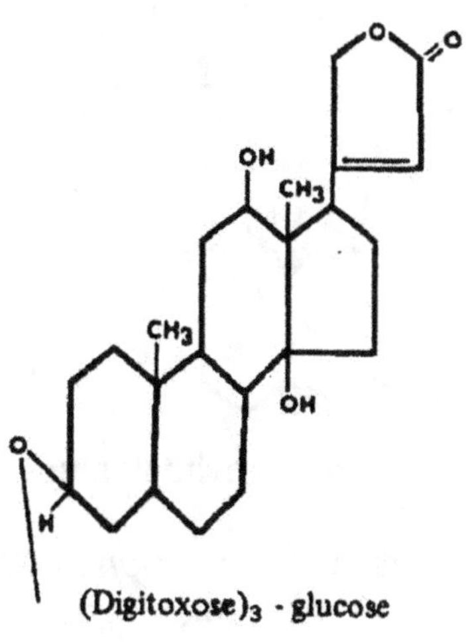

Lanatocide C is a cardiotonic glycoside from *Digitalis lanata.* As you can see, the aglycone is identical with that of digoxin.

(2) Cathartic glycosides. The cathartic glycosides or the anthroquinone purgatives, as they are sometimes called, are contained in such official drugs as cascara and senna. Upon ingestion, these drugs are assimilated in the GI tract, circulated through the blood stream, and are carried to the large intestine where, through their irritant action, they produce catharsis.

(a) Cascara sagrada.
(b) Senna (senna leaf).
(c) Danthron (Dorbane).

Danthron is a synthetic cathartic derived from anthraquinone.

27. Steroids. The steroids are a class of compounds found in both plants and animals with cyclopenta-phenanthrene as their basic structure. These include sterols, bile acids, sex hormones, adrenocortical hormones, and some miscellaneous substances.

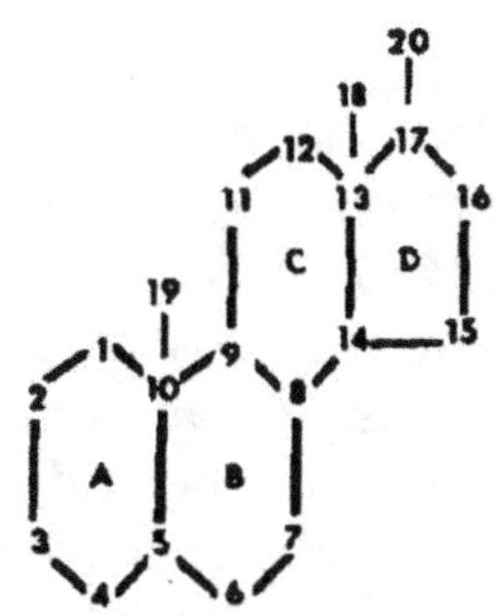

Perhydro-cyclopenta-phenanthrene

a. Sterols. The sterols have been previously mentioned in the discussion of fats, fixed oils, and waxes. Chemically, they have the cyclopenta-phenanthrene nucleus, with an aliphatic side chain at the 20 position, a CH_3 at the 18th and 19th carbon, and an alcohol (OH) group at the 3d carbon. They are secondary alcohols. The most important sterol is cholesterol (or cholesterin), a zoosterol. It is a component of gallstones and brain and spinal cords. The brain and spinal cords of animals are first saponified; the remaining unsaponifiable matter yields cholesterol. In recent years there has been much concern over the significance of cholesterol in the body and human diet. Normal human blood contains cholesterol in colloidal solution. If the concentration becomes too high, the cholesterol precipitates out of its colloidal solution and deposits on the walls of the arteries and heart to cause a type of sclerosis.

b. Bile salts. The bile salts are a group of very similar acids, the bile acids, chemically joined to glycine and taurine (amino acids). The parent compound of this group is cholic acid, shown below.

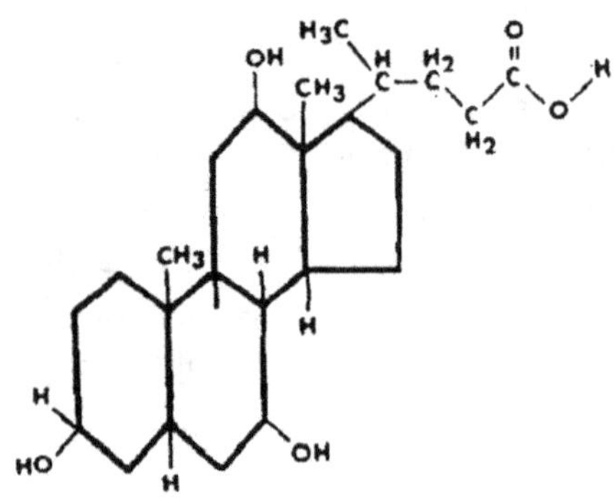

Bile salts emulsify the fats consumed in our diet and make them more readily reactive with the natural enzymes. The bile salts are necessary for the proper absorption of the fat-soluble vitamins. Dehydrocholic acid (Decholin) is the oxidation product of cholic acid. It causes an increase in biliary secretion when given in the form of a tablet, or the soluble salt (sodium dehydrocholate) by injection.

c. Sex hormones. Hormones are secreted by glands into the blood stream. They regulate other organs. The anterior lobe of the pituitary gland secretes a gonadotropic substance which causes the gonads to develop, both in the male and in the female. These glands, in response, manufacture and secrete their own hormones.

(1) Female hormones.

(a) Estradiol.

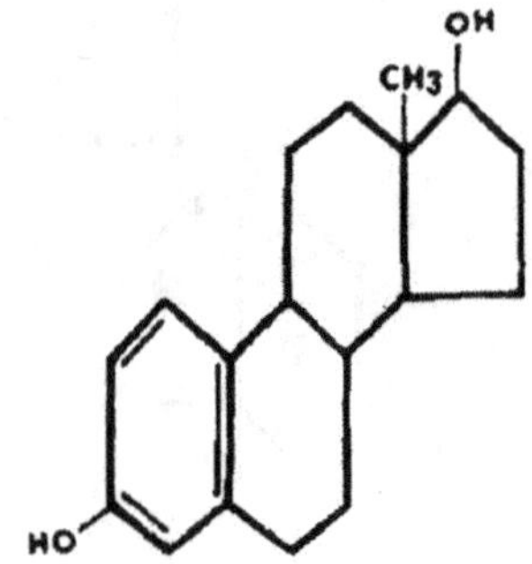

Estradiol is the basic female hormone. Notice that the A ring in this tetracyclic compound is aromatic and thus the OH group is a phenolic, rather than an alcohol group, giving the compound the stability and chemical reactivity of a phenol.

(b) Estrone. Estrone is closely related chemically to estradiol.

(c) Diethylstilbestrol (Stilbestrol).

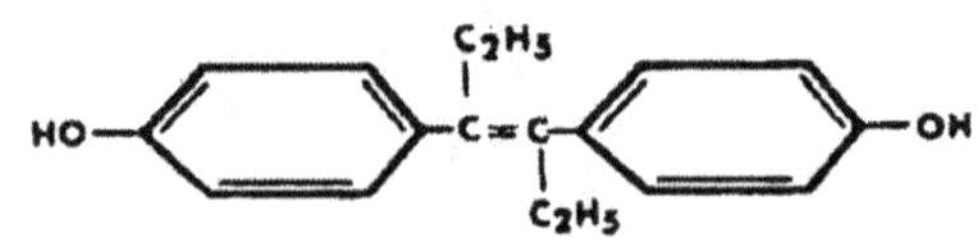

Diethylstilbestrol is one of the most popular and most widely used of preparations of this type. It is frequently used after childbirth to treat engorgement of the breasts and suppress lactation. Diethylstilbestrol is synthetic.

(2) Male hormones. The male hormones, called androgens, are also steroids. Testosterone is the basic hormone of this group of agents and is graphically represented below.

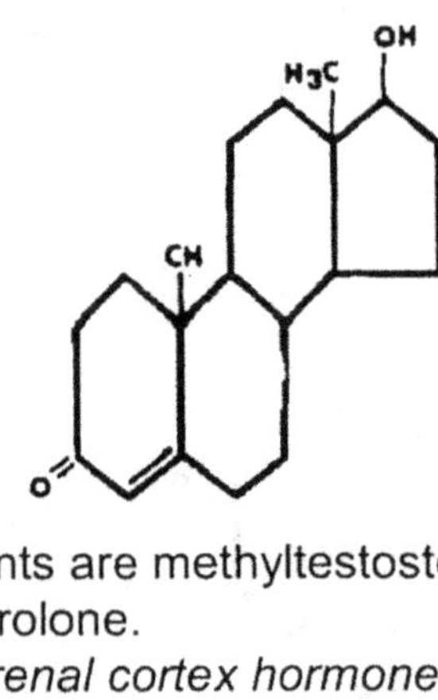

Other agents are methyltestosterone and norethandrolone.

d. Adrenal cortex hormones. Although it is possible for the human to survive without the adrenal cortex and the hormones produced by it, serious repercussions are displayed. Over 44 steroids have been isolated from the adrenal cortex, 7 of which elicit a biological effect. Notice the structural similarity between the corticosteroids below and in the opposite column.

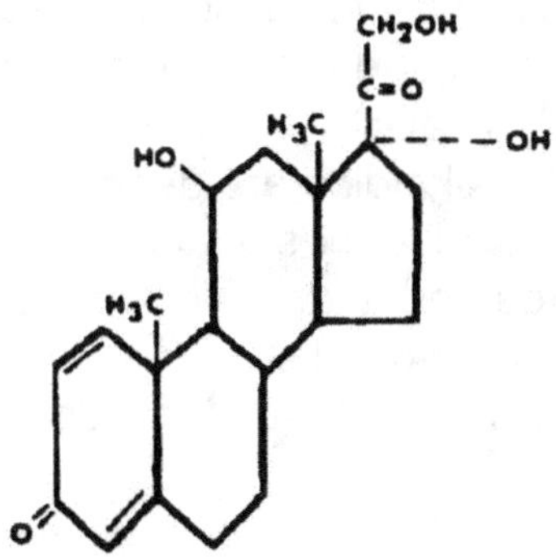

Prednisone

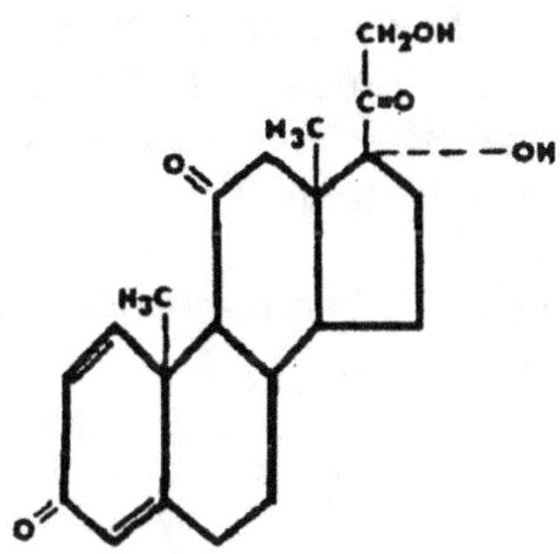

Prednisolone

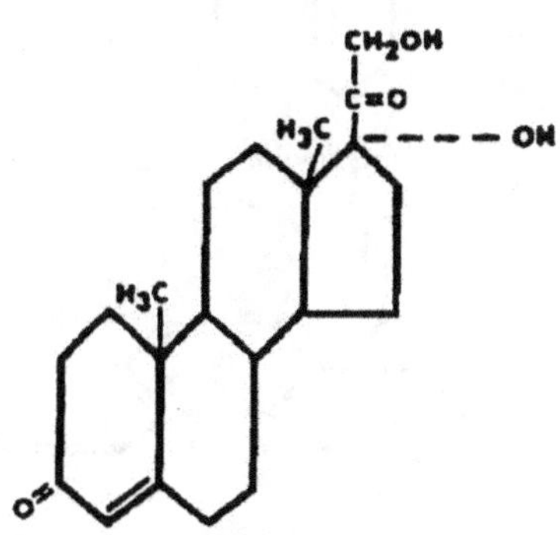

Cortisone

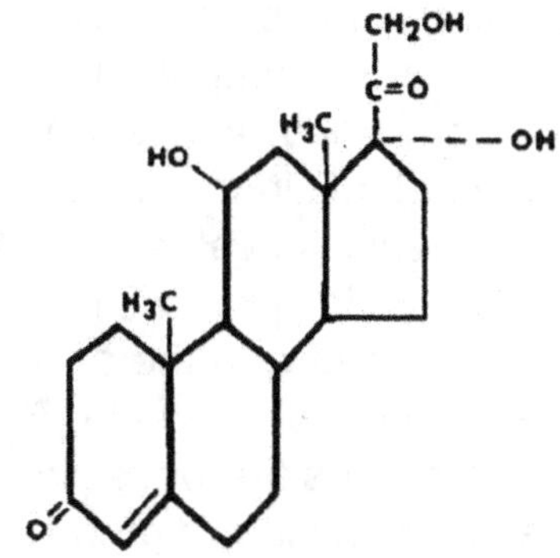

Hydrocortisone

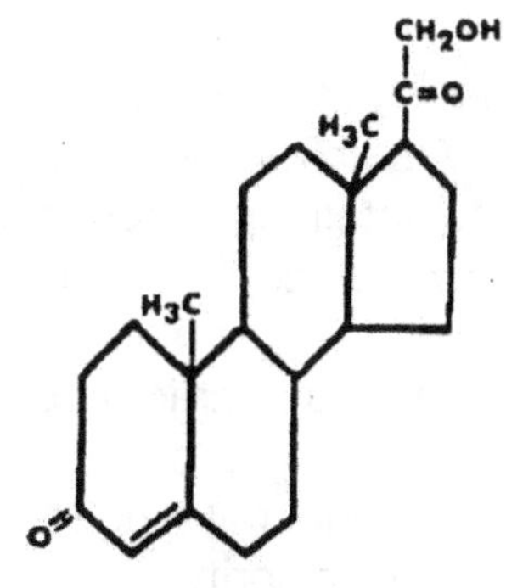

Desoxycortisone

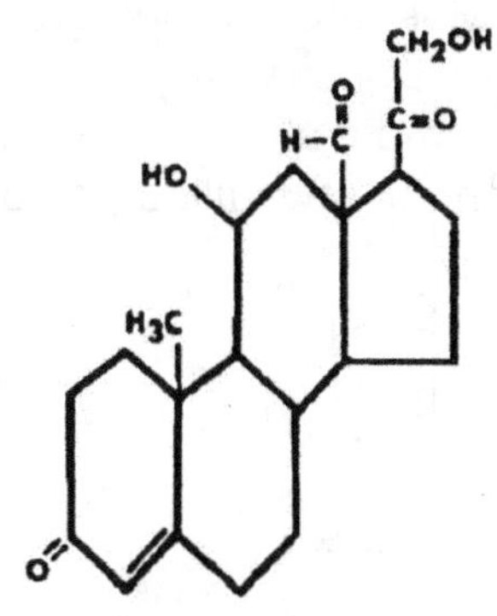

Aldosterone

28. Plant drugs. The plant drugs were first called vegetable alkalies, but later renamed alkaloids, meaning alkali-like. These are the active principles in plants. Centuries ago, crude plants were used as poisons; these included plants such as poison hemlock and deadly nightshade. Others were made into teas and extracts for curative uses. In the early 1800's, it was found that the alkaloidal content was the effective ingredient of these plants. Since then hundreds of alkaloids have been iso-

lated, including some of the most important pharmaceutically. Despite the large number of alkaloids already in use, only about 5 percent of the plant kingdom has been explored for medicinal value. At present a systematic screening process has been initiated to identify new and therapeutically useful agents in the plant world. Although most of the alkaloids are physiologically active, their responses are greatly varied. Some depress, while others stimulate. Some are miotic, others mydriatic. Some raise blood pressure, others lower it.

a. General properties of the alkaloids.

(1) Alkaloids are complex organic compounds containing nitrogen and it is the nitrogen which confers the alkali-like property to them.

(2) The vast majority of the alkaloids are of plant origin, but a few are derived from the animal kingdom.

(3) The majority are naturally occurring. A few, however, are either completely or partially synthetic.

(4) Most are physiologically active; their responses vary.

(5) Almost all of the alkaloids are white or colorless crystalline powders. Nicotine is a liquid; sanguanarine and berberine are red and yellow, respectively.

(6) Most of the alkaloids are chemical compounds which are comprised of carbon, hydrogen, nitrogen, and oxygen. The liquid alkaloids contain no oxygen.

(7) Alkaloidal solutions are alkaline in reaction and therefore react with acids to form salts.

(8) Alkaloids are generally insoluble in water, but their salts are water soluble. Sulfates and hydrochlorides are the most widely used salts.

(9) Most of the alkaloids are optically active.

(10) Most have a bitter taste, and many are violently poisonous.

(11) The alkaloids have many incompatibilities. Preparations containing them should be carefully scrutinized for the possibility of incompatibility. Some alkaloidal precipitants are the heavy metals, tannic acid, and the tannins.

b. Nuclei (or fragments of nuclei) common to the alkaloids.

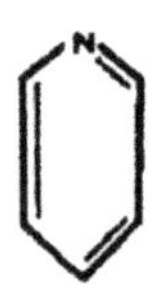

Pyridine

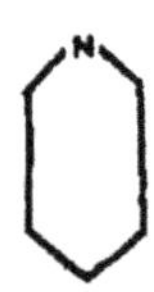

Piperidine

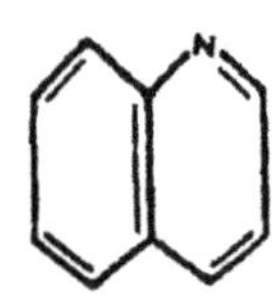

Quinoline

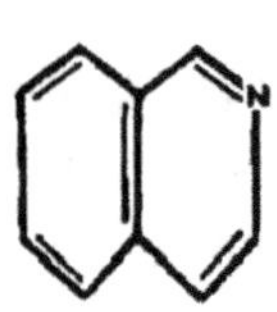

Isoquinoline

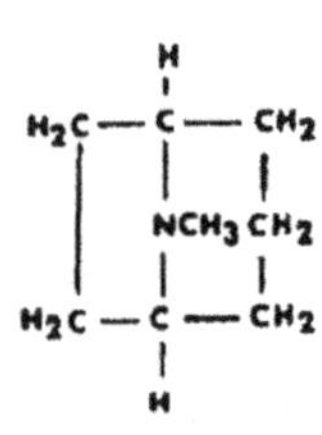

Tropane

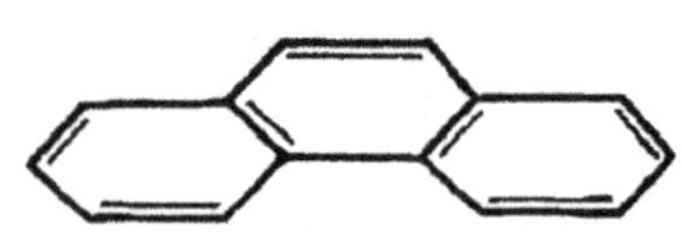

Phenanthrene

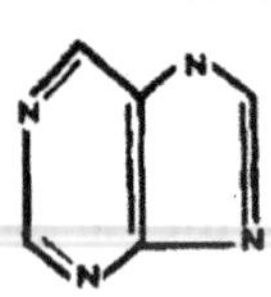

Purine

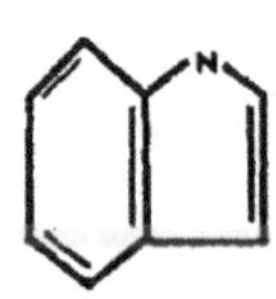

Indole

c. Pharmaceutically important alkaloids. The pharmaceutically important alkaloids can be conveniently divided into seven subcategories: opium alkaloids, cinchona alkaloids, tropane alkaloids, xanthine alkaloids, ergot alkaloids, rauwolfia alkaloids, and miscellaneous alkaloids.

(1) Opium alkaloids. Opium is one of the oldest medications known to man. The plant from which it is obtained has long been cultivated in the Orient where, in many areas, it grows wild. The capsules of the Papaver somniferum (opium poppy) are slit and the exudate collected, air-dried, and powdered to yield opium. From the opium plant can be extracted more than 20 different alkaloids, of which only a few are important to the physician and pharmacist. Powdered opium contains 9.5 percent of anhydrous morphine. It is used mainly in the manufacture of the two more commonly prescribed forms, opium tincture and paregoric. Opium is firmly regulated by the Controlled Substances Act.

(a) Morphine.

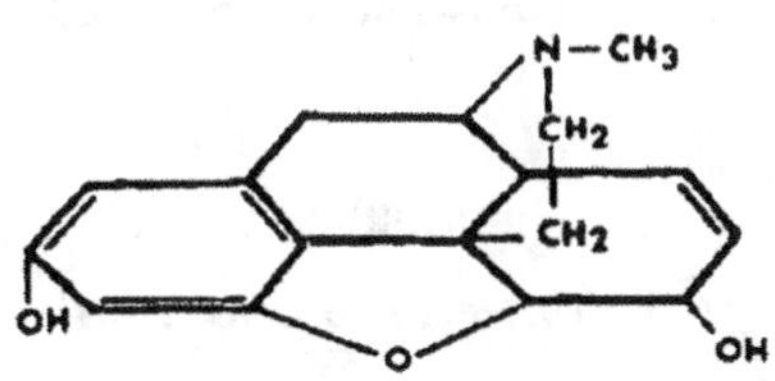

Morphine, the first opium alkaloid to be discovered, is a member of the phenanthrene group. It is of tremendous importance to the physician and the patient and, used properly, is an effective analgesic, sedative, hypnotic, and respiratory depressant. However, addiction is one of its drawbacks. Morphine is generally used in the form of soluble salts, particularly the sulfate. It cannot be stressed too often that morphine is a potent, addicting drug which must be rigidly controlled. The penalties for mishandling this and related drugs are very severe.

(b) Codeine.

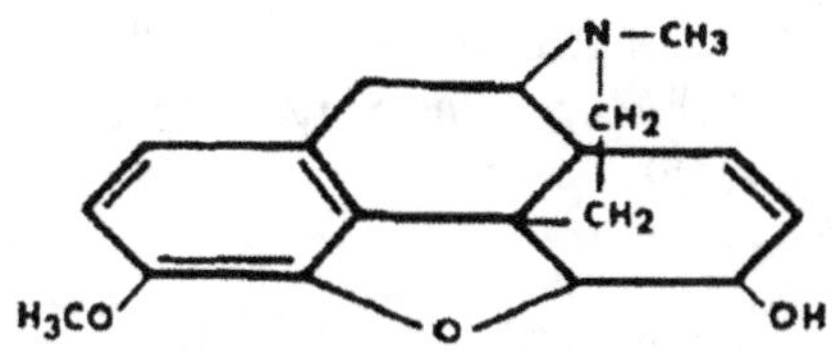

Codeine may be obtained either from the opium plant or made by methylating morphine. It is also official in the form of its phosphate and sulfate salts. The phosphate is more soluble. It is used as an analgesic and cough suppressor.

(c) Dihydrocodeinone bitartrate (Hydrocodone; Hycodan). Dihydrocodeinone is a semisynthetic agent prepared from codeine. It has the same antitussive qualities as codeine and is equally addicting.

(d) Dextromethorphan hydrobromide (Romilar).

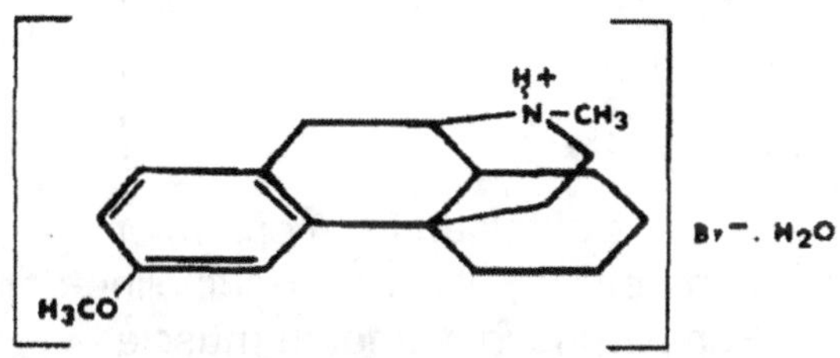

Dextromethorphan is a synthetic morphine derivative with no addicting qualities. It is effective against the cough reflex for which it is used exclusively. Dextromethorphan has no analgesic action.

(e) Propoxyphene hydrochloride (Darvon).

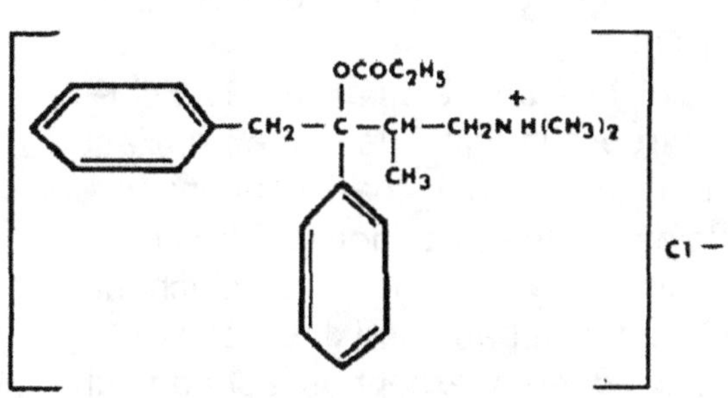

Dextropropoxyphene is a synthetic analgesic which is not addicting and has no antitussive properties.

(f) Levopropoxyphene (Novrad). Levopropoxyphene, an isomer of d-propoxyphene, has been recently found to

have excellent antitussive properties and no analgesic or antipyretic properties.

(g) Meperidine hydrochloride (Demerol HCl).

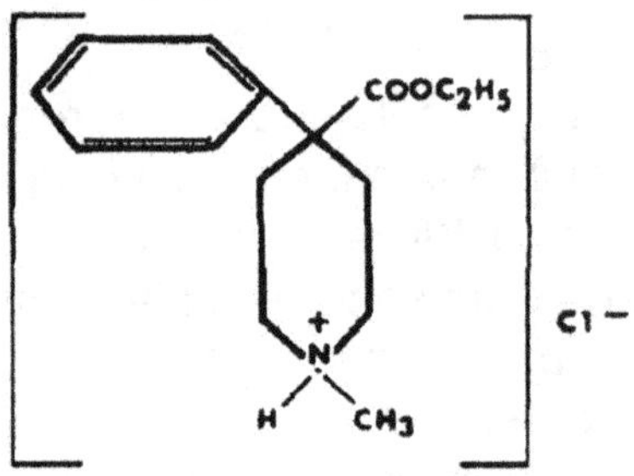

Meperidine produces sedation and analgesia.

(h) Papaverine hydrochloride.

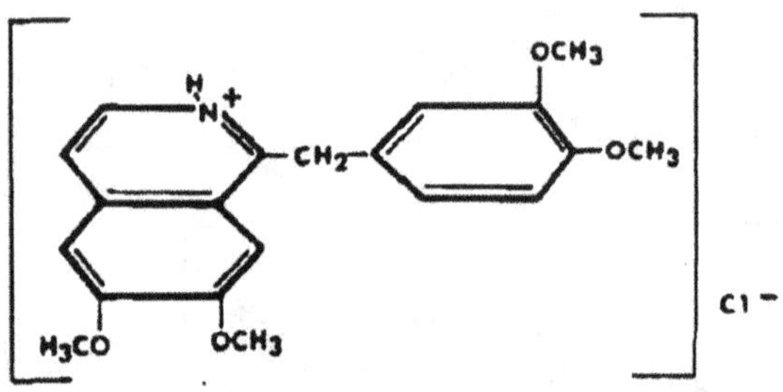

Papaverine is obtained from opium or prepared synthetically. It is an isoquinoline derivative. Papaverine is a smooth muscle relaxant. It is nonaddicting and not controlled as a narcotic drug.

(i) Other natural and synthetic derivatives.

- Hydromorphone (Dilaudid).
- Diacetylmorphine (heroin).
- Apomorphine hydrochloride.
- Methadone hydrochloride (Dolophine HCl).

(2) Cinchona alkaloids. The cinchona tree is indigenous to the Far East and Latin America. Its bark contains useful alkaloids related to quinoline. The crude drug, cinchona, also known as cinchona bark, Peruvian bark, and Jesuitsí bark, is rarely used today except as a cheap substitute for the alkaloids it contains. It is antimalarial, antipyretic, and analgesic in action. It contains the following pharmaceutically important alkaloids:

(a) Quinine. Over 100 salts of quinine have been listed. The actions and uses of this drug are more thoroughly considered in chapter 9.

(b) Quinidine sulfate. Quinidine is the stereoisomer of quinine but is a heart drug rather than an antimalarial.

(c) Quinacrine hydrochloride (Atabrine).

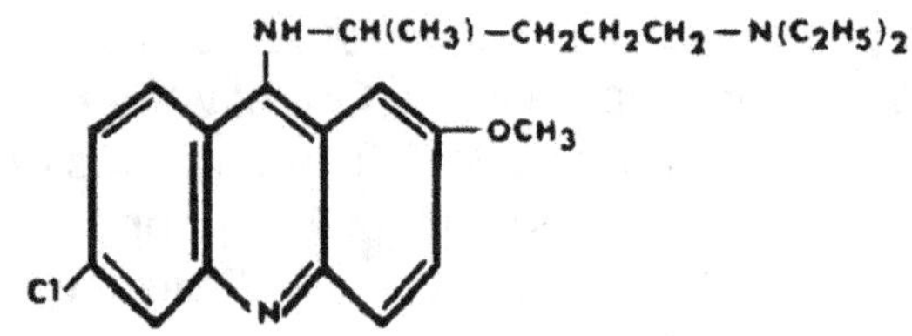

Quinacrine

(d) Chloroquine phosphate (Aralen phosphate).

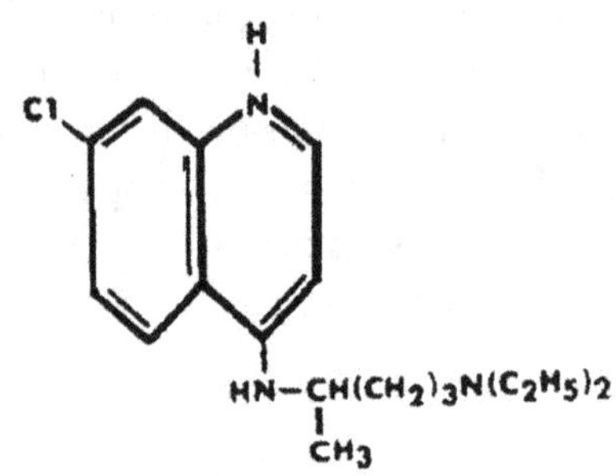

Chloroquine

(e) Primaquine phosphate.

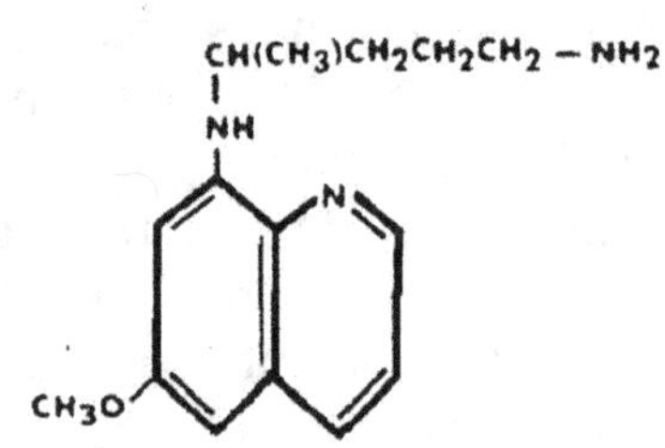

Primaquine

(f) Comparison of cinchona alkaloid structures. In the comparison of the cinchona alkaloid structures below, notice the relationship between the agents; quinine and quinidine are structurally identical but stereoisomers of each other.

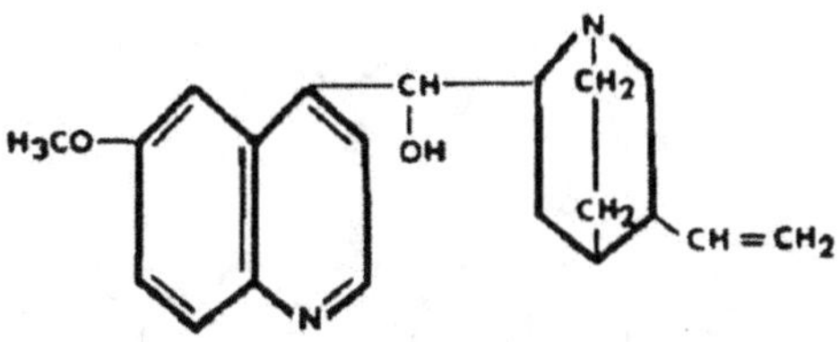

Quinine

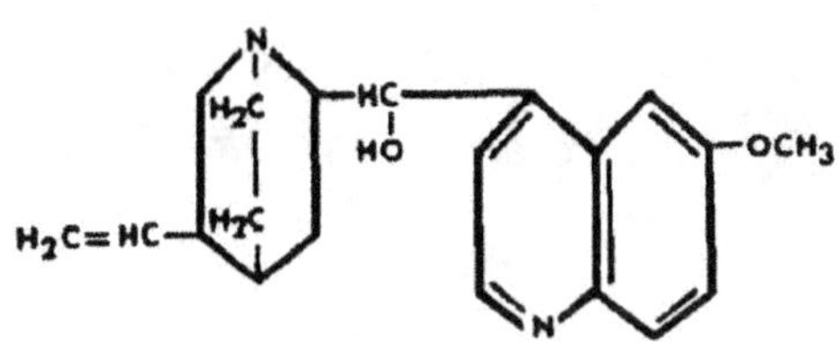

Quinidine

(3) The tropane alkaloids. The tropane alkaloids actually consist of two groups: the solanaceous (nightshade) members which are atropine and related substances, and cocaine which is derived from the coca leaf. Although these two terms are used together, you should understand the difference between them.

(a) Cocaine.

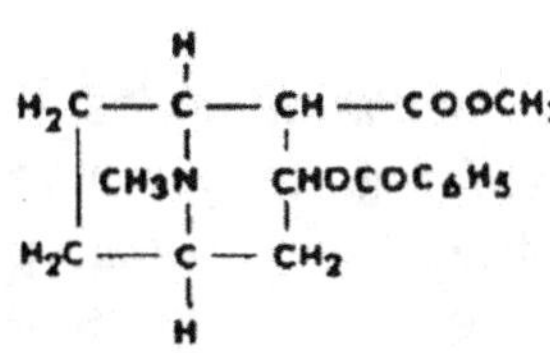

Cocaine is an alkaloid from the coca leaf. Compare its structure with that of the members of the nightshade family which follow.

(b) Tropane alkaloids from the nightshade family. The tropane alkaloids from the nightshade family are referred to as the solanaceous alkaloids. Of this group, atropine is the most important and is the prototype. Below are the formulas for these alkaloids. The nightshade or solanaceous family consists of belladonna plant (deadly nightshade), hyoscyamus, stramonium, and other plants. Belladonna derives its name from Italian ìbella + donnaî meaning ìbeautiful lady,î because squeezings from this plant were used by the elegant women of the time as an eye wash to dilate the pupils.

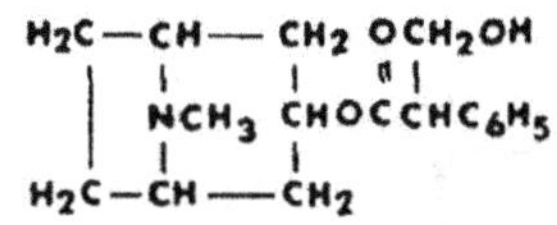

Atropine
(l-hyoscyamus)

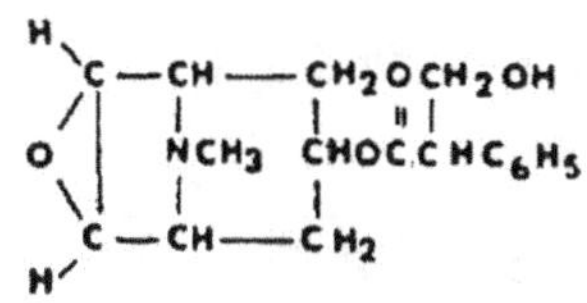

Scopolamine
(Hyoscine)

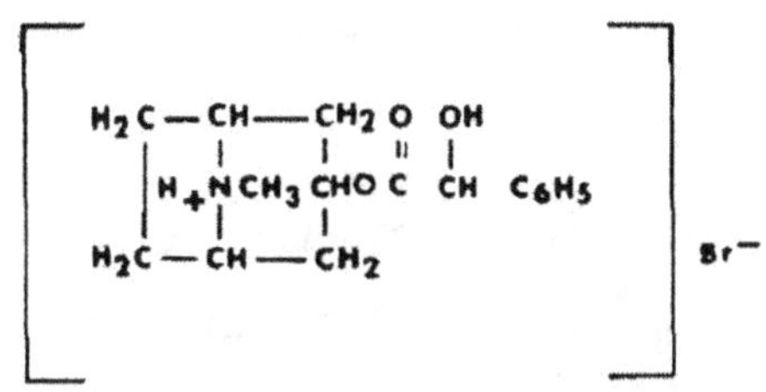

Homatropine Hydrobromide

(4) Xanthine alkaloids. The xanthine alkaloids and their derivatives all contain the parent molecule, purine, which is graphically depicted below.

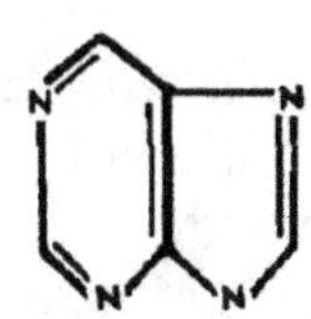

Caffeine, theophylline, and theobromine all contain the same (purine) base, but occur naturally in different plants. Generally, all the xanthine derivatives can be said to be central nervous system stimulants, diuretics, and smooth muscle relaxants.

(a) Theophylline.

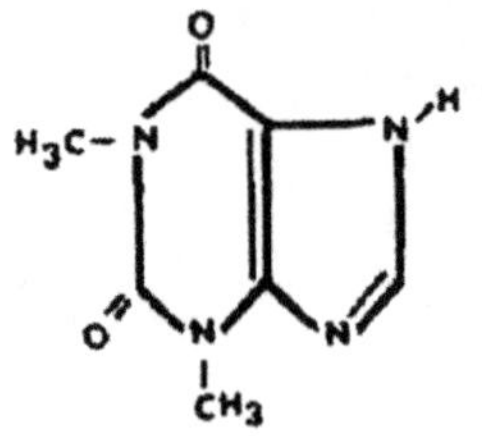

Theophylline

(1, 3-Dimethylxanthine)

(b) Caffeine.

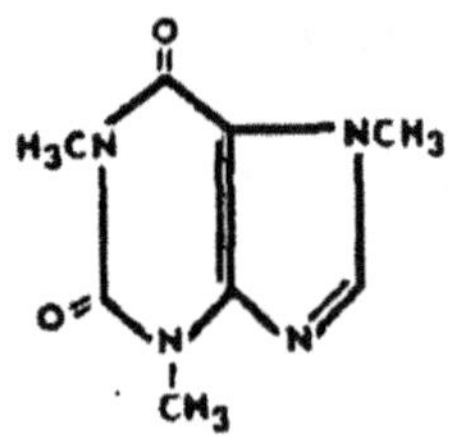

Caffeine

(1, 3, 7-Trimethylxanthine)

(c) Theobromine.

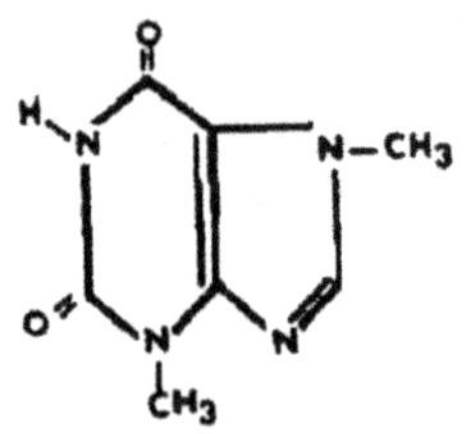

Theobromine

(3, 7-Dimethylxanthine)

(5) Ergot alkaloids. Ergot is a growth produced by a fungus growing on grains such as rye, wheat, oats, barley, and rice. The official ergot is that growth from the rye plant.

(a) Constituents. Ergot is made up of a number of different chemical substances which include alkaloids, carbohydrates, sterols, glycerides, amino acids, and coloring principles. Of these constituents, we will be concerned only with the alkaloidal principles, all of which are substituted amides of lysergic acid.

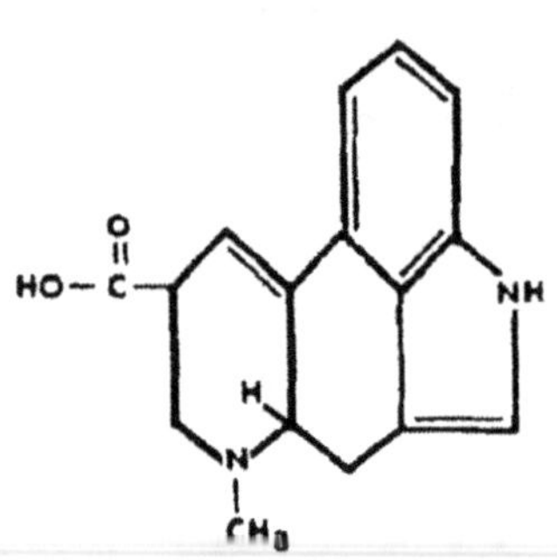

Lysergic Acid

(b) Ergonovine maleate (Ergotrate maleate).

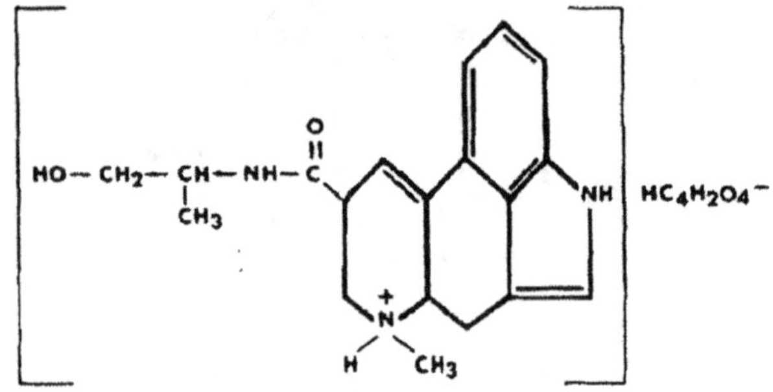

(c) Ergotamine tartrate (Gynergen).

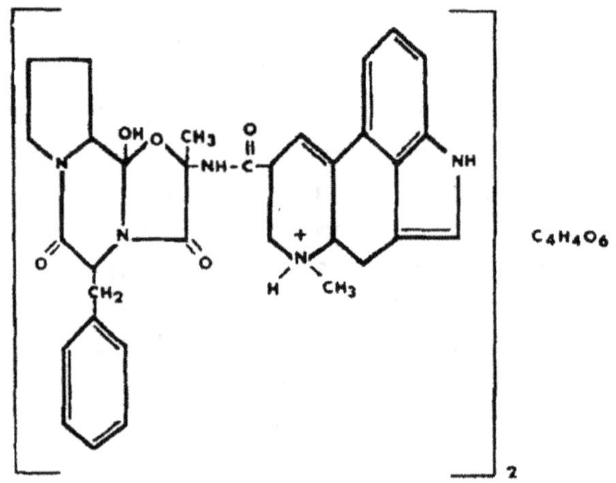

(6) Rauwolfia alkaloids. It was not until 1931 that the first crystalline alkaloid was isolated from the rauwolfia plant, a plant used since ancient times as a remedy. With the recognition of this alkaloid, reserpine, an entirely new field of endeavor sprang into operation. It is through research on rauwolfia, reserpine, and other similar agents that the entire field of tranquilizers and psychotherapeutics has emerged. The rauwolfia alkaloids are intended primarily for reducing high blood pressure.

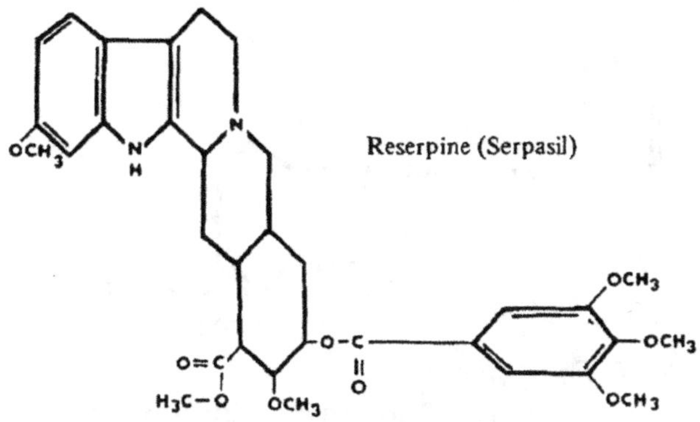

Reserpine (Serpasil)

29. Antibiotics. In a broad sense, and from the derivation of their name, antibiotics are agents against life. From a more restricted medical and pharmaceutical sense, however, they are chemical substances produced by microorganisms and are capable of inhibiting the growth of or destroying other bacteria and microorganisms. Before the birth of Christ, the Chinese used moldy soybean curd as a curative application for boils and furuncles, and yet it was not until 1929 that Sir Alexander Fleming discovered penicillin. Even then antibiotic investigation was slow because of the considerable attention being paid to the sulfonamides. It was not until the 1940is that they really began to find their place in medicine.

a. Methods of antibiotic production. Antibiotics which cannot as yet be synthesized, or are too costly to obtain by synthesis, may be produced by two methods: the surface process and the submerged process.

(1) Surface process. In this method, the organisms producing the antibiotic grow in pad-like formation on the surface of a liquid or divided solid medium. This process is adequate only for producing the small amounts required for laboratory use.

(2) Submerged process. The submerged process is the only natural method for producing antibiotics in the vast quantities necessary for clinical use. It is a much faster and more efficient process than the surface method. Steel tanks, with capacities up to 30,000 gallons, are filled with a sterilized nutrient medium and inoculated with a master culture. After 50 to 90 hours of culturing under rigid temperature and sterile controls, the batch is extracted and concentrated.

b. Penicillins. By substituting various groups for the R in the following general formula, we arrive at a number of different penicillins.

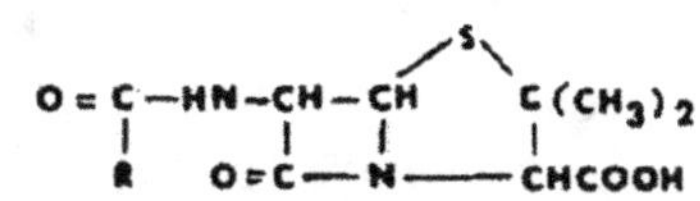

(1) Penicillin G (Benzyl penicillin). The R =

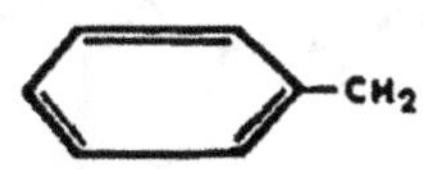

(2) Penicillin V (phenoxymethyl penicillin). The R =

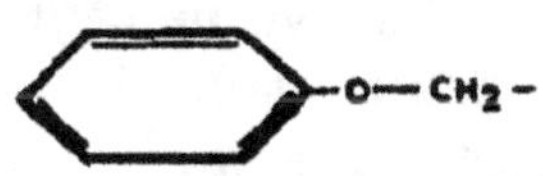

(3) Methicillin (Staphcillin). The R =

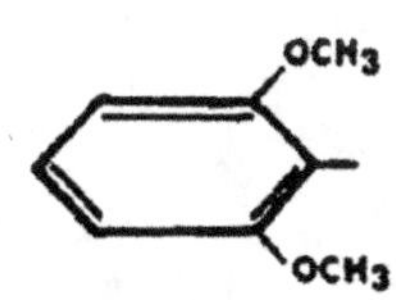

(4) Oxacillin (Prostaphlin). The R =

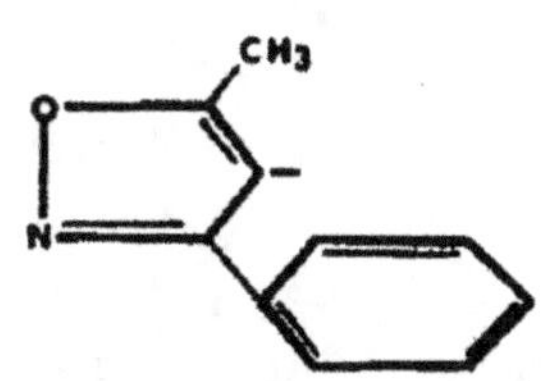

(5) Ampicillin(Polydllin).rnieR =

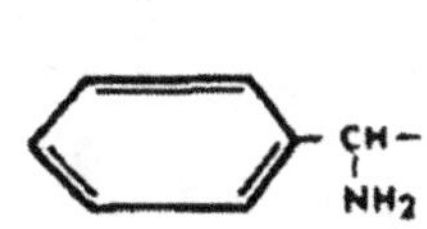

(6) Carbenicillin (Geopen).

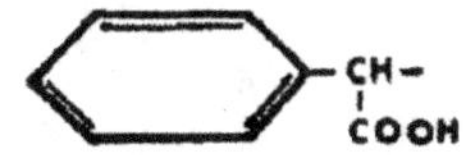

c. Chloramphenicol (Chloromycetin).

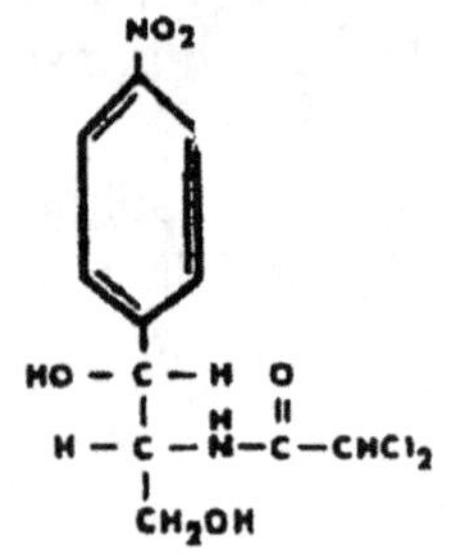

d. Tetracyclines.

(1) Tetracycline (Achromycin).

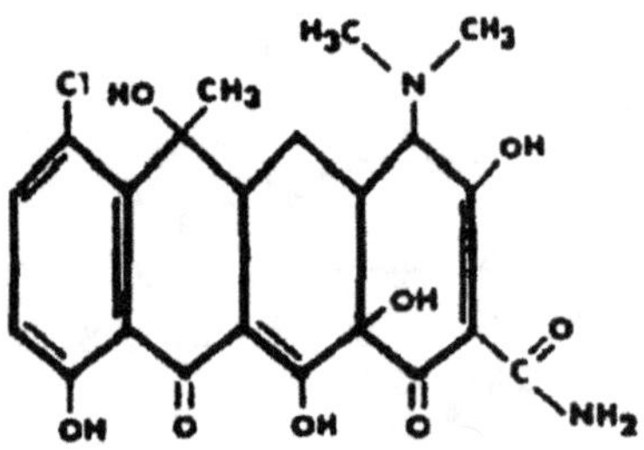

(2) Chlortetracycline (Aureomycin).

(3) Oxytetracycline (Terramycin).

e. Cephalothin (Keflin).

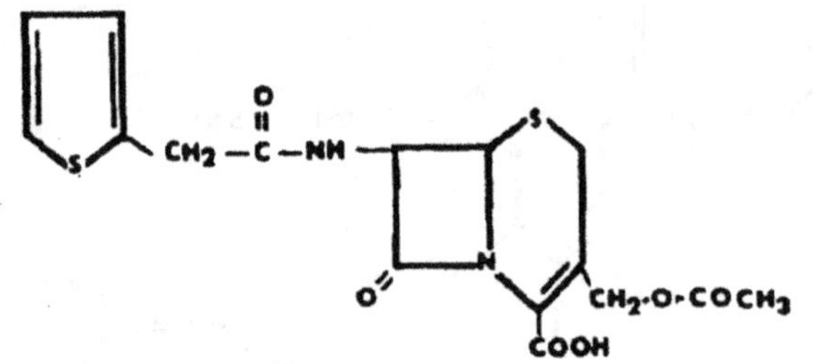

f. The "Mycins."

(1) Gentamicin(Garamycin).

(2) Kanamycin (Kantrex).

(3) Neomycin.

(4) Streptomycin.

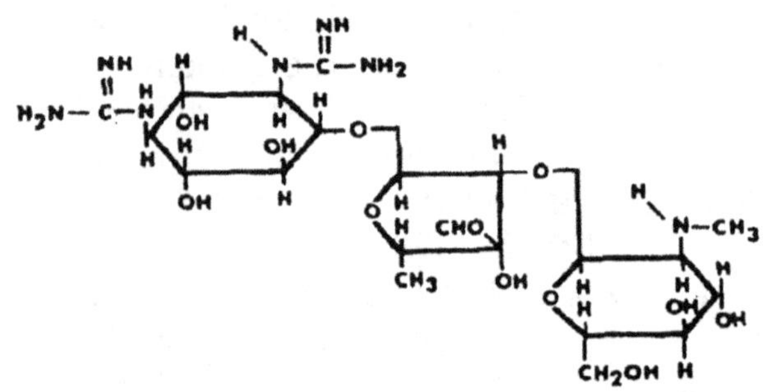

www.ingramcontent.com/pod-product-compliance
Lightning Source LLC
LaVergne TN
LVHW080027210926
848481LV00011B/3119
9781799350477